Sheep Medicine

SECOND EDITION

Sheep Medicine

SECOND EDITION

PHILIP R SCOTT

BVM&S, DVM&S, MPhil, DSHP, CertCHP, FHEA, DiplECBHM, DiplECSRHM, FRCVS

Royal (Dick) School of Veterinary Studies
Large Animal Hospital
University of Edinburgh
Roslin, Midlothian, UK

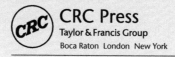

CRC Press
Taylor & Francis Group
Boca Raton London New York

CRC Press is an imprint of the
Taylor & Francis Group, an **informa** business

CRC Press
Taylor & Francis Group
6000 Broken Sound Parkway NW, Suite 300
Boca Raton, FL 33487-2742

First issued in paperback 2020

© 2015 by Taylor & Francis Group, LLC
CRC Press is an imprint of Taylor & Francis Group, an Informa business

No claim to original U.S. Government works

ISBN 13 : 978-0-367-57578-6 (pbk)
ISBN 13 : 978-1-4987-0014-6 (hbk)

Visit the Taylor & Francis Web site at
http://www.taylorandfrancis.com

and the CRC Press Web site at
http://www.crcpress.com

CONTENTS

The major objective of this second edition is to update the important diseases of sheep encountered by veterinary surgeons in general practice in the United Kingdom and worldwide, their diagnosis (**Figs 1, 2**), treatment (**Fig. 3**), prognosis (**Fig. 4**), control and, where appropriate, postmortem features. Almost all of the high-quality colour images used in the first edition have been replaced and take the reader through all stages of the disease process, highlighting the critical clinical features important in the diagnosis (**Fig. 5**). The book has been written for veterinary undergraduate students undertaking their clinical rotations, but many of the techniques and treatments described may be new to practitioners too busy to read scientific journals; only key references are listed.

The book is divided into chapters based upon body system. It is not possible to describe every disease that can affect sheep worldwide; therefore, it is essential that a thorough and systematic clinical

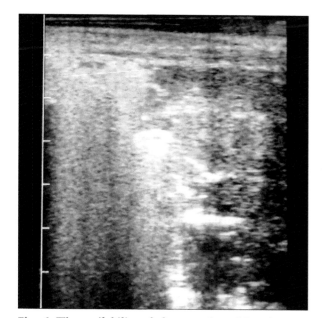

Fig. 1 The availability of ultrasound machines in farm animal practice allows ready confirmation of ovine pulmonary adenocarcinoma (OPA).

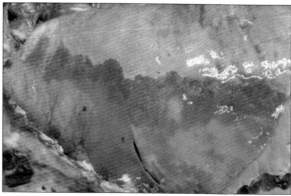

Fig. 2 Necropsy confirms the diagnosis of OPA.

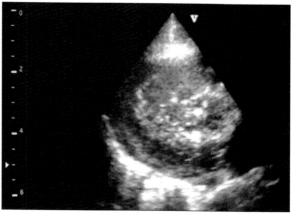

Fig. 3 Ultrasonographic demonstration of pleural abscesses guides specific antibiotic therapy.

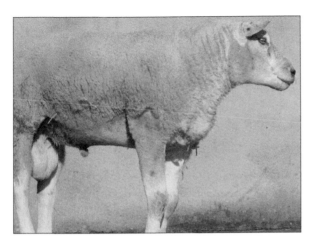

Fig. 4 Ultrasonographic assessment of superficial lung pathology provides a more accurate prognosis than thoracic auscultation.

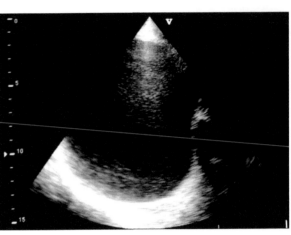

Fig. 5 Marked bladder distension is the best guide to urethral obstruction.

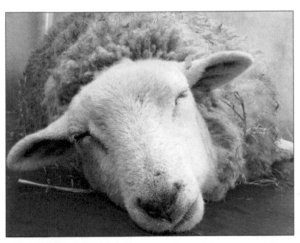

Fig. 6 Systematic assessment of cranial nerves will assist localization of the lesion in this sheep and the possible causes (see Fig. 7).

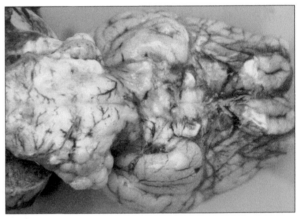

Fig. 7 Necropsy of the sheep featured in Fig. 6 showing the ventral surface of the brain. Systematic assessment of cranial nerve function localized the lesion as basilar empyema.

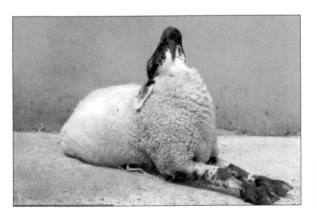

Fig. 8 A 6-month-old lamb presents with bilateral lack of menace response, dorsiflexion of the neck and hyperaesthesia.

examination of each organ/body system is undertaken noting the limitations of physical examination alone. Each chapter opens with a recommended approach to clinical examination of that body system (**Figs 6, 7**) rather than simply listing the disorders and diseases. Ancillary tests available to veterinary practitioners are detailed, emphasizing their practical applications and cost limitations where appropriate. The radiographic equipment and ultrasound machines used by the author and featured in this book are those used every day in large animal practice. Specialized

techniques, such as magnetic resonance imaging (MRI) and computed tomography (CT), have not been included because they are rarely available and cost-prohibitive in sheep practice.

Self-assessment exercises featuring typical clinical cases (**Fig. 8**) affecting each body system are collected in a revision chapter at the end of the book, primarily for undergraduate veterinary students. Diseases and disorders are included with the common differential diagnoses followed by the specific diagnosis and recommended treatment(s).

INTRODUCTION

ANIMAL WELFARE

The Animal Welfare Act 2006 (England and Wales), and similar legislation elsewhere in the world, includes a duty of care to provide for the needs of protected animals for which humans have permanent or temporary responsibility. Article 9(2)(e) of the Animal Welfare Act 2006 sets out an animal's 'need to be protected from pain, suffering, injury and disease'. Where applicable in the book, the author has discussed the likely animal welfare implications of diseases based upon the Farm Animal Welfare Council's (FAWC) Five Freedoms. FAWC reports and opinions on key areas of sheep farming, compiled by experts and available free of charge at http://www.defra.gov.uk/fawc/, provides interpretation and guidance on welfare concerns and issues and is a very useful resource for veterinary practitioners, as well as agricultural and veterinary undergraduates, when confronted with contentious issues.

The FAWC's Five Freedoms:

Freedom from hunger and thirst: by ready access to fresh water and a diet to maintain full health and vigour (**Figs 1.1, 1.2**).

Freedom from discomfort: by providing an appropriate environment including shelter and a comfortable resting area (**Figs 1.3–1.5**).

Freedom from pain, injury or disease: by prevention or by rapid diagnosis and treatment (**Fig. 1.6**).

Freedom to express normal behaviour: by providing sufficient space, proper facilities and company of the animals' own kind (**Figs 1.7, 1.8**).

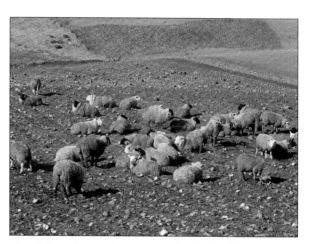

Fig. 1.1 Is this a diet to maintain full health and vigour?

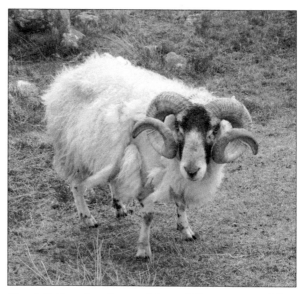

Fig. 1.2 Emaciated ram with woolslip – poor nutrition is the likely cause.

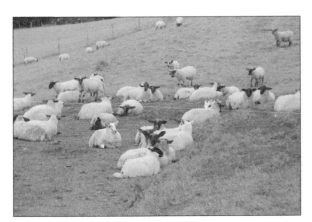

Fig. 1.3 These weaned lambs prefer bare earth to clean pasture.

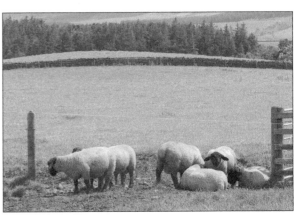

Fig. 1.4 These ram lambs prefer wet bare earth to hectares of clean pasture.

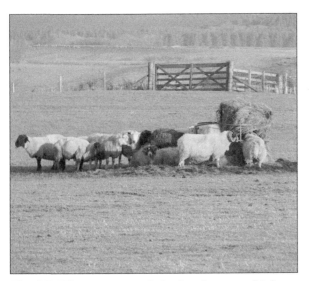

Fig. 1.5 These rams are sheltering from very high winds in the lea of the feeder; shelter appears more important than space allowance.

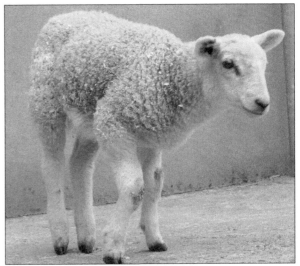

Fig. 1.6 Freedom from pain, injury or disease by prevention or by rapid diagnosis and treatment most concerns the veterinary practitioner.

Freedom from fear and distress: by ensuring conditions and treatment to avoid mental suffering (**Fig. 1.9**).

Of the Five Freedoms, freedom from pain, injury or disease by prevention or by rapid diagnosis and treatment most directly concerns the veterinary surgeon in farm animal practice.

The Codes of Recommendations for the Welfare of Livestock: Sheep provide a succinct and perceptive interpretation of the Five Freedoms: 'In acknowledging these freedoms, those who have care of livestock should practise:

- caring and responsible planning and management;
- skilled, knowledgeable and conscientious stockmanship;
- appropriate environmental design (e.g. of the husbandry system);
- considerate handling and transport;
- humane slaughter.'

Veterinary surgeons are experts in animal health but it is the consideration of the mental wellbeing of farm animals that differentiates animal welfare from animal health. The concept of mental

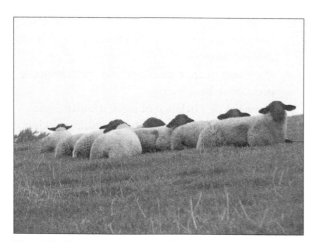

Fig. 1.7 Sheep often prefer close contact with other sheep.

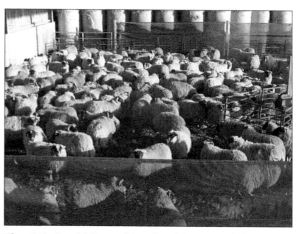

Fig. 1.8 Are high stocking densities stressful to sheep?

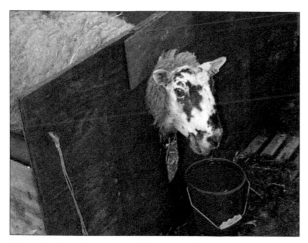

Fig. 1.9 Confinement of the ewe during cross-fostering neonatal lambs may cause fear and distress.

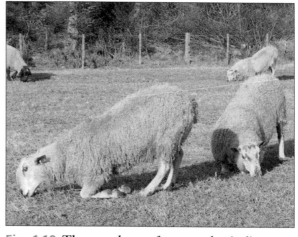

Fig. 1.10 The prevalence of many endemic diseases in sheep in the UK (footrot in this example) is too high.

wellbeing is addressed in the 2012 FAWC publication 'Farm animal welfare: Health and disease' which discusses the impact of disease on the physical and mental wellbeing of farm animals. The report states that 'There is now a considerable body of scientific evidence that farm animals are sentient and can suffer and therefore the effects of disease on mental wellbeing, e.g. fear, distress, anxiety, do affect their welfare.' Furthermore, the report states that the prevalence of many endemic diseases in farm animals, including sheep in the United Kingdom (UK), is too high (**Fig. 1.10**) and that the

farm's veterinarian is the pivotal link to continual improvements in farm animal health and welfare.

The FAWC report concludes that key themes to improve farm animal welfare through improved health include:

- Greater use of preventive health planning and production management with the veterinarian as a key external advisor.
- Greater involvement of the veterinarian in diagnosis and appropriate treatment of sick animals.

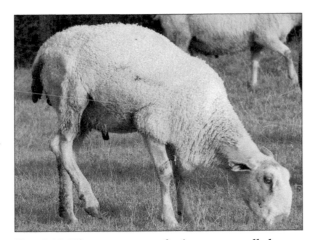

Fig. 1.11 The occurrence of pain can generally be more reliably identified than its intensity.

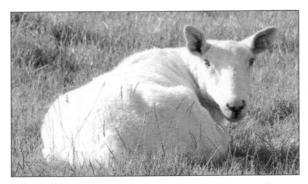

Fig. 1.12 Is it possible to distinguish an expression that suggests pain from fear?

- Continuing professional development of all connected with farmed livestock on health and disease issues.
- Provision of appropriate resources to improve preventive health care.
- Creation of a balance of legislation and self-regulation and effective partnership working that maximises the uptake of opportunities to improve health and welfare.
- An appreciation by all stakeholders that improved animal welfare through better health also delivers for other policy areas, e.g. productivity, emission reduction, food safety standards and reduction in energy consumption.

Freedom from pain is often considered a major indicator of good animal welfare by the veterinary profession; mental health is a lesser consideration because it is much more difficult to quantify. Pain is typically assessed by changes in behaviour and demeanour, stance, lameness, lowered food intake, and reduced use of the affected part. Ruminants experiencing pain often become subdued, spend more time lying down, spend less time eating and ruminating, and fail to clean the nostrils as frequently. Interpretation of multiple behavioural responses as an aggregate indicator of animal wellness status instead of

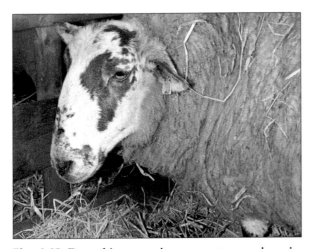

Fig. 1.13 Does this expression suggest toxaemia, pain or both?

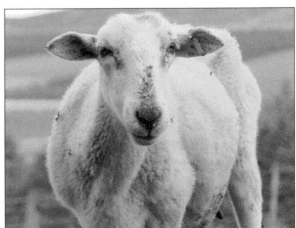

Fig. 1.14 Dullness, depression or lethargy may arise from disease where pain is not considered a cardinal feature, such as this case of paratuberculosis.

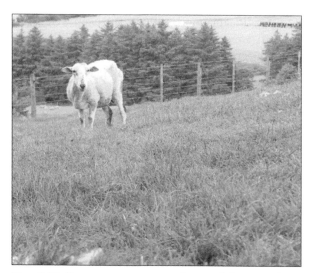

Fig. 1.15 Inappetence, not grazing, and decreased rumination rate are considered potential indicators of pain.

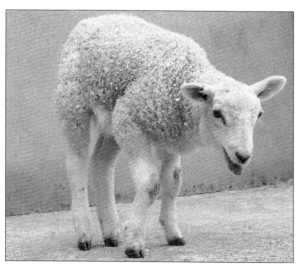

Fig. 1.16 Increased vocalization is considered a potential indicator of pain.

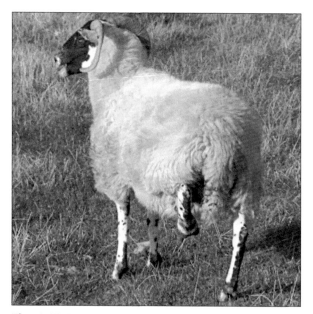

Fig. 1.17 Increased sensitivity is considered a reliable indicator of pain.

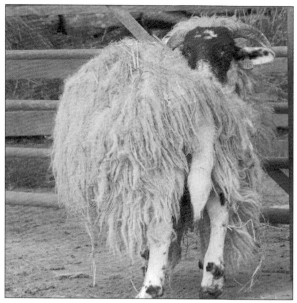

Fig. 1.18 Attention/nibbling/kicking is considered a potential indicator of pain at that site.

individual outcomes is regarded as the more accurate measure of true state of animal pain or wellness status.

It is generally stated that the occurrence of pain can be more reliably identified than its intensity (Figs 1.11–1.18). The common indicators of pain reported in the scientific literature are listed in *Table 1.1*, but much more work is necessary in this area, particularly when attempting to differentiate (endo-)toxaemia from pain.

Table 1.1 **Identification of pain in sheep**
• Facial expression • Dullness, depression, lethargy • Grunting, teeth grinding • Inappetance, isolation from others, not grazing, decreased rumination rate • Increased respiratory rate • Increased vocalization • Increased sensitivity (hyperalgesia) • Attention/nibbling/kicking at site of pain.

ALLEVIATION OF PAIN

Whilst nonsteroidal anti-inflammatory drugs (NSAID)s have benefits in small animal species, such as mitigation of pain, lessening of swelling, diminishing inflammation at the incision site and/or damaged tissues and more rapid patient recovery after the procedure, currently there are no NSAIDs approved for pain management in sheep in the UK and many other countries. Several NSAIDs are used in an extra-label manner in sheep but there is limited published evidence of any benefits. The concept of 'giving the animal the benefit of the doubt' with respect to NSAID administration is widely practised, including by this author prior to all surgical and obstetrical procedures; however, there are situations where corticosteroids may be more effective such as the treatment of infection of the atlanto-occipital joint.

Significant improvements in sheep welfare have been demonstrated after sacrococcygeal extradural injection of 0.5–0.6 mg/kg lignocaine in ewes with obstetrical problems attended by veterinary practitioners (**Figs 1.19, 1.20**). Inclusion of xylazine in these analgesic protocols has demonstrated effective analgesia of extended duration and these findings have been published in peer-reviewed scientific articles. This regimen has also been described as a 'leap forward in the alleviation of suffering in ewes'.

Sheep flock health planning – an example

A veterinary flock health plan to improve the welfare status of sheep flocks proposed the introduction of husbandry practices, anthelmintic treatments, and

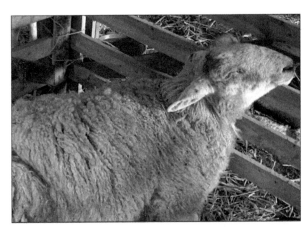

Fig. 1.19 **Pain can arise from unskilled assistance at lambing (see Fig. 1.20).**

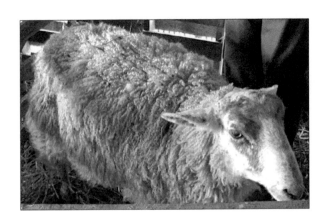

Fig. 1.20 **There is significant improvement in this sheep's welfare immediately after sacrococcygeal extradural lignocaine injection.**

Table 1.2 **Annual cost of operating a flock health plan for a 1000 ewe lowland flock in the UK producing 1,500 lambs sold for slaughter by 5 months old (adapted from Scott and Sargison, 2007)**

Chlamydophila vaccination (25% flock)	£500
Toxoplasmosis vaccination (25% flock)	£500
Clostridial diseases vaccination (all adult sheep)	£150
Sheep scab control (all purchased sheep – 25% flock)	£200
Parasitic gastroenteritis (diarrhoeic sheep)	£200
Quarterly veterinary visits (1.5 hours at £60 per hour)	£360
10 dystocia cases (at veterinary surgery)	£450
10 prolapse cases (at veterinary surgery)	£200
Examine 10 sheep (misc. problems at veterinary surgery)	£100
Antibiotics	£200
Treat/prevent PGE (1,500 lambs; two treatments)	£300
Cutaneous myiasis control (soiled lambs only; 10%)	£60
Footbath chemicals (1,500 lambs; two treatments)	£200
TOTAL	£3420

strategic vaccinations that could be achieved within industry costs of £3.50 per ewe per annum for veterinary fees and medicines; an updated version is reproduced in *Table 1.2*.

The proposed flock health plan tackles obstetrical problems, which the authors consider to be the most important animal welfare concern (**Fig. 1.21**), but also includes those diseases considered of major economic importance by industry. The estimated annual costs of gastrointestinal parasites in the UK (2005) were £84 million, £24 million for footrot, £8 million for sheep scab, £20 million for chlamydial abortion, and £12 million for toxoplasmosis.

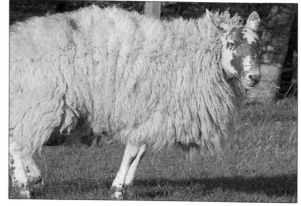

Fig. 1.21 Flock health plans must make specific provision to tackle obstetrical problems.

CHAPTER 2

HUSBANDRY

Flock management varies greatly worldwide and it is outwith the scope of this book to detail all production systems. This chapter describes typical semi-intensive flock management in the United Kingdom (UK) where the target is the seasonal production of two 40 kg lambs of good conformation by 4–8 months per ewe, achieved largely from pasture (**Fig. 2.1**).

HANDLING FACILITIES

Ewes pass through handling facilities on most farms between 12 and 20 times per annum. It is therefore essential that the permanent handling facilities function well, and are in good repair. The permanent handling facilities should be roofed to afford protection for the sheep and shepherd during adverse weather. A concrete base and galvanized metal partitions allow thorough cleaning and disinfection of the facilities at the end of the day's work.

Such precautions are essential when large numbers of sheep are handled over a few days. Too often handling facilities are poorly maintained (**Fig. 2.2**). Infections such as footrot, caseous lymphadenitis, contagious pustular dermatitis and sheep scab could persist in this environment and be transmitted between groups of sheep.

During the handling process the ewes should move around through 180° so that they head out of the pens in the direction from which they came, thus giving the sheep the impression that they are returning to the field. The pens should have solid sides to a level above the height of the sheep. With such a design the sheep cannot see through the pen partitions and are neither distracted nor frightened when moving through the facilities (**Fig. 2.3**). In this way the sheep will head towards daylight and move smoothly through the handling pens. Sheep quickly become familiar with a quiet and relaxed handling system where the shepherd's patience is rewarded by

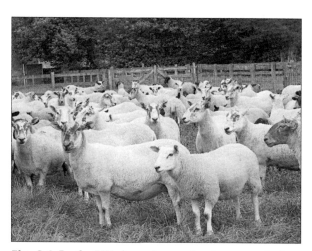

Fig. 2.1 In the UK the major production target is the seasonal production of two 40 kg lambs by 4–8 months per ewe, achieved largely from pasture.

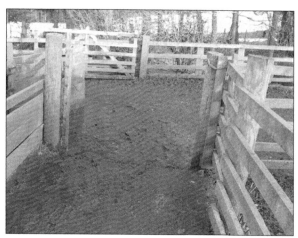

Fig. 2.2 These handling facilities cannot be properly cleaned and may act as a reservoir of pathogens causing footrot and other diseases.

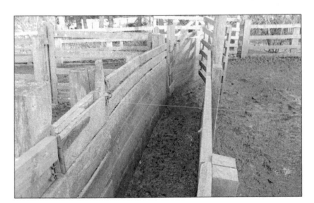

Fig. 2.3 Solid pen divisions aid movement of sheep through the facility and reduce the risk of injury.

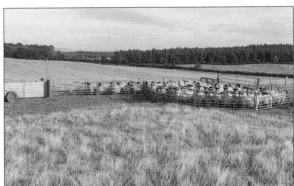

Fig. 2.4 Good quality handling pens reduce stress for sheep and shepherds and greatly improve efficiency.

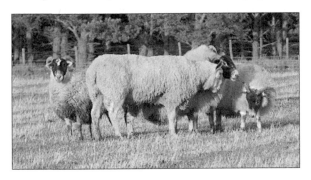

Fig. 2.5 All ewes should be mated during the first 17 days of the service period.

smooth movement through the pens. The presence of dogs around the handling pens invariably disrupts the smooth flow of sheep and increases workload unnecessarily, stressing both sheep and shepherd.

The pens must have smooth surfaces with no protruding hinges or latches which could cause injury. Limb fractures are not uncommon when growing lambs are caught in poorly-designed pens.

Good-quality mobile handling pens are essential for farmers who rent grazing land (**Fig. 2.4**) to ensure treatment of sheep as soon as signs appear.

MATING PERIOD/PREGNANCY

The mating period is timed such that lambing coincides with the start of rapid grass growth in the spring. Such timing approximates the natural breeding season of all sheep breeds.

Targets
- All ewes should be mated during the first 17 days of the service period (**Fig. 2.5**).

- Less than 5% of ewes should return to service.
- Rams should be removed after two oestrous cycles (5 weeks).
- No ewes should return for a third service (detected by vasectomised ram).
- At scanning time 98% (or greater) ewes should be pregnant.
- Abortions should total less than 2%.
- 95% (or greater) ewes should rear lamb(s) to weaning.

Selection of ewes for breeding

Ewes are usually culled from the breeding flock after six crops of lambs (voluntary culling) but this will vary depending upon geographical and husbandry practices. In addition, ewes with palpable mastitis lesions, poor dentition, chronic lameness and poor body condition are culled from the breeding flock (termed involuntary culling). This latter involuntary culling rate (**Fig. 2.6**) should be less than 5%; veterinary investigations are warranted if higher than this target.

Body condition scoring

Body condition scoring is a subjective but reliable method for determining the ewe's fat reserves, and to a lesser degree the amount of skeletal muscle. The amount of fat and muscle covering the transverse processes of the lumbar vertebrae are determined by palpation and subjectively graded 1 (very thin/emaciated) to 5 (obese) in 0.5 units. The target body condition score for lowground sheep during early pregnancy is 3–3.5 falling to around 2.5–3 during mid-gestation with little further loss, but ewes with a multiple litter may lose a further 0.5–1 unit during the last 6 weeks of gestation.

Mating period

One ram is introduced to 50–80 ewes on hill pastures in the UK. The ewes are not given improved grazing prior to mating because the desired litter size is one lamb.

In lowground flocks one ram is introduced to 30–50 ewes, or more commonly, three rams are added to a group of 100–120 ewes as an insurance policy in case one ram has poor fertility. While fighting amongst the groups of three rams may be briefly experienced in this type of breeding system, a pecking order rapidly becomes established amongst the rams. The competition and constant search for oestrous females during the breeding season causes the rams to lose body condition rapidly and supplementary grain feeding (0.5–0.75 kg/day) is strongly advised to prevent excessive weight loss. The rams are removed after two oestrous cycles.

Conception rate

The conception rate in mature sheep should be greater than 90%, preferably above 95%; therefore the breeding season can be restricted to two oestrous cycles. A poor conception rate is usually caused by subfertile ram(s). Infertility in individual ewes is uncommon unless the ewe is emaciated or there is a history of previous dystocia.

Flushing ewes

In the UK, and many other sheep-producing countries, the provision of improved nutrition by means of access to a good grass sward for up to 6 weeks before mating (**Fig. 2.7**) and during the breeding season ('flushing') increases ovulation rate and embryo implantation rate with a resultant increase in litter size. However, if we compare ultrasound scanning data during mid-gestation (often >200% for lowground flocks) to the weaning rate (often 155%),

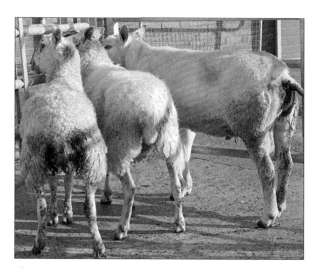

Fig. 2.6 The number of ewes culled should represent less than 5% of the flock per annum.

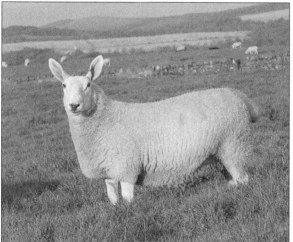

Fig. 2.7 Improved nutrition for up to 1 month before mating, and during the breeding season, increases ovulation rate and embryo implantation rate with a resultant increase in litter size.

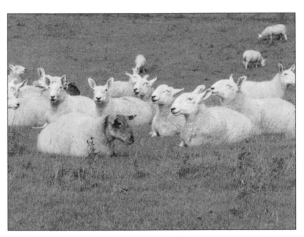

Fig. 2.8 Appropriate ewe condition score at mating can also be achieved by correct management after weaning.

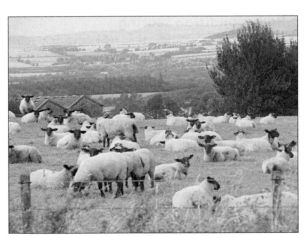

Fig. 2.9 Reserving grass for flushing ewes reduces grazing available for weaned lambs.

the question arises do sheep farmers really need more lambs at lambing time and is such nutritional management a sensible strategy?

Flushing can ensure appropriate ewe condition score at mating but can also be achieved by correct management after weaning (**Fig. 2.8**). It should also be remembered that triplet-bearing ewes are more prone to pregnancy toxaemia, vaginal prolapse and rupture of the prepubic tendon.

Advantages of flushing

- Flushing for 4–6 weeks should provide for a 0.5–1 unit increase of condition score at mating time.
- Flushing increases ovulation and implantation rates which is beneficial in hill breeds producing F1 hybrid females, i.e. twins on improved pasture compared to singles when maintained on hill ground. Litter size at the normal breeding season can be increased by approximately 15% by the use of melatonin implants.

Disadvantages of flushing

- Fields must not be grazed for 4–6 weeks to ensure a good (8 cm) grass sward for September/October.
- Extra fertilizer is needed which is costly.
- Reduced grazing for weaned lambs or purchased store lambs (**Fig. 2.9**).

- Flushing increases ovulation and implantation rates in hybrid ewes resulting in more triplet litters.
- Potential for more triplet lambs which suffer higher perinatal losses.
- Cost and labour involved with rearing orphan lambs.

PREGNANCY

Pregnancy can effectively be divided into three stages (*Table 2.1*).

Table 2.1 Three stages of pregnancy

		WEEKS
First trimester	Implantation	2–7
Second trimester	Placental development	8–14
Third trimester	Foetal growth and development	15–21

Implantation

In many management systems, pasture is reserved for the 5–6 week mating period and for 1 month or so thereafter. Dietary energy supply around the time of implantation, and during the first 6 weeks of gestation, is therefore adequate because sufficient autumn grass is still available (**Fig. 2.10**).

Placental development

While the effect of ewe undernutrition during mid-trimester on poor placental development, and subsequently reduced lamb birthweights, has been demonstrated under experimental conditions, it can prove difficult to be certain of such an influence in commercial flocks because many other factors influence lamb birthweights. Weather and/or grazing conditions need to be severe for at least 10 days during mid-gestation to impair placental development (**Fig. 2.11**).

However, reduced lamb birthweights can occur when placental development has been limited by competition in the uterus for caruncles, resulting in a reduced number of placentomes per foetus. This situation is not uncommonly encountered in multiple litters where the birth of twins with disproportionate weights, e.g. 5.5 kg versus 3.5 kg (**Fig. 2.12**), probably indicates that three embryos implanted and underwent early foetal development but one foetus failed to develop further and was resorbed.

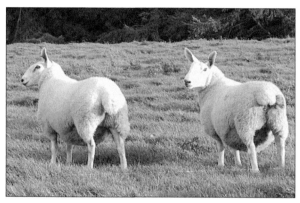

Fig. 2.10 **Dietary energy supply around the time of implantation, and during the first 6 weeks of gestation is adequate because there is still sufficient autumn grass available.**

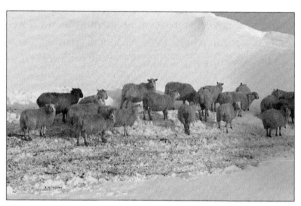

Fig. 2.11 **Weather and/or grazing conditions need to be severe for at least 10 days during mid-gestation to impair placental development.**

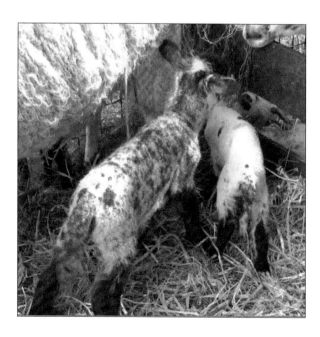

Fig. 2.12 **The birth of disproportionate twins can occur when placental development has been limited by competition for caruncles that results in a reduced number of placentomes for one foetus.**

The limited number of caruncles available to the remaining foetus in the ipsilateral horn results in poor growth and a reduced birthweight compared to the co-twin which developed without competition in the contralateral horn. While the placentomes can increase in size and blood flow, these compensatory mechanisms often fail to overcome their reduced number. Severe subacute fasciolosis has been associated with foetal resorption (**Fig. 2.13**) and a much reduced scanning percentage.

Real-time B-mode ultrasound scanning should be undertaken at 45–90 days of gestation to determine foetal number, thereby ensuring more accurate and selective concentrate feeding during the last 6 weeks of gestation when 75% of foetal growth occurs. This scanning process can be easily undertaken with up to 120 ewes scanned per hour, costing approximately 75 pence per ewe.

Foetal growth and development

Perinatal lamb mortality ranges from 10% to 15% on most UK farms but figures as high as 25% are still quoted. While many factors, including farm management, levels of flock supervision and infectious diseases contribute to such losses, correct lamb birthweight together with good ewe body condition and adequate passive antibody transfer remain fundamental to ensuring a good start for the lamb during the critical first 36 hours of life (**Fig. 2.14**).

The importance of adequate ewe energy supply during late gestation on lamb survival cannot be overemphasized (**Fig. 2.15**). Adequate ewe

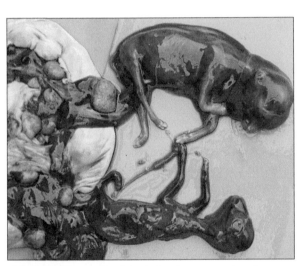

Fig. 2.13 Severe fasciolosis has been associated with foetal resorption and a much reduced scanning percentage.

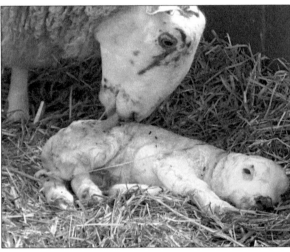

Fig. 2.14 Correct birthweight and adequate passive antibody transfer remain fundamental to ensuring a good start for the newborn lamb.

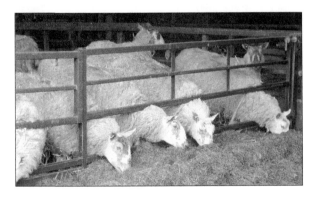

Fig. 2.15 The importance of adequate ewe energy supply during late gestation on lamb survival cannot be overemphasized.

nutrition during the last 6 weeks of pregnancy, when 75% of foetal growth occurs, is essential to ensure appropriate lamb birthweight.

The direct influence of dam energy undernutrition during late gestation on reduced lamb birthweight and inadequate accumulation of colostrum in the udder was established more than 40 years ago by Dr Angus Russel and co-workers. Many studies have found significantly higher lamb perinatal mortality in the progeny of underfed ewes, with the effects greater in triplet than twin lambs; singletons were largely unaffected by dam nutritional status. Reports have detailed lamb mortality rates in excess of 40% when their dams were underfed compared to 7% in lambs born to well-fed dams. The long-term health benefits of appropriate colostrum feeding in dairy calves, including fewer disease events, lower age at first breeding and higher first lactation yield, are now well established and should be equally applicable to neonatal lambs. It is likely that ingestion of adequate colostrum has long-term health benefits for the lamb with fewer disease events and, consequently, higher financial returns for the farmer.

Dietary energy supply relative to metabolic demands can be determined accurately during late gestation by measuring ewes' serum (or plasma) 3-OH butyrate concentration. Increased 3-OH butyrate concentrations (a ketone body) reflect inefficient fatty acid utilization caused by high glucose demand from the developing foetuses not matched by dietary propionate or glucogenic amino acid supply. Experimental studies have determined an energy supply, reflected in the serum 3-OH butyrate concentration, that results in the birth of healthy lambs of normal birthweight, and a dam with sufficient accumulation of colostrum in the udder. These factors combine to ensure the optimum start to the newborn lamb's life. The reader is directed to the excellent article written by Dr Angus Russel in *In Practice* (vol. 7, pp. 23–28; 1985) which describes the interpretation of the serum 3-OH butyrate concentration in relation to dam energy requirements. This article is the cornerstone of sheep preventive medicine programmes and has been used by this author since its publication, with numerous published studies of its practical application.

FARM VISIT TO ASSESS LATE GESTATION EWE NUTRITION

Ewes due to lamb during the first week should be body condition scored and blood sampled 4–6 weeks before the start of lambing time, thereby allowing sufficient time to implement dietary changes. Note that 75% of foetal growth occurs during the last 6 weeks of gestation. Primiparous sheep (ewe lambs and gimmers) should not be sampled as they have significantly more singletons and may give a skewed set of results. If the flock has been scanned to determine foetal number an equal number of twin- and triplet-bearing ewes should be sampled; there is little benefit in collecting samples from ewes with singletons other than to establish reference values. Sick ewes, thin ewes and those not representative of the flock must be investigated separately and not included as part of the nutrition assessment exercise.

Details of the diet, forage analyses, and future alterations should be noted. Feed allocations must be checked on weigh scales and the number of sheep per group accurately determined – approximations lead to unnecessary errors.

Results and interpretation

A range of 3-OH butyrate concentrations is often encountered in a flock test, largely in relation to foetal number; thus a more reliable interpretation of results can be afforded in those flocks which have determined foetal number by prior ultrasound scanning.

The target mean 3-OH butyrate concentration is below 1.0 mmol/l. 3-OH butyrate concentrations above 1.6 mmol/l in individual ewes represent severe energy underfeeding, with the likelihood of pregnancy toxaemia developing as pregnancy advances and foetal energy requirement increase unless dietary changes are implemented. 3-OH butyrate concentrations greater than 3.0 mmol/l are consistent with a diagnosis of ovine pregnancy toxaemia.

Once the mean 3-OH butyrate concentration has been determined, any alteration in the ration can be made with reference to Dr Russel's *In Practice* article and the farmer advised immediately by telephone, and in writing, regarding any dietary or management changes.

Example

During a flock visit to determine nutritional management 4 weeks before lambing commences the mean serum 3-OH butyrate concentration of 10 twin- and triplet-bearing ewes sampled at random on this farm is 1.5 mmol/l. This underfeeding situation necessitates an extra 4 MJ metabolizable energy (ME)/day (0.3 kg of concentrates as fed) to return the ewes to a satisfactory level of energy supply (mean 3-OH butyrate concentration below 1.0 mmol/l). The flock should be re-visited and blood samples collected 2 weeks later to check on progress and further monitor any changes in ewe body condition scores.

Evaluation of protein status

Blood samples can also be analysed for blood urea nitrogen (BUN) which indicates short-term protein intake, and albumin, which reflects longer-term protein status. Care must be exercised with the interpretation of these parameters as recent feeding can greatly influence BUN concentrations. Blood samples should be collected either before concentrate feeding or at least 4 hours later to avoid postprandial increases. Low BUN concentrations usually indicate a shortage of rumen degradable protein. Serum albumin concentrations fall during the last month of gestation as immunoglobulins are manufactured and accumulate in the udder; thus serum albumin concentrations in the region of 26–30 g/l are 'normal' during the last month of gestation. Plasma protein concentrations are often 10% higher than corresponding serum protein concentrations; therefore it is essential to be aware of what samples were submitted to the laboratory before interpretation.

VACCINATION PROGRAMME

Farmers are advised to vaccinate their ewes against the clostridial diseases 4 weeks before lambing. It is advisable to vaccinate the flock as two separate groups, with the later lambing ewes vaccinated 2 weeks later. Ewes' fleeces must be dry when they are vaccinated and care must be taken to ensure correct subcutaneous injection of every ewe. Subcutaneous injection of ewes when they are wet may result in contamination of the needle and abscess formation. Careful and gentle handling of the pregnant ewes is essential during the operation; speed is not important.

By ensuring ewes are in good condition at vaccination time, and receiving an appropriate level of supplementation as determined by the blood samples collected, a plentiful accumulation of protective antibodies in the ewes' colostrum at lambing time is guaranteed. Thus it is important that the farmer is reminded of the importance of ensuring passive antibody transfer within the first 2 hours of the lamb's life.

If there are few losses due to pasteurellosis in lambs less than 1 month old, consider using a multivalent clostridial vaccine only and not a vaccine containing the 'Pasteurella' components.

FOLLOW-UP VISIT DURING LAMBING TIME

A visit during lambing time is essential to discuss the results with the farmer and shepherd. Measurement (with a spring balance) and recording of lamb birthweights and ewe condition scores are essential to determine the success of the flock nutrition advice during late gestation. Particular attention should be paid to the triplet litters during a visit. Has the farmer witnessed any improvement in lamb viability, ewe milk supply, general health, reduced perinatal disease incidents, and mortality compared to previous years? Is the farmer happy with the advice; if not why not? Postmortem examination of any neonatal deaths will provide much useful information if the results contradict expectations.

It is essential to determine any benefit:cost ratio from this exercise. Have reduced losses and greater lamb growth rates more than compensated for any increased feed bills? What are the improvements, if any, in terms of animal welfare? What improvements can be made for next year? Remember always to provide written reports, to remove doubts over specific points and provide a record for future reference.

LAMBING FACILITIES

During farm visits, veterinarians should check whether pens are cleaned out between successive litters, the provision of food and water including roughage such as hay, and lamb navel treatments. Perinatal mortality will only be significantly reduced when all husbandry tasks are performed well by farm staff.

Housing

If there have been no previous problems on the farm with respiratory diseases such as ovine pulmonary adenocarcinoma or maedi, it is recommended that ewes are housed based upon foetal number and their due lambing date (keel marks). The critical dimensions of a sheep pen are 3 m wide and 450 mm trough space per ewe along one side, allowing 1.3 square metres of floor area per ewe (**Figs 2.16, 2.17**).

Individual pens

Individual pens must be well drained, a minimum size of 1.5 m by 1.5 m (**Fig. 2.18**) and have concrete floors with solid partitions whenever possible. These pens must be cleaned out and disinfected between every ewe but this practice is rarely achieved on most commercial farms. Each pen must be provided with a water bucket and feed container. Newly-lambed ewes will often drink more than 10 litres of water after lambing. Placentae must be removed from the individual pens and put into plastic sacks for burning or burial.

During an intensive lambing period (up to 15% of ewes lambing in a 24 hour period), the practice

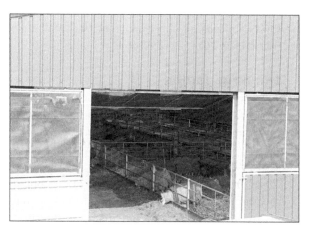

Fig. 2.16 **Modern purpose-built sheep shed.**

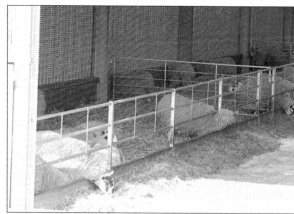

Fig. 2.17 **Sheep pens are 3 m wide with 450 mm trough space per ewe along one side, allowing 1.3 square metres of floor area per ewe.**

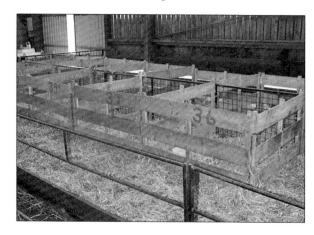

Fig. 2.18 **Individual lambing pens must be well drained, a minimum size of 1.5 m by 1.5 m, and have concrete floors and preferably solid partitions.**

of fostering lambs and in the likelihood of adverse weather, one pen per five ewes is essential to avoid accommodation shortages. During adverse weather farmers rarely have sufficient housing and overcrowding can lead to problems with infectious bacterial diseases.

FOSTERING

The perinatal lamb mortality rate is high in many sheep flocks and as a consequence triplet lambs are often fostered onto those ewes that have lost a lamb, whether stillborn or dead from other causes. In addition, lambs are commonly fostered onto those ewes which produce a single lamb. No large surveys have been undertaken to determine the number of attempted fosterings in lowground flocks, but it could conservatively be estimated at greater than 10–15%. Furthermore, this procedure is not as simple as would first appear and the long-term acceptance rate by the ewe is likely to be less than 70%. Numerous animal welfare concerns arise from the various methods employed to convince a ewe to accept another lamb.

Orphan lambs are usually triplet lambs removed because of poor dam milk yield. Often these lambs have failed to ingest sufficient colostrum and are therefore prone to a wide range of bacterial diseases during the neonatal period.

Transfer of foetal fluids

Rubbing an orphan lamb in the foetal fluids of the newborn single lamb before the ewe licks her own lamb is the most successful fostering method; good acceptance rates are achieved when the foster lamb is as young as possible and preferably newborn. It has been suggested that the shepherd should gently insert a well-lubricated gloved hand into the ewe's posterior reproductive tract to simulate birth of another lamb, but this practice is uncommon.

If the foster lamb is more than a few hours old and its coat is dry, it should first be immersed in a bucket of warm water to aid transfer of foetal fluids and associated odours onto the wet fleece. Many shepherds will place only the foster lamb in the pen with the ewe for a period of time before introducing her own lamb. Time spent ensuring initial acceptance by the ewe is well worthwhile. Some shepherds may elect to castrate and tail dock the foster lamb using elastrator rings at this time to delay its normal active behaviour and teat searching, because the ewe is suspicious of a 'newborn' lamb which is already ambulatory.

A variation on the fostering methods described above is to place both lambs in a cloth sack which is then tied at the neck and placed in the pen with the ewe for 1 hour. This practice facilitates mixing of odours and increases the foster lamb acceptance rate when the lambs are introduced to the anxious ewe.

Disparity in size of the new 'pair' of lambs frequently results (6–7 kg singleton and 3.5 kg triplet). The smaller foster triplet lamb may be unable to keep up with the much larger singleton when the litter is turned out to pasture, and careful supervision of fostered lambs is essential to achieve good results and ensure the welfare of the smaller lamb (**Figs 2.19, 2.20**).

'Skinning' lambs

Fostering lambs with the aid of the dead lamb's skin has good success depending upon the age of the dead lamb and age of the foster lamb (**Fig. 2.21**).

Foster crates

There are many designs of foster crates but it is essential that clean water and good quality roughage are always available, and that concentrates are fed at least twice daily where the ewe can reach them (**Fig. 2.22**). Inadequate ewe nutrition merely leads to poor milk production and poor long-term foster lamb acceptance rates.

Rope halters

The use of a rope halter affords greater freedom and improved comfort for the ewe (**Fig. 2.23**) than a foster crate, provided the halter does not tighten across the bridge of the ewe's nose. Halters should be made of soft rope and not a single strand of polypropylene baler twine. The rope should not be tied around the ewe's horns.

Rejection of foster lamb

The ewe and lambs must be carefully supervised to detect early rejection such as not letting the foster

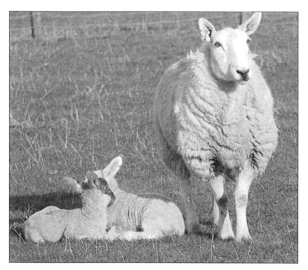

Fig. 2.19 Careful supervision of fostered lambs is essential when the litter is turned out to pasture.

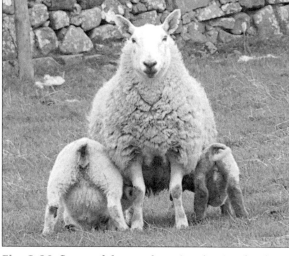

Fig. 2.20 Successful cross-fostering despite the size disparity of the lambs.

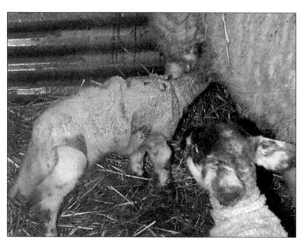

Fig. 2.21 Fostering lambs with the aid of the dead lamb's skin has good success although the development of a leather appearance in this case suggests otherwise.

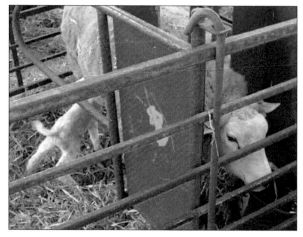

Fig. 2.22 It is essential that the ewe has plenty of fresh food and water whilst confined in a foster crate.

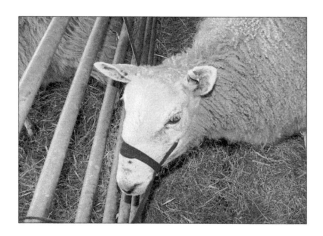

Fig. 2.23 A halter affords some degree of normal behaviour and freedom when cross-fostering lambs.

lamb suck, pushing the lamb away, and vigorous head butting, which can cause severe chest trauma and indeed death of neglected lambs. Ewes with foster lambs should be clearly marked and allocated to small paddocks for up to 1 week before re joining the main flock.

Rearing orphan lambs

Orphan lambs can be reared very successfully on artificial rearing systems using automatic milk dispensers. These achieve excellent growth rates and a low incidence of digestive disturbances such as abomasal bloat and/or volvulus.

PART 1 FEMALE REPRODUCTIVE SYSTEM

CLINICAL EXAMINATION

Clinical examination of the female reproductive system in sheep can be divided into five stages of the reproductive cycle:

1. Failure to become pregnant during a restricted breeding period.
2. Embryonic loss/abortion.
3. Vaginal/uterine prolapses.
4. Dystocia.
5. Metritis.

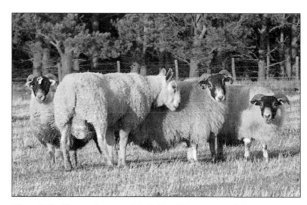

Fig. 3.1 Sheep have a high fertility rate with more than 90% of females conceiving during one cycle of the normal breeding season.

Failure to become pregnant during a restricted breeding period

Unlike cattle, sheep have a high fertility rate with more than 90% of females of appropriate bodyweight and body condition score conceiving during one cycle of the normal breeding season to a fertile ram (**Fig. 3.1**). This figure may be as high as 95% when approximately 40 ewes are run with one fertile ram. Less than 2% of females should be nonpregnant after a restricted breeding period of only 35–42 days (two reproductive cycles).

Investigations of infertility are rarely undertaken in individual commercial-value female sheep and these animals are simply culled. If commercial-value sheep do not breed during their first season they should be culled as most fail to become pregnant the following season. Infertility in older ewes is generally considered to arise from previous uterine infection and/or physical damage arising from dystocia, but there have been no detailed large scale studies.

Investigation of infertility in a pedigree female would include a history detailing previous breeding performance including any dystocia/caesarean operation(s), and diary of service dates and ram(s) used. A complete physical examination must be undertaken as infertility may be the result of disease in another organ system, e.g. chronic respiratory tract infection, causing weight loss and poor body condition. Investigation of the female reproductive tract is restricted to the external genitalia and transabdominal ultrasonography immediately cranial to the pelvic brim using a 5 MHz sector scanner, although this will not reveal the normal involuted uterus which is contained within the pelvic canal. Ultrasonography will only identify gross abnormalities such as pyometra when there are large accumulations of exudate within the uterus (**Fig. 3.2**).

More detailed examination of the uterus and ovaries could involve laparoscopy. Certain 'infertile' pedigree ewes undergo an embryo flushing programme with the laparoscopic examination undertaken at the time of surgical insemination or embryo collection if transcervical insemination is used. The cost of the

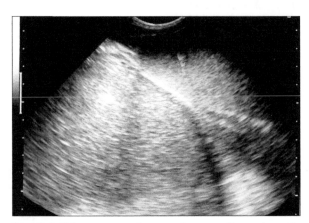

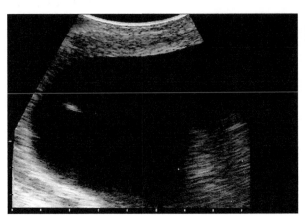

Fig. 3.2 Ultrasonography reveals gross distension of the uterine horns with pus as the cause of infertility in this ewe (5 MHz sector scanner).

Fig. 3.3 Ultrasound studies have demonstrated that the vaginal prolapse usually contains urinary bladder.

flushing programme is relatively inexpensive with embryos collected if no abnormalities are present. If there are abnormalities present preventing successful embryo collection, then the only added cost is that of the flushing programme.

Embryonic loss/abortion

Embryo/foetal loss from non-infectious causes is considered to be very low in sheep. Detailed investigations would generally not be undertaken unless the number of sheep returning to service after around 30 days exceeded 2%, more commonly 5% in commercial situations. In many situations, the rams are removed after a 35–42 day breeding period and embryo/foetal loss may not be detected until scanning time, which may be up to 90 days post service. Indeed, embryo/foetal loss may only become apparent when ewes are found to be barren at the end of the lambing period. Vasectomized rams can be returned to the groups of breeding ewes after removal of the rams to identify returns to service.

Vaginal/uterine prolapses

The investigation and treatment of vaginal and uterine prolapses are detailed in the relevant sections below. Ultrasound studies have demonstrated that vaginal prolapse may contain either urinary bladder (**Fig. 3.3**) or uterine horn. These studies are important because they highlight the risks of needle decompression to facilitate replacement.

Indeed, having identified that the vaginal prolapse contains urinary bladder effectively instructs the clinician to elevate the prolapse after low extradural block and relieve the kink in the urethra and allow urine to drain.

The interval from parturition to uterine prolapse is important; while uterine prolapse may occur spontaneously after prolonged second stage labour in a sheep with a singleton, prolapse 12–48 hours after parturition indicates excessive manual interference of a dystocia causing tensemus. In the latter group there is typically marked oedema/bruising/superficial infection of the posterior reproductive tract.

Dystocia

Normal parturition and the approach to dystocia cases are detailed below. This is an important area of veterinary work in many countries. The importance of a full clinical examination before attempting to correct the dystocia cannot be overemphasized because uterine rupture, and other iatrogenic trauma, are not uncommon.

Metritis

A diagnosis of metritis is not simple in sheep and largely involves ruling out other common diseases causing endotoxaemia. Manual vaginal examination for the presence of uterine discharges is not possible and vaginoscopic examination is rarely undertaken. Transabdominal ultrasonography of the caudal abdomen using a 5 MHz sector scanner will identify the uterus for 2–3 days after parturition, but interpretation of uterine diameter and fluid accumulations is problematic. There are no definitive data on the significance of bacteria isolated from vaginal swabs.

OBSTETRICS

Survey data on dystocia rates

Ewe deaths around lambing time in lowground flocks in the UK are estimated around 5% with 70% caused by dystocia, but there are few data from large commercial flocks.

Easy-care lambing system: In many countries, such as New Zealand and Australia, lambing takes place outdoors in carefully selected lambing paddocks which utilize natural shelter. Set stocking of paddocks is preferred to daily group movement as occurs in drift lambing. A stocking rate of around 18 ewes per hectare has been recommended, but this depends upon grazing conditions and other factors. Easy-care lambing systems allow supervision of lambing ewes without unnecessary disturbance (**Fig. 3.4**). Ewes may spend up to 6 hours at the selected birth site before the start of first stage labour and should not be disturbed during this period. Selection of breeding stock should be based upon the ability of ewes to rear at least one lamb depending upon the management system. Rams should be selected from families that show strong maternal instincts.

Hygiene/approach to dystocia cases: The basic hygiene approach to dystocia cases could be greatly improved on many UK sheep farms by farmers washing their hands and using arm-length disposable gloves prior to correction of all dystocia cases (**Fig. 3.5**). Such precautions should also be seen as a minimum standard to limit the risk of potential zoonotic infections.

Antibiotic therapy: All ewes should receive an antibiotic injection after an assisted lambing. Penicillin is the antibiotic most commonly used by sheep farmers and should be administered for a minimum of 3 consecutive days.

Euthanasia: Euthanasia of ewes with dystocia is a recent development in the UK sheep industry based solely upon economic considerations, because success rates exceeding 97% have been reported for caesarean operations undertaken in field situations (**Fig. 3.6**).

Animal welfare implications: There have been considerable advances in the provision of analgesia for ovine obstetrical conditions under field situations with visible improvements in the sheep's wellbeing. Such improved care and welfare of sheep can only be effected by veterinary involvement in obstetrical

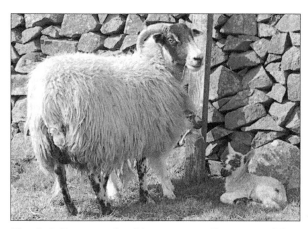

Fig. 3.4 Easy-care lambing systems allow supervision of lambing ewes without unnecessary disturbance.

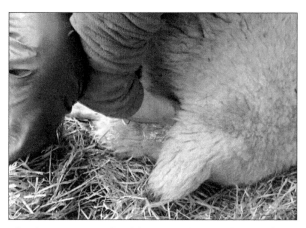

Fig. 3.5 Farmers should use arm-length disposable gloves prior to correcting all dystocias.

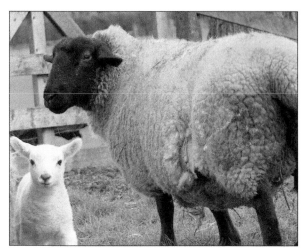

Fig. 3.6 Success rates exceeding 97% have been reported for caesarean operations undertaken in field situations.

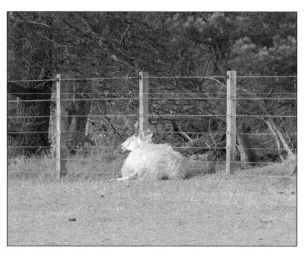

Fig. 3.7 During first stage labour the ewe will often select a secluded area of the field.

problems, something that is not requested on the majority of UK farms.

Definitions
- Presentation: signifies the relation between the long axis of the foetus and the maternal birth canal. It includes anterior or posterior longitudinal presentation or ventral or dorsal transverse presentation.
- Position: indicates the surface of the maternal birth canal to which the foetal vertebral column is applied. It includes dorsal, ventral and right or left lateral position.
- Posture: refers to the disposition of the moveable appendages of the foetus and involves flexion or extension of the cervical and limb joints, e.g. bilateral hip flexion.
- Foetal oversize:
  - Relative oversize: foetus normal dimensions, maternal pelvis is too small.
  - Absolute oversize: foetus abnormally large, maternal pelvis is normal.

Normal parturition in the ewe
Gestation length is from 143–147 days. Imminent parturition can be detected by changes in the ewe's behaviour, udder development, accumulation of colostrum and slackening of the sacro-iliac ligaments. The birth process is divided into three stages:

First stage labour
First stage labour is represented by cervical dilation which takes 3–6 hours but is more rapid in multiparous ewes.

There are various behavioural changes, including the ewe frequently does not come to the feed trough or leaves early before other sheep in the group. The ewe seeks a sheltered area of the field (**Fig. 3.7**) or corner of the barn and will paw at the ground, frequently sniffing at this area, and alternately lying/standing. These periods of increased activity often occur at 10–15 minute intervals with abdominal contractions lasting 15–30 seconds. A thick string of mucus is often observed hanging from the vulva. The bouts of straining then occur more frequently, usually every 2–3 minutes, coinciding with extension of the foetal forelimbs. The cervix is fully dilated at the end of first stage labour.

Second stage labour
Second stage labour is represented by expulsion of foetus(es), and typically takes about 1 hour. There is rupture of allanto-chorion often with a rush of fluid (**Fig. 3.8**). The amnion and foetal parts are then engaged in the pelvic inlet (**Fig. 3.9**).

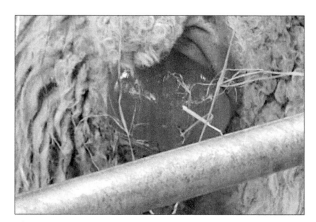

Fig. 3.8 **During first stage labour the allanto-chorion appears at the vulva.**

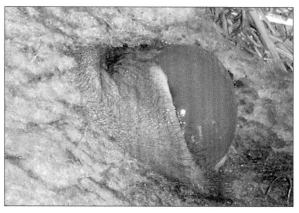

Fig. 3.9 **The amnion and foetal parts are now engaged in the pelvis.**

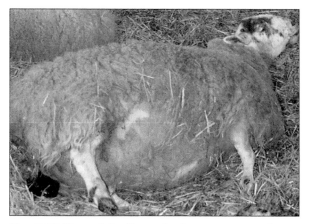

Fig. 3.10 **Powerful reflex and voluntary contractions of abdominal muscle and diaphragm ('straining') expel the foetus.**

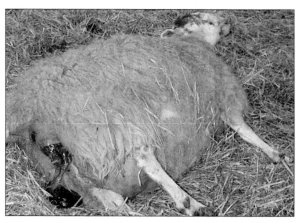

Fig. 3.11 **Progress from Fig. 3.10; there is no need to assist delivery of this lamb.**

The amniotic sac appears at the vulva and frequently ruptures at this stage. Powerful reflex and voluntary contractions of abdominal muscle and diaphragm ('straining') serve to expel the foetus (**Figs 3.10, 3.11**). However, the amniotic sac may not rupture until the ewe stands up after the lamb has been expelled. The delayed rupture of the amnion, referred to colloquially as the lamb being 'sheeted' or 'born with the skin over its nose', may result in death of the lamb due to asphyxiation. This scenario is not uncommon in multiple births, especially with later-born lambs. In multigravid ewes, the interval between birth of the lambs varies from 10 to 60 minutes (**Fig. 3.12**); intervention should be considered after 1 hour.

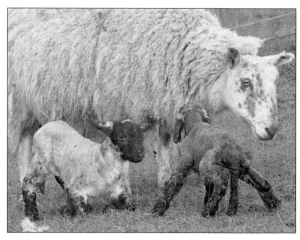

Fig. 3.12 **In multigravid ewes, the interval between birth of the lambs varies from 10 to 60 minutes.**

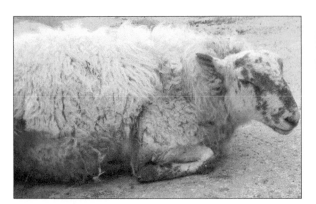

Fig. 3.13 It is essential to assess the patient in detail before attempting to correct the dystocia.

Third stage labour

Third stage labour is completed by expulsion of foetal membranes which usually occurs within 2–3 hours of the end of second stage labour.

Veterinary approach to every lambing case

As a veterinary surgeon it is essential to assess the patient in detail before attempting to correct the problem (**Fig. 3.13**). Inspection of the ewe will frequently give an indication of prolonged dystocia and/or toxaemia. Lateral recumbency with frequent abdominal straining and vocalization may result from engagement of the lamb within the pelvis or from excessive manual interference leading to trauma of the posterior reproductive tract. Bruxism (teeth grinding), and an elevated respiratory rate with abdominal component (panting) may indicate more serious concerns such as uterine rupture.

Attempted delivery by an unskilled shepherd frequently results in oedema, reddening and bruising of vulval labiae within 1–2 hours. There may be evidence of vaginal bleeding on the tail and perineum (**Fig. 3.14**) especially on the lower side when the ewe was recumbent. The ewe's mucous membranes must be checked for evidence of pallor. The presence of a foetid yellow-brown vulval discharge indicates the presence of autolytic lambs *in utero*. It is important to express any concerns with the client before attempting correction of the dystocia (**Fig. 3.15**), especially if significant trauma to the reproductive tract is suspected.

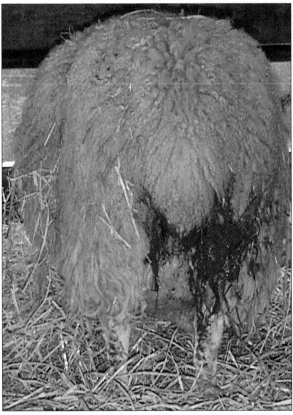

Fig. 3.14 Attempted delivery of the lamb may cause bleeding which will be present on the tail and perineum.

Caudal analgesia

Caudal analgesia is strongly recommended for all manipulations undertaken by the veterinary surgeon. This involves extradural injection of 0.5 mg/kg 2% lignocaine solution at the sacrococcygeal site (caudal block). Blockage of the ewe's reflex abdominal contractions greatly assists corrections/manipulations of dystocia cases and has obvious animal welfare benefits (**Figs 3.16, 3.17**). Reliance on strength by the shepherd to repel the foetus risks serious damage to the ewe, such as uterine rupture. Likewise, raising the ewe by the hindlimbs using an assistant or a pulley system is unacceptable as this merely transfers the full weight of the rumen, gravid uterus and other abdominal viscera onto the ewe's diaphragm. It is difficult to believe that there could be any possible benefit of gravity gained with the ewe in this position.

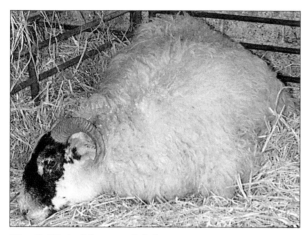

Fig. 3.15 A sick ewe – it is important to express any concerns with the client before attempting correction of the dystocia.

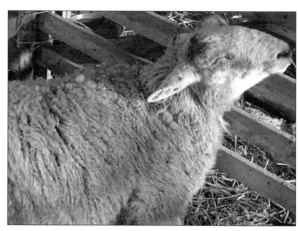

Fig. 3.16 Evidence of pain originating from attempted delivery of lambs – caudal analgesia is essential before attempting to correct any dystocia (see Fig. 3.17).

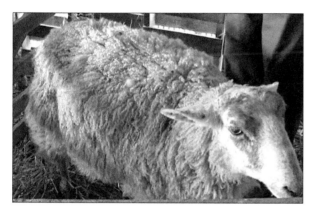

Fig. 3.17 Effective pain relief; this image shows the same ewe as in Fig. 3.16 after injection of 0.5 mg/kg of 2% lignocaine solution at the sacrococcygeal site.

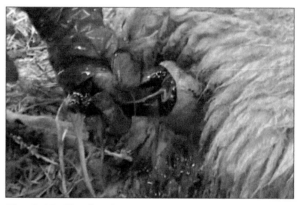

Fig. 3.18 Shepherds must use arm-length disposable gloves during the correction of all dystocia cases to reduce the risk of iatrogenic uterine infection.

The reader is directed to Chapter 17 (Anaesthesia) for the detailed approach to extradural analgesia in dystocia cases.

Hygiene

Farmers must wash their hands and then use arm-length disposable gloves during the correction of all dystocia cases to reduce the risk of iatrogenic uterine infection (**Fig. 3.18**). Obstetrical gel is then liberally applied to the hand of the shepherd's gloved arm; the fingers of the hand are forced together at their tips to form a cone-shape then gently introduced into the vagina. Careful examination is essential not only for welfare reasons but the likelihood of infection of the posterior reproductive tract is greatly increased by trauma.

Arm-length disposable plastic gloves are cheap and easily carried in pockets, thus there can be no excuse for non-compliance with such basic hygiene even under extensive flock management systems.

DYSTOCIA

Incomplete cervical dilation
(syn: ringwomb)

Definition/overview
The true incidence of ringwomb is difficult to determine because in most situations the onset of first stage labour has not been noted by the farmer especially in overcrowded, housed flocks and extensive pasture-managed systems. It is probable that most dystocia cases classified as ringwomb represent over-zealous interference during early first stage labour. A working definition of ringwomb could be 'the presence of an incompletely dilated cervix more than 3 hours after first appearance of the foetal membranes (allanto-chorion) at the vulva'.

Aetiology
Some authors refer to previous cervical trauma during previous births, but ringwomb has been described in primiparous sheep.

Pathophysiology
Numerous studies have failed to find a satisfactory explanation for this condition.

Clinical presentation
Foetal membranes (allanto-chorion) are present at the vulva for 3 or more hours with an incompletely dilated cervix detected upon digital examination of the posterior reproductive tract. Typically, the external cervical os is only 3–5 cm in diameter allowing passage of only two or three fingers. The cervix feels corrugated and is up to 1 cm thick.

Differential diagnoses
- Disturbed early first stage labour before full cervical dilation.
- Uterine torsion.
- Incomplete cervical dilation associated with lamb in posterior presentation with hip joints extended (breech).

Diagnosis
Diagnosis is based upon digital examination of the reproductive tract and failure of the cervix to dilate under digital pressure applied for up to 10 minutes. The cervix feels approximately 1 cm thick with obvious radial corrugations.

Treatment
Digital pressure applied for 5–10 minutes will gradually dilate the cervix in some cases, but such cases may well represent those ewes disturbed during early first stage labour. If the cervix feels 2–3 mm thin with no obvious corrugations at first presentation then it will probably dilate under digital pressure. It is not uncommon for a farmer to diagnose ringwomb but the condition to have largely resolved by normal progression when the veterinary surgeon attends the case 1–2 hours later.

If no progress has been made in 10 minutes, continued manual interference will simply lead to contamination of the foetal extremities, posterior reproductive tract and uterus, with an attendant risk of contamination of the peritoneal cavity when the lamb is delivered during the corrective caesarean operation. Trauma to the posterior reproductive tract frequently results in reflex abdominal contractions which may complicate the caesarean operation, although this complication is resolved following the routine extradural injection given by the veterinary surgeon. Various smooth muscle relaxants have been used in ringwomb sheep but there is no convincing evidence that these are effective.

Management/prevention/control measures
Too early/frequent human interference may delay normal progression of first stage labour by inhibiting the ewe's normal behavioural patterns. Shepherds should be encouraged to leave sheep undisturbed for 3 hours after the appearance of a mucus string or allanto-chorion at the vulva, especially in primiparous animals. However, frequent bouts of powerful abdominal contractions occurring more frequently than every 5 minutes or so must be investigated because of the likelihood of foetal malposture.

Economics
Failure to deliver the lamb(s) *per vaginam* in cases of ringwomb requires veterinary assistance. Correction of dystocia at the veterinary surgery costs £25–40 and a further £40–85 if a caesarean operation is necessary. A visit charge could add a further £25–45 to the invoice.

Welfare implications

Excessive unskilled interference in cases of ring-womb results in trauma to the posterior reproductive tract. Trauma may cause continued straining after the end of second stage labour and uterine prolapse could occur. Unhygienic conditions and failure to wash hands and use disposable arm-length gloves increase the risk of metritis.

While extradural sacrococcygeal lignocaine injection has been routinely employed by veterinary surgeons prior to bovine obstetrical procedures, the adoption of this technique for ovine obstetrical problems in general practice has only recently been recommended. Manual correction is made easier and the combined score of abnormal behaviours is significantly reduced after sacrococcygeal extradural injection of 0.5–0.6 mg/kg lignocaine. Hindlimb paresis may persist for several hours in a small percentage of ewes after extradural injection.

Uterine torsion

Uterine torsion is very uncommon indeed in the ewe and is usually seen in single pregnancies (**Fig. 3.19**). The diligent shepherd will notice that the ewe does not progress beyond the behavioural signs of early first stage labour; careful manual examination of the posterior reproductive tract may reveal a torsion if the twist is distal to the cervix (which is uncommon). It is not possible to detect a twist proximal to the cervix. Correction of the torsion is usually made following delivery of the lamb(s) by caesarean operation; alternatively, the torsion can be corrected via an abdominal approach before uterine incision. This author has encountered only four cases of uterine torsion in a ewe in 36 years' clinical practice. However, in some countries, uterine torsion is considered a relatively common cause of dystocia presented to veterinary surgeons.

Uterine inertia

Primary uterine inertia is very uncommon in the ewe. Unlike cattle, hypocalcaemia is very uncommon around the time of parturition in sheep.

Rupture of the prepubic tendon

Rupture of the prepubic tendon occasionally occurs in older multigravid ewes during the last 2 weeks of pregnancy. A large swelling appears immediately cranial to the pubis (**Fig. 3.20**). The ventral abdominal wall may be close to the ground and there is extensive subcutaneous oedema. Rupture of the ventral body wall results in an altered position of the uterus in relation to the pelvic inlet and assistance is frequently necessary because the lambs are not correctly presented. While the ewe will survive with such a rupture, affected sheep should be euthanased for welfare reasons following delivery of the lambs.

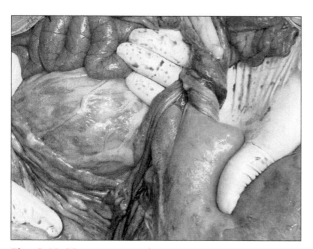

Fig. 3.19 Necropsy reveals a 720° torsion of the uterus. The devitalized uterine wall, secondary to vascular compromise, is shown to the bottom right of the image.

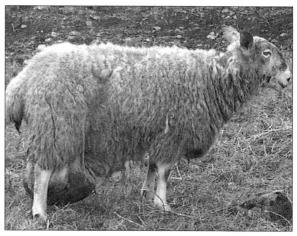

Fig. 3.20 Rupture of the prepubic tendon occasionally occurs in older multigravid ewes during the last 2 weeks of pregnancy.

Foetal dystocia
Overview

Presentation and postural abnormalities are very common but are generally simple to correct, provided that they are identified during early second stage labour. Congenital abnormalities, while usually rare on individual farms, appear common to the veterinary practitioner because of the large number of sheep within the practice area. Arthrogryposis caused by *in utero* Schmallenberg virus infection is reportedly a common cause of dystocia in many countries within Europe.

Anterior presentation

When the lamb is presented in anterior presentation (head and both forelimbs presented normally) the lamb is often born after 5–10 minutes of vigorous abdominal straining (**Figs 3.21–3.23**).

In the case of a large single lamb, the forelimbs protrude as far as the hooves or fetlock joint while the muzzle and swollen tongue only become visible when the ewe strains. If no progress is made within 30 minutes the ewe should be cast into lateral recumbency and patient assistance given. When both forefeet are present at the vulva and the muzzle can be touched within the pelvic canal, each forelimb should be extended in turn. One forefoot is held between the thumb and forefinger and steady traction is applied when the ewe strains. Such traction should extend the elbow and the forelimb protrudes to the carpus (knee). A sudden 'clunk' sensation is often appreciated when the elbow is

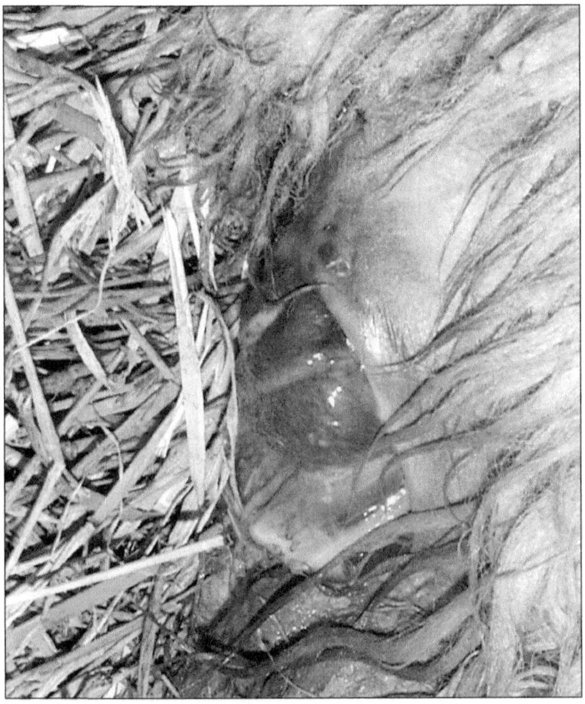

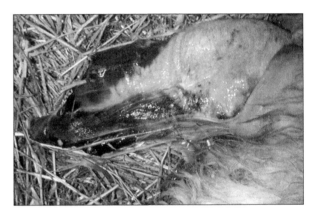

Fig. 3.22 The head, shoulders, forelimbs and chest are delivered.

Fig. 3.21 First in a sequence of three images showing the birth of a lamb in anterior presentation; the nose and forefeet present at the vulva.

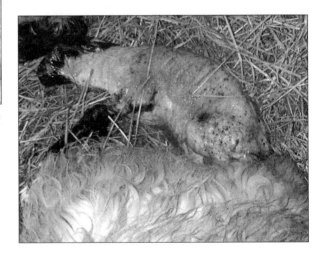

Fig. 3.23 Delivery of the lamb; the ewe will remain lying for 1–2 minutes after the birth of the lamb.

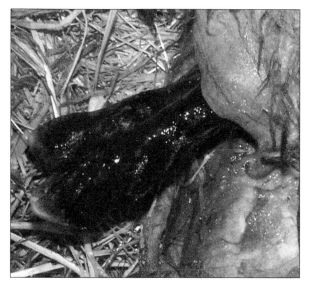

Fig. 3.24 Traction has extended the elbows, and the forelimbs protrude from the vulva to the carpus.

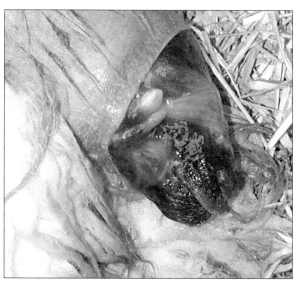

Fig. 3.25 Leg back; the retained forelimb lies alongside the lamb's chest and must be brought forward before any traction is applied.

extended (Fig. 3.24). The other forelimb is extended in the same manner ('clunk'). Slight traction on both forelimbs should cause the head to protrude from the vulva. At this stage the poll of the head is grasped and slow, steady traction is applied to the poll and both forelimbs. The lamb should be delivered in a downward arc without undue force over 10–30 seconds. Note that the traction is applied in an arc and the lamb is pulled 'down and around' and not 'straight out'.

The lamb should be left for a about 1 minute with the umbilical vessels still intact (Fig. 3.23) and not instantly be snatched away and placed at the ewe's head. It may take up to 30 seconds before the lamb takes its first deep breath. There are few indications to swing the lamb around by the hindlimbs – any fluid which appears at the mouth or nostrils during these aeronautics originates from the lamb's stomach not its lungs.

Take time to observe a ewe which lambs unaided. She will always lie for 1–2 minutes before regaining her feet and licking her lamb. Parturition is a feat of great physical exertion and the ewe should not be expected to leap instantly to her feet as soon as the first lamb hits the straw. After delivery of one lamb

it is usual to ballot the abdomen gently, which readily reveals whether there is another lamb(s) *in utero*. Opinion is divided whether to deliver the second lamb or to leave well alone. Unnecessary interference in unhygienic conditions increases the likelihood of uterine infection (metritis). It is reasoned, however, that the second lamb may be born in the intact amnion ('skin over its nose', 'sheeted') and therefore all remaining lambs should be delivered at this time to avoid such risks. Delivery of the remaining lambs allows the ewe and her lambs to be penned together and may simplify management.

Head and only one forelimb presented

In this situation (Fig. 3.25), the retained forelimb lies alongside the lamb's chest and must be brought forward before any traction is applied to the lamb. Correction of this malposture involves flexing the shoulder and elbow joints, and then carefully extending the carpus (knee) and fetlock joints in that order, which presents the foot at the pelvic inlet. Gentle traction applied to both forelimbs should result in delivery of the lamb.

Some shepherds will attempt to deliver a lamb with only one foot presented at the vulva, after checking that the other foot is not within the pelvic canal (this implies that the other limb lies alongside the lamb's chest). This practice will usually be successful if the lamb is a twin (see mark on ewe if previously scanned for litter size) but must never be undertaken if the lamb is a singleton.

Bilateral shoulder flexion (hung lamb)

The head is presented through the vulva (**Fig. 3.26**) but both forelimbs are retained alongside the chest. Correction of this malposture involves repulsion of the head into the vagina, flexing the shoulder and elbow joint of one forelimb, and then carefully extending the carpus (knee) and fetlock joint in that order, which presents the foot at the pelvic inlet. These manipulations are then repeated for the other forelimb.

The lamb's head and tongue may remain swollen for a few hours and it is prudent to stomach tube these lambs to ensure that they receive sufficient colostrum before 6 hours old, if not sooner.

Repulsion of the lamb's head is greatly facilitated after sacrococcygeal extradural lignocaine injection, which blocks the reflex abdominal contractions of the ewe. This technique is routinely employed by veterinary surgeons and greatly improves ewe welfare as well as rendering the various foetal manipulations much easier to perform (**Figs 3.27, 3.28**). The more traditional means of repelling a lamb is to enlist the help of an assistant who suspends the ewe by the pelvic limbs while the lamb is forced back against the ewe's strong abdominal contractions. This procedure causes considerable distress to the ewe because the weight of the pregnant uterus, rumen and other abdominal viscera are forced against the diaphragm. The risk of trauma to the uterus and vagina are greatly increased if the lamb is forced back into the body of the uterus against such powerful opposition.

Posterior presentation

First stage labour proceeds normally but there is much reduced straining during second stage labour because the lamb does not become fully engaged within the ewe's pelvis to stimulate the powerful reflex abdominal contractions. The shepherd examines the ewe because it has made no progress since being noted in first stage labour 2–3 hours previously. Digital examination of the vagina reveals the lamb's hooves facing the roof of the vagina (not the floor) and the hocks can be felt by progressing forward; sometimes the tail can be felt (**Fig. 3.29**).

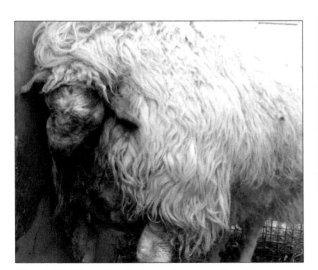

Fig. 3.26 Hung lamb; the oedematous head is presented through the vulva but both forelimbs are retained alongside the chest.

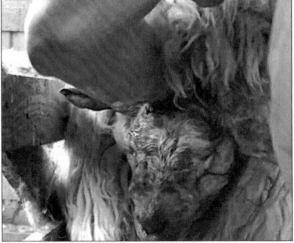

Fig. 3.27 Sacrococcygeal extradural lignocaine injection blocks the reflex abdominal contractions of the ewe allowing the lamb's forelimbs to be drawn forward.

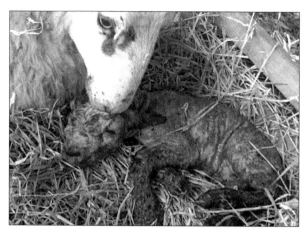

Fig. 3.28 Safe delivery of the hung lamb shown in Figs 3.26, 3.27.

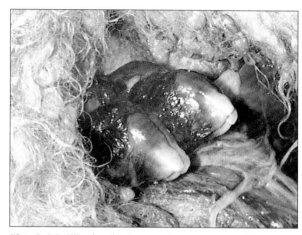

Fig. 3.29 The lamb's hooves face the roof of the vagina in posterior presentation; the ewe's tail is visible at the top of the image.

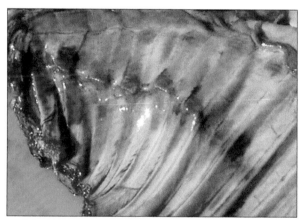

Fig. 3.30 Fractures of the ribs caused by excessive traction revealed at necropsy.

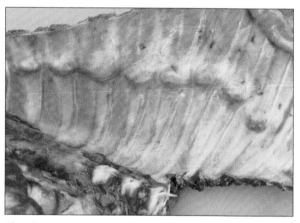

Fig. 3.31 Necropsy reveals healing of rib fractures with considerable callus formation; the lamb was euthanased for an unrelated disease (polyarthritis).

Trauma to the rib cage at the costochondral junctions (fractures) is a risk for large lambs (especially singletons) delivered in posterior presentation. Fractures of the ribs can severely impair respiratory function and may cause death (**Fig. 3.30**). It has been suggested that lambs that sustain rib fractures during assisted delivery (**Figs 3.31, 3.32**) are more prone to respiratory disease. Excessive traction can also cause rupture of the liver, although this more commonly occurs in breeds such as the North Country

Fig. 3.32 Lateral chest radiograph reveals callus formation at the site of multiple rib fractures.

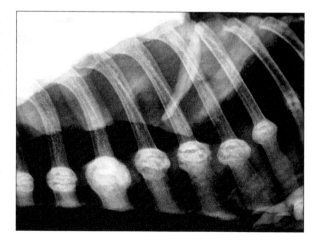

Cheviot and Texel that have a relatively short sternum, thus exposing the liver to potential trauma. In valuable pedigree sheep the prudent decision is to perform a caesarean operation when presented with a large single lamb in posterior presentation, but the client may not always be prepared to pay for surgery in commercial-value sheep.

In most situations a twin lamb in posterior presentation can be delivered without trauma by steady traction. If one twin is in posterior presentation, it is likely that the other twin will also be in posterior presentation; therefore, it may be prudent to check the presentation of a second lamb immediately after delivery of the first lamb.

Posterior presentation with bilateral hip extension (breech presentation)

Signs of second stage labour, such as powerful abdominal straining, are not observed when the lamb is in breech presentation because the lamb does not engage in the maternal pelvis; instead the lamb's pelvis/tailhead becomes lodged at the pelvic inlet. Occasionally, the lamb's tail may protrude several centimetres through the ewe's vulva (**Fig. 3.33**).

Ewes with lambs in posterior presentation are detected by the shepherd recognizing that the ewe has not progressed to second stage labour. Sometimes these dystocia cases are not detected until 24–48 hours after the lambs have died and the ewe has become sick (**Figs 3.34–3.36**).

Correction of a breech presentation involves flexing the hips while the distal limb joints (stifle, hock and fetlock joints) are fully flexed. In this manner a breech presentation is first converted to a posterior presentation and then the lamb is delivered as described above. Singleton lambs are rarely presented as a breech delivery.

Correction of the breech presentation is facilitated by gently repelling the lamb into the body of the uterus. Great care must be taken during flexion of the hip joints, especially if the uterus is clamped down around the lamb. It is not uncommon for an unskilled person to rupture the uterus during these manipulations, and veterinary assistance must be called if there is any doubt regarding correction of the presentation. Extradural lignocaine injection facilitates

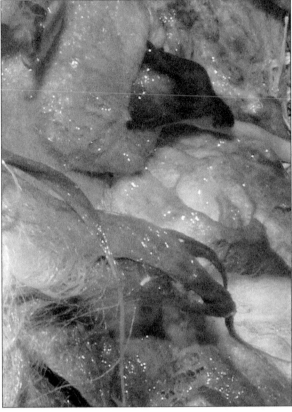

Fig. 3.33 In a posterior presentation with bilateral hip extension, the lamb's tail may protrude through the ewe's vulva.

the various manipulations during correction of a breech posture by blocking the powerful abdominal contractions.

Prolonged second stage labour

Ewes that appear to have stopped straining after 2 or more hours should be examined. Reasons for cessation of abdominal straining include fatigue, a lamb in either posterior presentation or posterior presentation with bilateral hip extension (breech presentation), simultaneous presentation of two lambs, the ewe being continually disturbed or other reasons.

Simultaneous presentation of two lambs

There are many possible combinations of heads and limbs when two lambs are presented simultaneously. It is necessary to identify which limb corresponds to which head by tracing the limb to the shoulder region,

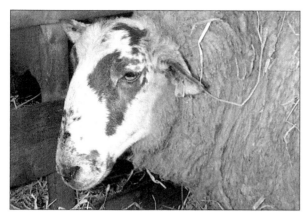

Fig. 3.34 Toxaemic ewe caused by death of the lambs *in utero* because the dystocia has not been recognized.

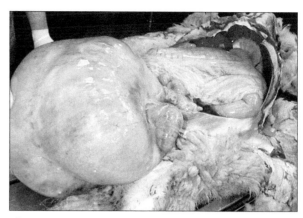

Fig. 3.35 Death of the ewe from toxaemia following foetal death from a dystocia, not recognized in time.

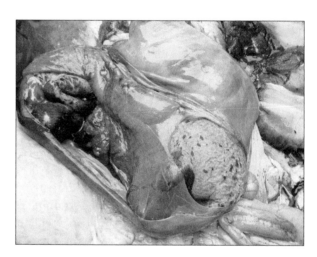

Fig. 3.36 Necropsy, undertaken immediately following euthanasia of a toxaemic ewe where the dystocia was not recognized in time, reveals a compromised uterus and dead lambs showing early autolysis.

and then to the neck and head. Once both forelimbs and head have been correctly identified, one lamb is gently repelled as traction is applied to the other. Only gentle traction should be necessary to deliver a twin lamb in this situation; if little progress is being made it is essential to check that the correct anatomy has been selected. Unlike cattle, congenital abnormalities such as schistosoma reflexa are rare in sheep.

Lateral deviation of the head

Both feet are presented in the pelvis with lateral deviation of the head; the lamb is often dead. The foetal limbs and neck are gently repelled and a wire head snare is placed behind the lamb's ears around the poll and through the mouth. The head is then drawn into the pelvic inlet just after the forefeet

enter the pelvis. Plenty of lubrication is needed if the lamb is dead and its fleece is dry.

Rupture of the uterus

Excessive manual interference can cause rupture of the uterus with subsequent shock, acute peritonitis and death of the ewe. This unfortunate event is more common in situations where lambs are presented in breech posture and/or where excessive unskilled force has been used. The ewe presents in shock, with fast shallow abdominal breathing and a rapid pulse. There is frequent odontoprisis. The ewe may show frequent abdominal straining with arterial blood at the vulva. In these cases, signs of excessive manual interference should be obvious and an emergency caesarean operation is the only treatment. Repair of the uterine tear is often possible.

Vaginal prolapse

Definition/overview

The diameter of the prolapsed vaginal wall varies from 8 cm to 20 cm, and the prolapse may contain urinary bladder, uterine horn(s) or both of these structures (**Figs 3.37, 3.38**). Preparturient vaginal prolapse occurs in mature ewes during the last month of gestation, with an average annual incidence around 1%, although this rate can vary from 0–15%.

Aetiology

Many factors have been implicated in the aetiology of vaginal prolapse including: excess body condition (body condition score 3.5 and above; scale 1–5); multigravid uterus; high-fibre diets, particularly those containing root crops; limited exercise in housed ewes; lameness leading to prolonged periods in sternal recumbency; steep fields; and subclinical hypocalcaemia. Short-docked tails (**Fig. 3.39**) have been implicated in vaginal prolapse but the condition also occurs in the UK in hill breeds with undocked tails.

Studies of ovine vaginal prolapse have reported that abdominal straining is an important feature of the aetiopathogenesis. Although it was not determined whether vaginal prolapse was initiated by straining, it is apparent that prolonged straining following vaginal prolapse could result in premature onset of labour, general debility with increased susceptibility to ovine pregnancy toxaemia and rupture of the dorsal vaginal wall and evisceration.

Clinical presentation

Extra care is needed when checking ewes with undocked tails and long fleeces as vaginal prolapse is easily overlooked. In extensively managed systems, vaginal prolapse may not be noted for some days with resultant gross contamination, vascular compromise of prolapsed tissues and secondary bacterial infection (**Fig. 3.40**). Good lighting is essential to examine housed sheep during the hours of darkness.

Ewes with vaginal prolapse may show many behavioural signs consistent with first stage labour, including isolation from the remainder of the flock, failure to come forward for concentrate feeding and periods spent in lateral recumbency with repeated, short-duration, forceful abdominal contractions and associated vocalization. This behaviour does not include frequent periods spent sniffing the ground characteristic of first stage labour, and the abdominal contractions may be more correctly termed tenesmus. An increased respiratory rate is also noted during this period of distress accompanied by a marked abdominal component ('panting'). Frequent attempts to urinate, with no urine voided, is often noted when the ewe raises herself. Neither cervical mucus plug nor foetal membranes are visible at the vulva; instead a red spherical prolapse measuring 8–20 cm is present.

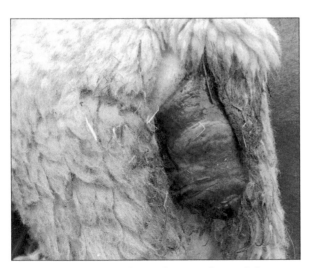

Fig. 3.37 Vaginal prolapse shows oedema of the vaginal wall and vulva.

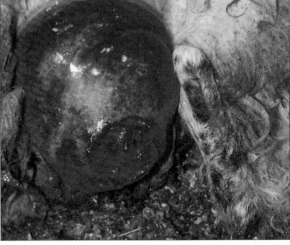

Fig. 3.38 The vaginal prolapse may contain urinary bladder, uterine horn(s) or both of these structures.

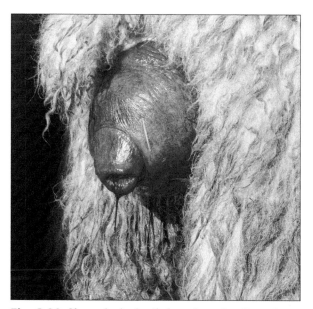

Fig. 3.39 Short-docked tails have been implicated as a risk factor for vaginal prolapse.

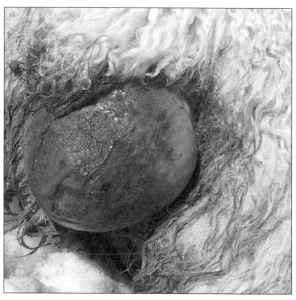

Fig. 3.40 Gross contamination, vascular compromise and secondary bacterial infection of prolapsed vaginal tissues afford a guarded prognosis after replacement.

The duration of prolapse directly affects the degree of contamination with faeces, bedding material and soil, and this compromises the integrity of the vaginal mucosa. The vaginal wall quickly becomes oedematous and turgid, greatly increasing the risk of rupture during manual replacement, especially if this procedure is attempted without effective caudal analgesia. The vaginal prolapse may become damaged when the ewe is transported to the veterinary practice or confined in a pen while awaiting veterinary attention.

Vascular compromise of the vaginal mucosa, trauma and faecal contamination may also greatly increase toxin uptake across the vaginal mucosa (**Fig. 3.40**). Fibrin exudation on the surface can be pronounced, particularly when the vaginal prolapse has occurred post partum; however, this material can be carefully removed after soaking with warm water, causing only capillary bleeding.

A full clinical examination must be undertaken as clinical signs indicating toxaemia (inappetance, reduced ruminal contractions, rapid pulse and congested mucous membranes) may be consistent with foetal death, associated metritis and impending abortion. Particular attention should be paid to the cervix and

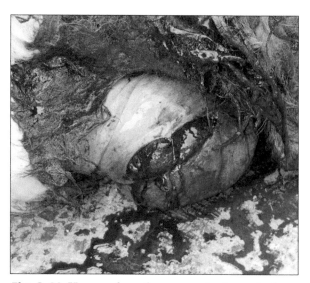

Fig. 3.41 Haemorrhage from a tear in the vaginal wall (see also Fig. 3.42).

the nature of any discharges. Haemorrhage may be visible externally from tears in the vaginal wall (**Fig. 3.41**) and revealed as pale mucous membranes (**Fig. 3.42**), but significant internal bleeding may also result (**Fig. 3.43**). The accumulation of colostrum in the udder may give some approximation of the due lambing date.

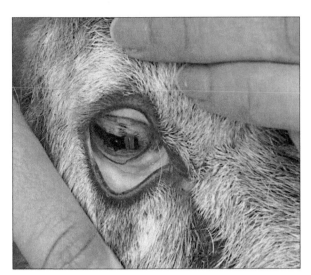

Fig. 3.42 Haemorrhage from a tear in the vaginal wall has caused anaemia.

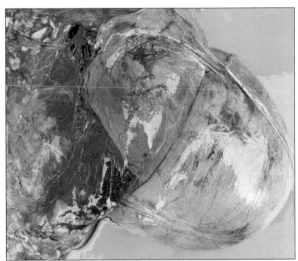

Fig. 3.43 Necropsy of the ewe featured in Figs 3.41, 3.42 reveals significant haemorrhage into the broad ligament and a distended urinary bladder.

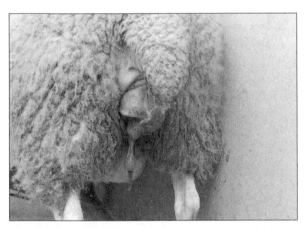

Fig. 3.44 Immediate action is necessary when the foetal membranes protrude through the cervix, indicating impending abortion/parturition.

If there is doubt regarding the viability of the foetus(es) after the vaginal prolapse has been replaced, foetal movement can be reliably demonstrated in near-term sheep using a transabdominal real-time B-mode ultrasound machine with a 5 MHz sector transducer. Foetal heart beat can prove more difficult to detect in near-term foetuses even after searching for 5 minutes. It must be remembered that ultrasonographic findings only indicate the presence of one or more live foetuses at the time of examination; foetal death may occur subsequent to the examination. If no foetal movement is detected after 5 minutes, it is highly probable that the foetuses are dead and very close supervision of the ewe is essential to detect signs of impending abortion. However, it is unlikely that consecutive daily ultrasound examinations to monitor pregnancy would be undertaken except for valuable pedigree ewes.

The presence of foetal membranes protruding through the cervix indicates impending abortion/parturition (**Fig. 3.44**) and immediate action is necessary. Caesarean operation is only indicated when the foetal membranes appear normal; surgical outcome is hopeless when there is a foetid vaginal discharge.

Differential diagnoses

Differential diagnoses include:

- Rectal prolapse.
- Eversion of the bladder.
- Evisceration of intestines through a tear in the dorsal vaginal wall.
- Impending parturition.

Diagnosis

The diagnosis of vaginal prolapse is easily confirmed on clinical inspection. The contents of the vaginal prolapse can be readily determined using real-time B-mode ultrasonography with a 5 MHz transducer and either linear array or sector scanners. Portable linear array scanners are available in most large animal practices and provide good quality images of the vaginal prolapse contents. After thorough cleaning with warm dilute antiseptic solution, contact gel should be applied to the vaginal prolapse to ensure good contact between the transducer and prolapsed tissue.

The vaginal prolapse may contain dorsal vaginal wall, urinary bladder, uterine horn(s) or both urinary bladder and uterine horn(s). Urinary bladder is readily identified as an anechoic (black) area on the sonogram, usually greater than 10 cm in diameter and compressed dorsoventrally (see **Fig. 3.3**). A fold in the bladder wall, which presents as a hyperechoic (white) line, is often visualized in the ventral one-third of the anechoic area.

Treatment

Emptying of the bladder can be readily achieved in the standing ewe after caudal block (**Fig. 3.45**). The prolapse is raised relative to the vulva, thereby reducing the fold in the neck of the bladder, at which point urine flows from the urethral orifice (**Fig. 3.46**).

It is essential to determine the contents of the vaginal prolapse if needle decompression of the suspected distended bladder is attempted before replacement. Puncture of the allanto-chorion would greatly increase the risk of introducing infection and thus cause subsequent abortion. Furthermore, puncture of a major blood vessel may occur if uterine horn is contained within the prolapsed tissues.

Effective caudal analgesia is essential before replacement of the vaginal prolapse is attempted (**Fig. 3.47**). Sacrococcygeal extradural injection is much more easily undertaken in standing sheep than when in sternal recumbency. Please refer to Chapter 17 (Anaesthesia) for a detailed description of this technique.

The 5–10 minute interval between extradural injection and prolapse replacement affords the veterinarian time to remove gross contamination from the mucosal surface of prolapsed tissues using warm dilute antiseptic solution. However, it may prove difficult to remove all impacted soil and faeces from desiccated areas of vaginal mucosa. Vigorous attempts to remove all superficial

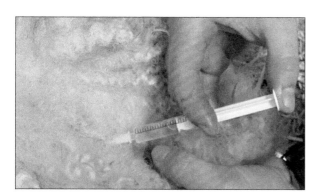

Fig. 3.45 Sacrococcygeal extradural injection is essential before replacing the prolapse.

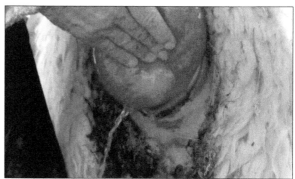

Fig. 3.46 Emptying of the bladder can be readily achieved in the standing ewe under caudal block.

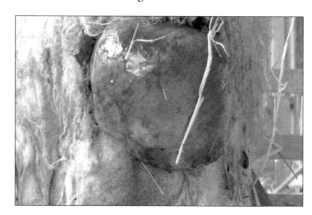

Fig. 3.47 Effective caudal analgesia is essential to aid replacement of an oedematous vaginal prolapse.

contamination may be counter-productive and simply increase toxin uptake across the compromised mucosa.

The vaginal prolapse should be replaced with the ewe standing; in fact, the vaginal prolapse will frequently return to the normal position within 5 minutes once caudal analgesia has commenced and tenesmus has ceased. This is especially so if the prolapse contains urinary bladder, which can be decompressed before replacing the much-reduced prolapse. There is no reason to suspend the ewe by the hindlimbs.

Overdosage with xylazine/lignocaine may cause hindlimb paresis 10–15 minutes after sacrococcygeal extradural injection (**Fig. 3.48**) but no adverse sequelae have been observed. If hindlimb paresis occurs, the ewe can be placed in lateral recumbency and the prolapse replaced.

Methods of retention after replacement of vaginal prolapse

Buhner suture: A Buhner suture of 5 mm nylon tape is placed in the perivulvar subcutaneous tissue 1–2 cm from the labia (**Fig. 3.49**) and is tightened to allow an opening of 1.5 cm diameter (**Fig. 3.50**). Parenteral penicillin should be injected once daily for 3–5 consecutive days. The ewe is clearly marked and the shepherd instructed to observe her closely for signs of impending parturition (**Fig. 3.51**). The Buhner suture

can easily be untied to allow examination of the cervix for signs of dilation. Oedema surrounding the vulva often results following placement of the Buhner suture but this rarely causes significant problems and no specific treatment is necessary except for monitoring that the ewe can urinate freely.

Sutures which penetrate the vaginal mucosa, such as single interrupted or mattress sutures, must be avoided as urine scalding of vaginal mucosa around the suture material, in conjunction with secondary bacterial infection, forms large diphtheritic areas, which cause considerable discomfort and tenesmus. Furthermore, single interrupted and mattress sutures must be removed to permit digital examination of the posterior reproductive tract during periods of suspected first stage labour.

Hindlimb paresis occasionally results 10–15 minutes after extradural injection of combined lignocaine and xylazine solution and may persist for up to 36 hours. The shepherd must be warned of this possibility in advance and affected sheep should be confined to well-bedded pens until ambulatory. Fresh food and clean water must be within easy reach of recumbent sheep. Recumbent ewes must be observed regularly for signs of first stage labour and this will involve raising the tail and examination of the vulva for the presence of foetal membranes.

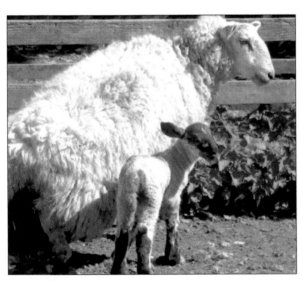

Fig. 3.48 Over-dosage with xylazine/lignocaine may cause hindlimb paresis 10–15 minutes after sacrococcygeal extradural injection.

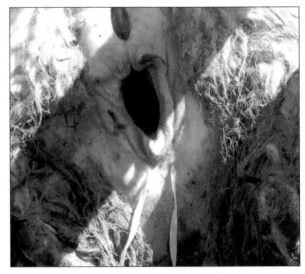

Fig. 3.49 A Buhner suture of 5 mm nylon tape is placed in the perivulvar subcutaneous tissue.

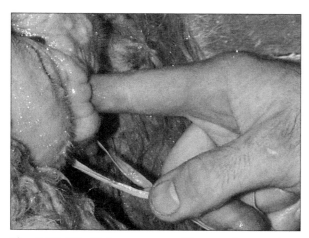

Fig. 3.50 The Buhner suture of 5 mm nylon tape is tightened to allow an opening of 1.5 cm diameter.

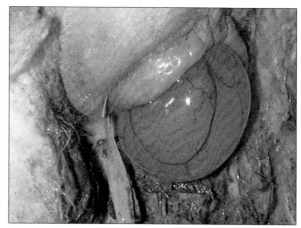

Fig. 3.51 Early first stage labour – the Buhner suture must be untied and slackened to allow birth of the lambs.

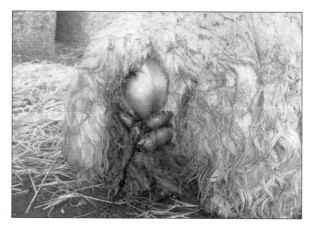

Fig. 3.52 Death of this ewe resulted because the farmer did not notice that lambing had started; the lambs died and the ewe became toxaemic.

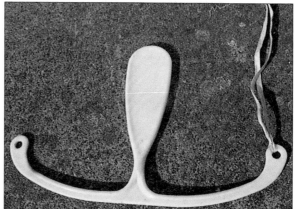

Fig. 3.53 Plastic retention devices are shaped such that the central loop is held within the vagina by the two side arms tightly tied to the fleece of the flanks.

All ewes with retention sutures for vaginal prolapse must be clearly identified and staff notified that there could be problems at lambing with this group of sheep (**Fig. 3.52**). Permanent ewe identification is essential to ensure culling before the next breeding season.

Analgesia: There are no analgesic agents licensed for use in sheep in the UK; however, there are sufficient clinical data that non-steroidal anti-inflammatory drugs (NSAIDs) are helpful in the treatment of endotoxaemia, and possibly pain, in sheep to support their use after replacement of vaginal prolapse. Daily monitoring of ewes after replacement of vaginal prolapse under combined xylazine and lignocaine extradural injection has revealed that tenesmus is significantly reduced for up to 36 hours, with any further problems limited to parturition some days or weeks later.

Plastic retention devices: Plastic retention devices are shaped such that the central loop is held within the vagina by the two side arms tightly tied to the fleece of the flanks (**Figs 3.53, 3.54**). These devices work well in early cases but can cause irritation and secondary infection of the vaginal mucosa, resulting in frequent tenesmus (**Fig. 3.55**).

Harnesses or trusses: Harnesses and trusses are useful in situations where the prolapse is detected early and there is little superficial trauma/contamination

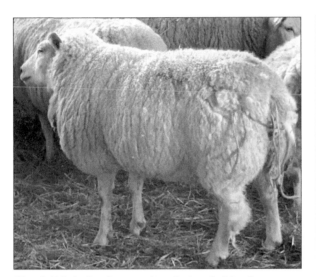

Fig. 3.54 A plastic retention device tied in place.

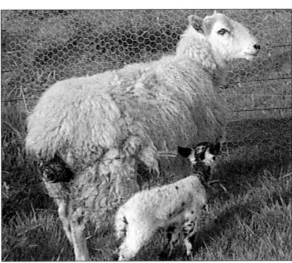

Fig. 3.55 Plastic retention devices work well in early cases but can cause irritation and secondary infection of the vaginal mucosa, resulting in frequent tenesmus leading to reprolapse.

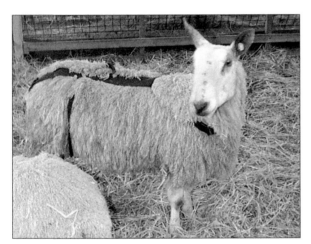

Fig. 3.56 Harnesses and trusses are useful in situations where the prolapse is detected early and there is little superficial trauma/contamination.

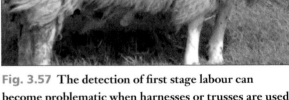

Fig. 3.57 The detection of first stage labour can become problematic when harnesses or trusses are used.

(**Figs 3.56, 3.57**). However, these devices may prove difficult to fit and may give rise to pressure sores if too tight and not inspected regularly. Faecal staining of the perineum and detection of first stage labour can become problematic when harnesses or trusses are used.

Plastic retention devices, harnesses or trusses are often employed because there is no need for veterinary attendance of vaginal prolapse cases. However, as no caudal analgesia is given the cycle of pro-

lapse/trauma/superficial infection/tenemsus continues, and indeed may be aggravated by poorly-fitted retention devices. Many shepherds only present those vaginal prolapse cases for veterinary attention that have failed to be controlled by other methods.

Impending parturition: In most ewes tenesmus is not observed after replacement of the vaginal prolapse and, under these circumstances, it is recommended that the Buhner suture be untied and slackened after an interval of 3–4 days. If re-prolapse occurs it will be quickly detected due to the increased group supervision, and the tissues cleaned and replaced and the suture tightened and re-tied.

In most situations the retention suture is not untied by the shepherd until signs of first stage labour (including separation from the remainder of the group, frequent getting up and lying down, sniffing at the ground and abdominal straining with foetal membranes present at the vulva) have been observed. If the cervix is already fully dilated, and first stage labour completed, a lamb may be forcefully expelled as soon as the retention suture has been slackened. Unfortunately, if the ewe has not been closely supervised the forceful abdominal and myometrial contractions may force the lamb(s) through the vaginal wall before the suture has been slackened, causing perineal laceration.

The Buhner suture should be untied well before the expected lambing date. If effective analgesia has been achieved after replacement of the prolapse, and infection controlled by a course of broad spectrum antibiotic injections, then the prolapse should not recur. It is a much simpler procedure to replace a vaginal prolapse that has just recurred as a consequence of premature slackening of the Buhner suture, than it is to repair the vaginal and perineal lacerations that may result if an unsupervised lambing occurs when the sutures are still tightly in place.

Complications of vaginal prolapse

Abortion: Abortion may occur 24–48 hours after replacement of the vaginal prolapse. It is not known whether this event is a consequence of trauma to the foeto-placental unit during prolapse, or due to other factors. Ewes must be confined and carefully supervised after replacement of the prolapse for signs of impending abortion.

Incomplete cervical dilation: Considerable trauma, superficial infection and oedema of the vaginal prolapse at the time of replacement may result in incomplete cervical dilation during first stage labour. Typically, the foetal membranes are presented through the external cervical os and vulva.

Digital pressure for 5–10 minutes may result in partial cervical dilation in ewes that present with incomplete cervical dilation associated with prior vaginal prolapse; however, trauma to an inadequately dilated cervix during delivery of the lambs results in tenesmus post partum, and uterine prolapse is not an uncommon sequela. Prolonged manual interference during attempted delivery of the lambs also greatly increases the risk of metritis, and affected ewes often fail to nurse their lambs.

There are numerous advantages in favour of performing a caesarean operation when presented with a ewe with incomplete cervical dilation and a history of vaginal prolapse, including much improved prognosis for both ewe and lambs, and greatly improved animal welfare.

Management/prevention/control measures

Great care must be exercised by the shepherd when transporting sheep with vaginal prolapse due to the friable nature of the oedematous and congested mucous membranes. Wherever possible the veterinarian should visit the farm to deal with such cases. Cases that cannot be successfully managed using either harnesses or plastic retainers should be sutured using a Buhner pattern. Economics dictate that many farmers may elect to undertake this task, but they must first have received practical instruction from their veterinary surgeon, and the suture inserted under local field infiltration with procaine.

Economics

The farm visit comprises the major component of the veterinary fee (*Table 3.1*) but lacerations to the friable vaginal wall caused during transport can prove very difficult to repair and the welfare aspects of such transport may be difficult to support on economic grounds alone.

If it is necessary to transport a ewe with vaginal prolapse to the veterinary surgery, the prolapse should be covered with a towel soaked in warm water to prevent further trauma and desiccation. A caesarean operation will cost a further £45–85 (plus visit charge where applicable), thus the total invoice for veterinary services may well exceed the commercial value of the sheep. However, there are no other

Table 3.1 **Cost of vaginal prolapse replacement by veterinary surgeon**	
Visit farm	£25–45
Replace vaginal prolapse	£15
Drugs (xylazine, lignocaine, penicillin)	£3
Total	£43–63
Purchase of breeding sheep (Autumn 2014 prices)	
Gimmer	£100–180
Draft ewe	£65–85
Value of breeding sheep (Spring 2015 prices)	
Ewe with twin lambs at foot	£220–240

options if the welfare of the ewe and lambs is the sole consideration. In a UK survey, fewer than 10% of ewes with vaginal prolapse received veterinary attention.

Uterine prolapse

Definition/overview

Uterine prolapse results from prolonged and powerful abdominal straining. It may occur either immediately after lambing or after an interval of 12–48 hours. In the first instance, prolapse usually results as a consequence of prolonged second stage labour culminating in the delivery of a large singleton lamb. Uterine prolapse occurring after an interval of 12–48 hours generally results from tenesmus caused by pain arising from infection and swelling of the posterior reproductive tract, which has developed consequent to excessive and unskilled interference by the shepherd during delivery of the lamb(s).

Clinical presentation

The everted uterus is readily identifiable by its large size (up to 50 cm long and 25 cm in diameter) extending from the vulva to below the level of the hocks, with prominent caruncles and adherent foetal membranes (**Fig. 3.58**).

Differential diagnoses

- Vaginal prolapse.
- Eversion of the bladder.
- Evisceration of intestines through a tear in the dorsal vaginal wall.

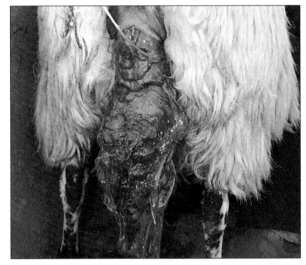

Fig. 3.58 The everted uterus is readily identifiable by its large size, prominent caruncles and adherent foetal membranes.

Treatment

Unless the uterus is replaced correctly and fully inverted to its normal position within the abdomen, the ewe will continue to strain causing considerable distress and suffering, and re-prolapse. For welfare reasons uterine prolapse must only be replaced by a veterinary surgeon using extradural anaesthesia (see Chapter 17 for caudal caudal injection technique). Such analgesia greatly facilitates return of the uterus into the abdominal cavity.

A Buhner suture of 5 mm umbilical tape affords the best means of retaining the uterus, but the shepherd must be aware that partial eversion may still occur, with the tip of the uterus still retained within the vagina. This situation will cause vigorous straining; therefore, any discomfort shown by a ewe after replacement of a uterine prolapse must be carefully investigated and veterinary assistance sought.

Antibiotics, either procaine penicillin or oxytetracycline, should be administered intramuscularly daily for 3–5 consecutive days after replacement of the uterine prolapse, to limit bacterial infection of the traumatized tissues. There are no analgesic drugs licensed for use in sheep but there have been numerous published studies undertaken in sheep to recommend the injection of a NSAID if only to counter endotoxaemia.

The ewe's milk yield will be reduced for a number of days after replacement of the uterine prolapse and her lambs may require supplementary feeding. Unlike vaginal prolapse, it is unusual for a ewe to prolapse the uterus the following year; therefore, there is no indication to cull such ewes prematurely.

Management/prevention/control measures

While it may prove difficult to prevent sporadic uterine prolapse following delivery of a large singleton lamb, uterine prolapse after protracted unskilled interference can be avoided by timely correction of the dystocia by a veterinary surgeon.

Welfare implications

Replacement of a uterine prolapse should only be undertaken by a veterinary surgeon.

Evisceration through vaginal tear

Evisceration of intestines, caecum and omentum through a tear in the dorsal vaginal wall occurs spontaneously in heavily pregnant ewes during the last month of gestation, often within 30 minutes of concentrate feeding. There is usually no history of prior vaginal prolapse or tenesmus. Excess body condition, triplet pregnancy and high-fibre diets are thought to be risk factors but the precise mechanism is not known. Affected ewes must be destroyed immediately for welfare reasons (**Fig. 3.59**). An emergency caesarean operation undertaken to salvage the lambs is rarely successful. If attempted, this is best undertaken after shooting the ewe, because the lambs can be recovered alive up to 5 minutes after the ewe has been rendered senseless.

Rectal prolapse

Very occasionally sheep may present with both vaginal and rectal prolapses (**Fig. 3.60**). In most situations when the rectal prolapse extends for 2–3 cm, provision of effective caudal analgesia to block tenesmus will allow the rectal prolapse to return to its normal position (see Chapter 17, Anaesthesia). If the rectal prolapse does not return it should be replaced under caudal analgesia and a purse string suture of 5 mm umbilical tape placed subcutaneously around the anus and tightened to reduce the internal diameter to approximately 1.5 cm. However, it

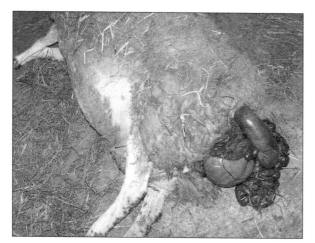

Fig. 3.59 Sheep with evisceration of intestines, caecum and omentum through a tear in the dorsal vaginal wall must be euthanased immediately.

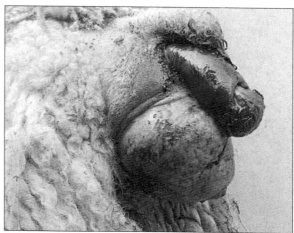

Fig. 3.60 Very occasionally sheep may present with both vaginal and rectal prolapses.

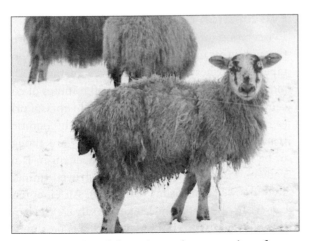

Fig. 3.61 Delayed detection and presentation of rectal prolapse adversely affects prognosis.

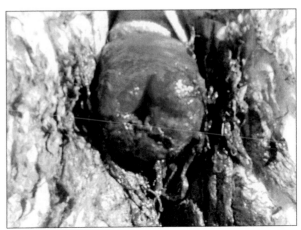

Fig. 3.62 It may prove difficult to judge whether the sheep will be able to defaecate yet retain the prolapsed oedematous rectal wall.

may prove difficult to judge if the sheep is still able to defaecate yet retain the previously prolapsed rectal tissue (**Figs 3.61, 3.62**). A single soluble corticosteroid injection, such as dexamethasone at normal dose rates, will reduce oedema of the rectal wall and does not result in abortion/premature birth. On rare occasions the rectal prolapse may extend to more than 15 cm; under these circumstances the prolapsed rectum should be amputated under caudal analgesia, although such surgery should be carefully considered.

In the USA rectal prolapse presents as a problem in over-conditioned show lambs with very short-docked tails. It is a legal requirement in the UK that sufficient tail must be left to cover the anus of male lambs and vulva of female lambs, including the caudal skin folds. Notwithstanding such anatomical differences, rectal prolapse has been effectively treated after caudal extradural injection of xylazine and lignocaine and placement of a Buhner suture of 5 mm umbilical tape. There is no justification for percutaneous injection of irritant substances around the serosal surface of the rectum in order to effect intrapelvic inflammation and adhesion formation.

An alternative regimen for inhibition of tenesmus causing prolapse in calves has been to effect temporary damage to the cauda equina by caudal extradural injection of isopropyl alcohol. This treatment regimen often fails to produce a successful outcome. Accurate dose calculation and injection technique is essential to block tenesmus but not compromise the lumbosacral outflow to the hindlimbs; this can cause prolonged posterior paralysis and its consequences. There are no published studies describing sacrococcygeal isopropyl alcohol injection in sheep but there is no indication for such a regimen when timely veterinary management employing extradural injection of lignocaine and xylazine proves successful, even in advanced cases. Where necessary, it is recommended that the extradural injection of lignocaine and xylazine can be repeated after 36–48 hours in problem cases.

Caesarean section

Caesarean section to correct dystocia has been routinely performed and with excellent success rates in general veterinary practice. Emphasis on sheep meat production and carcass conformation within Europe has resulted in development of breed characteristics which directly increase the likelihood of absolute foetal oversize (**Fig. 3.63**). Sire selection is still based upon phenotype, with little attention given to the possibility of dystocia. In many countries worldwide careful selection of sheep for ease of lambing under pastoral management systems, such as practised in New Zealand and Australia, has greatly reduced the dystocia rate so that caesarean section is rarely necessary. In addition, other factors such as cost and proximity to veterinary services preclude surgery on sheep of low financial value.

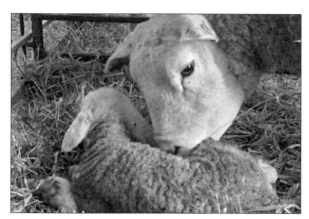

Fig. 3.63 Absolute foetal oversize is not uncommon in singleton lambs of meat breeds.

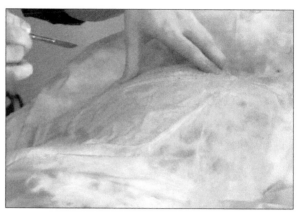

Fig. 3.64 A large area of the left flank is shaved and a sterile plastic disposable drape is fenestrated.

In the UK, the most common conditions necessitating delivery of lamb(s) by caesarean section are relative foetal oversize, particularly in the immature primiparous animal with a singleton foetus in posterior presentation, incomplete cervical dilation and vaginal prolapse. The incidence of caesarean section is often high in ewes that have been treated for prolapsed vagina, because gross oedema and trauma of the vagina, in association with incomplete cervical dilation, prevent normal delivery of the lambs.

Analgesia

- Caesarean sections are often performed after infiltration of the left flank incision site with 2% lignocaine solution, although the efficacy of this method in terms of animal welfare has been questioned. Analgesia of the left flank is best achieved by distal paravertebral injection.
- Xylazine at a dose rate of 0.07 mg/kg injected into the extradural space at the sacrococcygeal site affords analgesia of the flank approximately 30 minutes after injection.
- Excellent analgesia of flank for caesarean section can be achieved after lumbosacral extradural injection of 3–4 mg/kg of 2% lignocaine solution. This analgesic regimen is recommended when there is either considerable trauma to the posterior reproductive tract, a foetal monster *in utero* (for example arthrogryposis caused by in-utero Schmallenberg virus [SBV] infection) or a concurrent traumatized vaginal

prolapse resulting in tenesmus (see Chapter 17, Anaesthesia). Hindlimb paresis after lignocaine extradural injection causing recumbency in ewes for up to 3 hours could cause practical husbandry problems arising from lambs unable to suck colostrum, but this situation can be overcome by careful stockmanship and administration of colostrum by orogastric tube where necessary. Furthermore, such surgeries are often undertaken when the foetuses are dead.

Surgery

The ewe is positioned in right lateral recumbency. A large area of the left flank is shaved; under no circumstances should the wool be plucked from the skin. A plastic disposable drape is fenestrated over the incision site (**Fig. 3.64**).

Surgery is performed through a left flank incision midway between the last rib and the wing of the ilium, commencing 10–15 cm below the level of the transverse processes of the lumbar vertebrae. A 15 cm incision is made through the skin, external abdominal oblique muscle and internal abdominal oblique muscle using a scalpel blade. The transversus muscle and closely adherent peritoneum are grasped with forceps and raised. A small nick is made and subsequently extended (**Fig. 3.65**). Care is necessary at this stage to avoid puncturing an underlying viscus, especially if the ewe is bloated or shows tenesmus.

Care is necessary when exteriorizing the gravid uterine horn because of its thin wall and friable

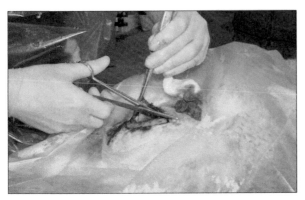

Fig. 3.65 The transversus muscle and closely adherent peritoneum are grasped with forceps and raised before a small nick is made and subsequently extended.

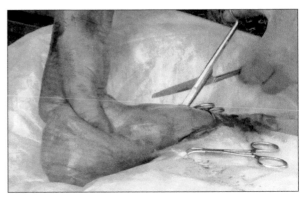

Fig. 3.66 An incision is made over the greater curvature in the exteriorized left uterine horn.

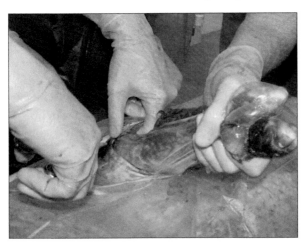

Fig. 3.67 The uterine incision is extended as necessary as the lamb is removed from the uterine horn. In twin pregnancies, the lamb in the left uterine horn is delivered hindlimbs first, when in anterior presentation.

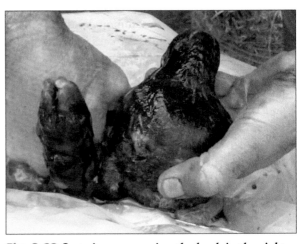

Fig. 3.68 In twin pregnancies, the lamb in the right uterine horn is delivered head first when in anterior presentation.

nature in many cases. In a multigravid uterus the left horn is always chosen (**Fig. 3.66**). The abdominal wound can be packed with sterile gauze swabs prior to the incision being made in the greater curvature of the uterus in an attempt to prevent leakage of uterine fluids into the abdomen, but this is not usually necessary. The incision is made using scissors, starting 6–8 cm from the tip of the uterine horn (at the level of the lamb's fetlock joints in those lambs in anterior presentation) and extending towards the cervix as necessary (**Fig. 3.67**). The uterine incision is normally extended to just over the lamb's tailhead. When the lamb in the left uterine horn is

presented in anterior presentation it will be delivered hindlimbs first. If present, lamb(s) in anterior presentation within the right uterine horn are delivered head first (**Figs 3.68, 3.69**). It is easier to use the right hand to manipulate the lamb's head within the right uterine horn. The lamb should first be drawn forward into the body of the uterus, then around into the left horn so as not to damage the uterine wall. The lamb's forelimbs are extended once the lamb's head is resting at the abdominal incision (**Fig. 3.68**).

Considerable difficulty may be encountered when manipulating and attempting to exteriorize part of

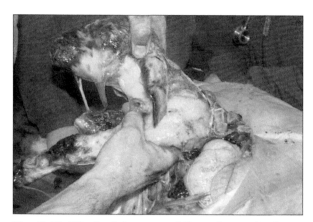

Fig. 3.69 The lamb is removed from the uterine horn after both forelimbs have been extended.

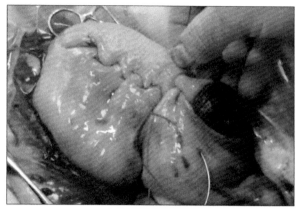

Fig. 3.70 A continuous inversion suture pattern is used to close the uterine incision, ensuring that closure is watertight and that no foetal membranes protrude through the suture line.

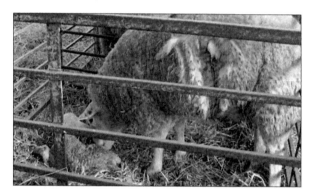

Fig. 3.71 Success rates should be 100% when the lambs are alive.

the uterine horn when emphysematous lambs are present *in utero* due to the oedematous and friable nature of the uterus.

The uterine incision is closed with a Connell suture of 7 metric chromic catgut or equivalent suture material (**Fig. 3.70**). The suture line is carefully checked for leakage of uterine contents; a second suture line is rarely necessary. The peritoneum and transverse abdominal muscles are closed with a continuous suture of 7 metric chromic catgut. The internal and external abdominal oblique muscle layers are then closed with a continuous suture of 7 metric chromic catgut. The skin incision is closed with interrupted horizontal mattress sutures of 6 metric monofilament nylon or similar. Success rates should be 100% when the lambs are alive and there has been little/no interference before surgery (**Fig. 3.71**).

Supportive therapy

Procaine penicillin is injected intramuscularly before surgery and for 3 consecutive days thereafter. Ewes are also injected intravenously with a NSAID before surgery. In toxaemic sheep, where costs permit, supportive therapy may include up to 3 litres of isotonic saline at a dose rate of 50 ml/kg/h administered intravenously during surgery. Extradural xylazine injection produces effective analgesia for up to 36 hours.

Metritis
Definition/overview

Metritis commonly affects ewes after unhygienic manual interference to correct foetal malpresentation/malposture, after delivery of dead lambs and following infectious causes of abortion. Metritis is also common following replacement of uterine prolapse.

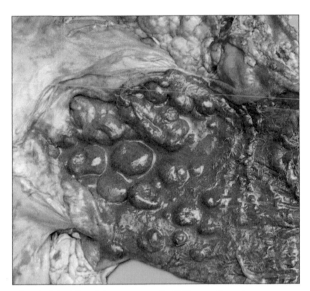

Fig. 3.72 Metritis commonly follows abortion as shown in this necropsy specimen.

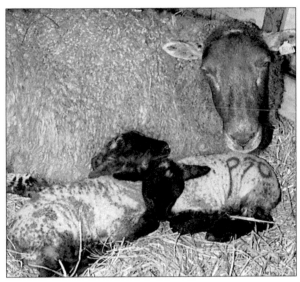

Fig. 3.73 Metritis often presents 2–3 days after unhygienic and excessive manual interference to correct foetal malpresentation/malposture.

Aetiology

Illness follows bacterial entry and multiplication within the uterus, with the production of toxins which are absorbed across the damaged endometrium. The likelihood of metritis increases in proportion to the duration of manual intervention in dystocia cases. Metritis commonly follows abortion caused by *Salmonella* spp. and other abortifacient agents (**Fig. 3.72**).

Clinical presentation

Metritis often presents 2 days after unhygienic and excessive manual interference to correct foetal malpresentation/malposture (**Fig. 3.73**). The likelihood of metritis is increased if the lambs are dead, and further increased if the lambs are autolytic. Unlike cattle, metritis in ewes is not commonly associated with retained foetal membranes.

The ewe shows little interest in her lambs and spends long periods in sternal recumbency. The ewe is depressed and inappetent, with a poor milk yield as evidenced by hungry lambs who attempt to suck whenever the ewe stands. Often lamb(s) have been 'fostered-on' to replace dead lamb(s), and their gaunt appearance may be masked by the covering dead lamb's skin. The ewe's rectal temperature is often only marginally elevated (40°C). The mucous membranes are congested. There are reduced/absent ruminal sounds and the sublumbar fossae may be sunken, reflecting reduced rumen fill. The vulva is usually swollen and oedematous consequent to manual interference during second stage labour, with evidence of a red/brown foetid discharge on the wool of the tail and perineum (**Fig. 3.74**). The vulval discharge may appear more purulent with an increasing postpartum interval. The posterior reproductive tract can be examined digitally but not the cervix or uterus. Digital examination frequently provokes forceful straining and vocalization. Abdominal ballotment fails to detect evidence of a retained foetus.

Differential diagnoses

It is difficult to ascertain that the cause of illness/endotoxaemia is metritis (**Fig. 3.75**) because the uterus cannot be examined in detail and a scant vulval discharge is present on the tail and perineum of many postpartum ewes. Diagnosis of metritis is based upon the history of dystocia and exclusion of other diseases of the postpartum ewe.

Other differential diagnoses to consider for inappetent recumbent ewes could include:

• Ruptured uterus if considerable difficulty is encountered during delivery of the foetus.

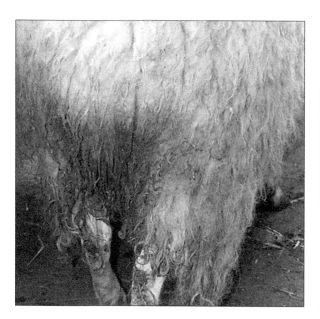

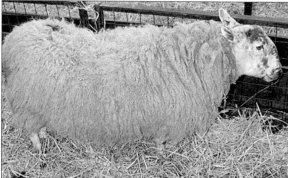

Fig. 3.75 It proves difficult to be certain that the cause of illness/endotoxaemia is metritis.

Fig. 3.74 In metritis cases there is evidence of a red/brown foetid discharge on the wool of the tail and perineum.

- Retained foetus.
- Acidosis if overfed concentrates post lambing.
- Peritonitis.
- Mastitis.
- Hypocalcaemia.

Diagnosis

The provisional diagnosis is based upon history, clinical findings and elimination of other common diseases.

Treatment

The common agents causing abortion in sheep are sensitive to a wide range of antibiotics. Typically, there is dramatic improvement in the sheep's demeanour and appetite within 12 hours of intravenous injection of oxytetracycline and dexamethasone. The inclusion of dexamethasone in the treatment regimen achieves a more rapid response than antibiotic injection alone. Other antibiotics (e.g. procaine penicillin) can also be administered. Deterioration in the clinical presentation in a small percentage of metritis cases results from development of septic peritonitis associated with a uterine tear or compromised uterine wall, rather than from treatment failure.

Management/prevention/control measures

Farmers should wash their hands and use arm-length disposable gloves prior to correction of all dystocia cases. In the case of infectious causes of abortion, such precautions would be seen as a minimum standard to limit the risk of zoonotic infections such as *Salmonella* and *Chlamydophila* spp. In multigravid litters, delivering all lambs, not just the lamb in malpresentation/malposture, increases the likelihood of introducing infection deep within the uterus.

Economics

Death of the ewe is uncommon, but poor milk production results in hungry lambs that require supplementation until the ewe recovers fully. This check in lamb growth during the critical first few days of life is often not recovered over the next few weeks to months, with a consequent extended period to market.

Welfare implications

Metritis in ewes results in poor milk production and hungry lambs which may die if not given supplementary milk.

ABORTION

Definition/overview

Infectious causes of abortion are most common after day 100 of pregnancy. While sporadic losses are variably attributed by farmers to handling, overcrowding during housing/feeding (**Fig. 3.76**), or movement,

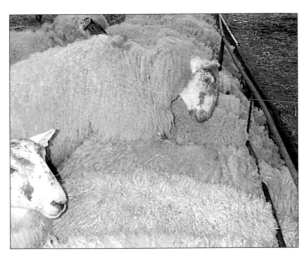

Fig. 3.76 Overcrowding during housing/feeding is an uncommon cause of abortion.

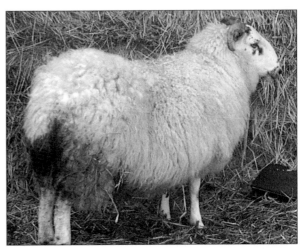

Fig. 3.77 All aborted sheep must be isolated and all aborted material disposed of.

an abortion rate in excess of 2% is suggestive of an infectious aetiology and laboratory investigation is strongly recommended. A standard set of samples will allow laboratory identification of the abortifacient agent(s) in most situations. The farmer must isolate all suspect aborted sheep and remove all aborted material (**Fig. 3.77**). The zoonotic potential of many abortifacient agents must be stressed to those tending the sheep. Appropriate hygiene precautions must also extend to the household, where infection could arise from contaminated clothing and footwear.

Sample collection
The minimum requirements for laboratory submissions for abortion investigation include the foetus(es) or foetal stomach content, a piece of placenta and a maternal serum sample. Instructions regarding safe packaging of pathological material can be obtained from the veterinary laboratory. While the first submission may identify a recognized abortifacient agent, it is important to continue submitting aborted material during the outbreak as more than one agent may be present within the flock and such knowledge is essential when formulating treatment, control and prevention strategies.

Chlamydial abortion
(syn. enzootic abortion of ewes [EAE], *Chlamydophila abortus* infection)

Definition/overview
Chlamydial (*Chlamydophila abortus*) abortion is a major cause of abortion and ewe and lamb deaths in many countries, with the exceptions of Australia and New Zealand, and is the main cause of ovine abortion in the UK. Pregnant women are at serious risk from *C. abortus* infection, because this organism is able to colonize the human placenta causing abortion, stillbirth and maternal illness.

Aetiology
Disease is transmitted by the oral route following exposure of susceptible females to high levels of infected uterine discharges/aborted material. Such exposure and transmission is greatly increased when sheep are intensively managed during late gestation and during the lambing period (**Fig. 3.78**). Infection does not result in clinical signs unless the ewe is more than 6 weeks from the due lambing date, infection remaining latent until the subsequent pregnancy.

Colonization of the placenta takes place from about day 90 of gestation, coinciding with rapid foetal growth. Rapid bacterial multiplication takes place within the placentome, with resultant inflammatory response and infection and reaction spreading to the intercotyledonary areas of the chorion. Impaired nutrient transfer across diseased placentomes result in foetal debility. Abortion may be triggered by reduced progesterone synthesis by damaged

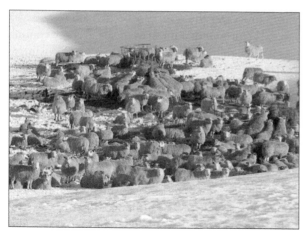

Fig. 3.78 Exposure and transmission of abortifacient agents is greatly increased when sheep are intensively managed during late gestation.

chorionic epithelial cells, and altered concentrations of oestradiol and prostaglandin.

Live lambs born to infected ewes, and lambs fostered on to aborted ewes, may acquire infection during the neonatal period and develop placental infection and/or abort if bred during their first year.

The role of venereal transmission of *C. abortus* is generally assumed to be uncommon but may occur in certain situations. *Chlamydophila abortus* infection can also result in abortion in goats.

Clinical presentation

Infection typically results in the abortion/birth of fresh dead and/or weakly lambs during the last 3 weeks of gestation. The ewe is not sick and may only be identified by a red/brown vulval discharge staining the wool of the tail/perineum, and a drawn-up abdomen. Aborted lambs have a sparse short coat and a distended abdomen due to accumulation of fluid within the abdominal cavity. Live lambs rarely survive more than a few hours despite supportive care. Retention of foetal membranes may lead to metritis and a sick ewe.

Differential diagnoses

Other common causes of abortion including:

- *Salmonella* serotypes.
- *Campylobacter fetus intestinalis.*
- *Listeria monocytogenes.*
- *Pasteurella* spp.
- Toxoplasmosis.

Diagnosis

A provisional diagnosis is based upon abortion of fresh lambs during the last 3 weeks of gestation and an associated necrotic placentitis; the ewe is not sick. Laboratory submissions for abortion investigation should include foetus or foetal stomach content, a piece of placenta and a maternal serum sample. Chlamydial abortion is confirmed following demonstration of large numbers of elementary bodies in placental smears stained by the modified Ziehl-Neelsen method. Serology involves the complement fixation test but may not distinguish between recent field infection and vaccination, and is therefore undertaken in conjunction with placental examination. It is important to continue to submit abortion material throughout the outbreak in case more than one abortifacient agent is involved, which may impact upon future control strategies.

Treatment

With abortions typically occurring within the last 3–4 weeks of gestation, prompt action is necessary if any benefit is to be gained from antibiotic therapy. Metaphylactic long-acting oxytetracycline injection (20 mg/kg) may reduce the number of abortions from *C. abortus* infection but cannot reverse placental damage. As a result, lambs are carried closer to term but are weakly at birth with consequent high mortality. From a practical standpoint, while such antibiotic metaphylaxis may not save the litter of infected sheep, it allows healthy lambs to be fostered onto ewes that abort much closer to term and consequently have reasonable udder development and sufficient milk to nurse a single lamb.

Management/prevention/control measures

In common with all infectious causes of abortion, aborted ewes must be isolated and aborted material and infected bedding removed and destroyed. Ewes that give birth to dead/weakly full-term lambs should also be isolated. Lambs fostered on to aborted ewes should not be retained for future breeding.

Freedom from *C. abortus* infection is best achieved by maintaining a closed clean flock with strict biosecurity, although there have been situations where infected material has been transmitted between neighbouring farms by birds and foxes.

Various accreditation schemes operate in some countries. These offer breeding female replacements from flocks declared free of *C. abortus* infection. Accredited status is achieved by serological surveillance of a statistically representative sample of the whole flock, and all aborted and barren ewes. Careful consideration must be given to establishing a clean but susceptible flock when the health status of neighbouring flocks cannot be guaranteed.

Purchase of *C. abortus*-infected carrier sheep presents the greatest risk to a clean flock, with infection transmitted following abortion. Infection of susceptible sheep, typically occurring following direct contact with aborted material or uterine discharges, can lead to an abortion storm the following year, with up to 30% of ewes aborting. Once infection becomes endemic in a flock, losses are largely confined to one-crop ewes that acquired infection at their first lambing, and this may give an annual abortion rate of 5–10% thereafter.

Ewes that have aborted or given birth to weakly lambs as a consequence of *C. abortus* are solidly immune and will maintain a normal pregnancy subsequently. In view of the possible venereal transmission from carrier ewes to clean ewes, it would be prudent to maintain the former as a distinct group at mating time.

Vaccination offers an excellent means of control for farms buying breeding replacements from non-accredited sources and in those flocks with an endemic *C. abortus* problem. In the UK, for example, there is a choice of either inactivated or live *C. abortus* vaccines, with administration before the start of the mating period. Vaccination of sheep already infected with *C. abortus* will not prevent abortion but may reduce the incidence. It is recommended that vaccination is repeated after 3 years.

Economics

Vaccination against *C. abortus* is expensive (£4 per dose). In many commercial situations, re-vaccination is not performed (without appreciable loss of immunity) so the cost can be divided over 3 years (i.e. the productive lifespan of the average commercial ewe), thereby reducing the cost to approximately £1 per annum. This cost is still approximately five times the cost of annual clostridial vaccination; however, it must be viewed against the average cost of female breeding replacements in the UK of £80 for 6 month-old sheep and £150 for 18 month-old sheep (2014 prices). The cost of abortion is variably quoted as £65–105 per aborted ewe.

Female breeding replacements generally command a premium of £2–5 although this can be variable. The 'gold standard' would be to purchase accredited stock and vaccinate them against *C. abortus*.

Welfare implications

Welfare concerns arise from the loss of weakly lambs and confinement of ewes during fostering procedures.

Toxoplasmosis

Definition/overview

Toxoplasma gondii infection during pregnancy can result in embryo/early foetal loss, foetal death and abortion/mummification and birth of weakly lambs. The parasite has a worldwide distribution and is the second most common cause of ovine abortion in the UK. Toxoplasmosis is a zoonosis with seroprevalence up to 30% in some human populations, although clinical illness is rare. People with an immunosuppressive illness are at most risk of illness. Infection of susceptible women during pregnancy can result in infection of the foetus.

Aetiology

Toxoplasmosis results from infection of susceptible sheep with the protozoon parasite *T. gondii*. The sexual cycle takes place in cats while the asexual cycle can occur in a range of species, including sheep.

Clinical presentation

Infection during early pregnancy may manifest as embryo/early foetal loss, with an increased number of returns to service after irregular extended periods. As the ram is often removed after a breeding period as short as 5–6 weeks, these returns to service are not noted unless a vasectomized ram is present with the ewes. Embryo/early foetal loss is then manifest as an increased barren rate, often above 8–10%; a 4% rate is acceptable and 2% the target after a 6 week breeding period. Typically, the highest number of barren sheep is within the youngest age group.

T. gondii infection during mid-pregnancy results in abortion or production of weakly live lambs near term, often with a mummified foetus. The mummified foetus has a dark brown leathery appearance with a crown–rump length of approximately 8–10 cm.

Differential diagnoses

The irregular and extended intervals of return to oestrus in the ewe suggest that ram infertility is unlikely to be the cause of a high barren rate. Other common abortifacient agents cause abortion during the last trimester and do not cause infertility in this manner.

The birth of a normal lamb and a mummified foetus is highly suggestive of toxoplasmosis but the other causes of abortion should also be considered:

- *C. abortus.*
- *Salmonella* serotypes.
- *Campylobacter fetus intestinalis.*
- *Listeria monocytogenes.*
- *Pasteurella* spp.
- Border disease.

Diagnosis

Serological testing merely indicates past infection; therefore, a single positive titre is not diagnostic for embryo/foetal death caused by toxoplasmosis.

It may prove difficult to establish a definitive role of toxoplasmosis in an increased barren rate in a group of sheep. Blood samples should be collected from six to 10 barren ewes and their serological titres compared with an equal number of pregnant sheep; the former group should show higher titres and a higher seroprevalence when the cause is toxoplasmosis. However, the pregnant ewes may have encountered infection just prior to mating or during late pregnancy and therefore have high titres themselves.

Toxoplasma-induced abortion is confirmed following histopathological examination of placentas and a high serology titre. The cotyledons appear dark red, with numerous white foci that become more visible under pressure from a microscope slide; the remainder of the placenta is unaffected. Antibody may also be present in the foetal fluids.

Antibody can also be detected in precolostral blood samples from newborn lambs but such samples are more difficult to acquire during a single farm visit.

Treatment

While effective treatment has been reported with a combination of pyrimethamine and sulphadimidine, this is unlikely to have practical application because the timing of infection has passed before evidence of barren or aborting ewes appears. Rather than treatment, efforts are directed at prevention through vaccination.

Management/prevention/control measures

All feed should be stored in vermin-proof facilities to prevent contamination by cats and other vermin (**Fig. 3.79**). Oocyst excretion is much greater in young cats and those with debilitating viral infections such as feline leukaemia virus and feline infectious enteritis. Maintaining a healthy adult cat population by appropriate vaccination and neutering policy, and controlling the feral cat population, should limit active excretion and contamination on the farm. However, prevention of toxoplasmosis is more readily and effectively achieved by vaccination of replacement breeding sheep. In common with all infectious causes of abortion, all aborted material must be collected and disposed of in an appropriate manner.

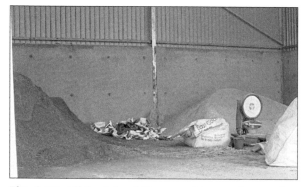

Fig. 3.79 All feed should be stored in vermin-proof facilities to prevent contamination by cats and other vermin.

In-feed medication with decoquinate, a commonly used coccidiostat, from mid-gestation at 2 mg/kg bodyweight daily, has been shown to reduce perinatal lamb losses from toxoplasmosis significantly. However, this is rarely practicable under farm situations and proves more expensive than vaccination when fed throughout every pregnancy, as challenge and immunity cannot be guaranteed during the first pregnancy. Monensin sodium has also been shown to be effective when fed at 15 mg/kg per head daily but this is no longer licensed for sheep in many countries.

Vaccination using a live attenuated vaccine is available in many countries and provides excellent immunity to natural infection and is administered at least 3 weeks before the breeding season. Care should be taken when administering the vaccine and safety instructions provided by the manufacturer must be followed.

Economics
The vaccine is expensive (£3 per dose) but as a single vaccination effectively provides lifelong immunity, this cost should be divided over the sheep's productive life, resulting in a more realistic cost of 50–60 pence per pregnancy.

Welfare implications
Abortion and the birth of weakly lambs can be prevented by timely vaccination which is cost effective under all production systems.

Neosporosis
Definition/overview
While *Neospora caninum* is recognized as an important abortifacient in cattle worldwide, there are few data indicating a similar role in sheep.

Aetiology
N. caninum has a broadly similar life cycle to *T. gondii* except the sexual cycle is in the dog not cat. In cattle, vertical transmission is an important route of infection that can result in abortion or birth of a congenitally-infected, but clinically normal, calf.

Management/prevention/control measures
There are no published reports detailing a field outbreak of neosporosis in sheep, although this situation may change with increased surveillance.

Salmonella abortus ovis
Definition/overview
Salmonella abortus ovis is a sheep-adapted serotype which is a major cause of abortion and neonatal lamb deaths in many countries worldwide. *S. abortus ovis* is not a zoonosis.

Aetiology
S. abortus ovis is introduced into a clean flock by apparently healthy carrier sheep, with bacterial shedding greater after stressful events. Subsequent bacteraemia leads to invasion of the pregnant uterus in susceptible ewes and foetal death and abortion or birth of full-term lambs depending upon gestational age. Abortion rates may exceed 50%, with ewe deaths in susceptible flocks encountering infection for the first time. Thereafter, females pregnant for the first time, and purchased susceptible sheep, are most at risk.

Clinical presentation
The major clinical presentation is abortion during the last trimester, which may not be detected. However, metritis following abortion is common and this may lead to septicaemia and death. Infection close to term leads to stillbirths and increased lamb losses during the neonatal period, some of which show prior respiratory disease.

Differential diagnoses
Differential diagnoses include other causes of abortion, especially other *Salmonella* spp. serotypes.

Diagnosis
Foetal stomach contents provide the best material for bacterial culture but vaginal swabs can be taken for up to 1 week after abortion.

Treatment
By the time the cause of abortion has been identified, infection is widespread throughout the group and metaphylactic antibiotic injection is unlikely to be economically justifiable. Metaphylactic long-acting oxytetracycline injection (20 mg/kg) may reduce the number of deaths from metritis following abortion during an outbreak of *S. abortus ovis*. Most *Salmonella* spp. serotypes causing abortion in

sheep remain sensitive to a wide range of antibiotics; most diagnostic laboratories routinely provide antibiotic sensitivity of bacterial isolates.

Management/prevention/control measures

Prevention is best achieved by maintenance of a high health status closed flock; where this is not possible, purchased sheep must be kept segregated until after lambing.

While mixing non-pregnant breeding replacement stock with aborted ewes may confer life-long protection against *S. abortus ovis*, this practice will also disseminate other abortion agents present within the flock and is not without considerable risk. Vaccines are available in certain countries against *S. abortus ovis*. The choice of which vaccine to use will depend upon the published literature relating to those available vaccines and knowledge of individual flock situations.

Economics

In endemic areas, vaccination is likely to prove necessary where a closed flock status cannot be assured. Introduction of *S. abortus ovis* into a susceptible flock could be financially disastrous.

Welfare implications

Prompt identification and antibiotic treatment of sick ewes and lambs should limit any welfare implications of this disease.

Other *Salmonella* species serotypes

Definition/overview

Numerous *Salmonella* spp. serotypes have been associated with abortion and death in pregnant ewes worldwide. Whilst the number of flocks affected is small, losses within a flock can be substantial.

Aetiology

In addition to *S. abortus ovis* described previously, a number of *Salmonella* spp. serotypes including *S. montevideo*, *S. dublin* and *S. typhimurium* have been associated with abortion and death in pregnant ewes. *S. brandenburg* is a particular problem in New Zealand where it is an important zoonotic pathogen. Other *Salmonella* spp. serotypes cause disease in different parts of the world.

Frequently, the interval between infection and abortion means that the source is not identified with certainty. Wild birds have been incriminated in the transmission of certain serotypes, particularly *S. montevideo* (**Fig. 3.80**). Cattle are frequently symptomless carriers of *S. dublin*. Cattle, especially calves, and human sewage are common sources of *S. typhimurium*.

Clinical presentation

Abortion is the main presenting feature with *S. montevideo* (**Fig. 3.81**). Affected sheep are dull and depressed and may be found standing isolated from the flock, often next to their aborted foetuses. The abdomen is drawn up in ewes that have aborted, which contrasts with the normal distended appearance of late gestation.

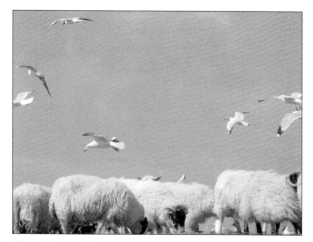

Fig. 3.80 **Wild birds have been incriminated in the transmission of certain *Salmonella* spp. serotypes, particularly *S. montevideo*.**

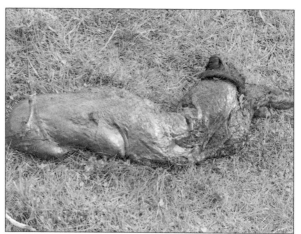

Fig. 3.81 **Abortion is the main presenting feature with *S. montevideo* infection.**

Abdominal ballotment fails to detect evidence of any foetuses. There is a foetid red/brown fluid vaginal discharge. The udder is poorly developed and there is no accumulated colostrum in the mammary glands.

Sheep affected with *S. typhimurium* may simply be found dead with autolytic lambs that have not been aborted *in utero*. Profuse dysentery is often observed in other sheep with *S. typhimurium*. These ewes are often heard tooth-grinding. The rectal temperature is elevated up to 41.0°C. The mucous membranes are very congested. No abnormal sounds are heard on auscultation of the chest and there are no ruminal sounds. Affected ewes rapidly develop severe metritis following abortion and deaths are not uncommon. The clinical picture of *S. dublin* is similar to that of *S. typhimurium* infection.

Differential diagnoses

Other common causes of abortion including:

- *Chlamydophila abortus*.
- *Campylobacter fetus intestinalis*.
- *Listeria monocytogenes*.
- *Pasteurella* spp.

Diagnosis

Foetal stomach contents provide the best material for diagnostic purposes. Where aborted foetuses are not available, vaginal and rectal swabs should be submitted. Blood samples can be collected for chlamydial and *T. gondii* serological testing but are not useful for *Salmonella* species. A provisional diagnosis of salmonellosis can often be given after culture for 24 hours.

Treatment

All aborted sheep must be isolated and not mixed with other sheep for at least 6 weeks. Sick ewes should be treated with intravenous oxytetracycline and intramuscular NSAIDs.

Despite supportive therapy including antibiotics, NSAIDs and oral fluids administered by orogastric tube, the prognosis for ewes with autolytic, often emphysematous lambs, is hopeless unless these lambs can be delivered. Death of the ewe may occur 5–7 days after delivery of rotten lambs because the devitalized uterine wall ruptures with the development of septic peritonitis.

Management/prevention/control measures

There are many potential sources of salmonellae in a group of sheep, including contaminated feedstuffs and watercourses (**Fig. 3.82**), sewage effluent overflow, other farmstock and carrion. All feed must be stored in vermin-proof bins but this is rarely achieved on many farms. Wherever possible, water should be supplied from a mains supply with ponds and surface water fenced off. Pregnant sheep should be managed separately from cattle.

The farmer must be advised regarding the zoonotic risk from suspected/confirmed salmonellosis and requested to adopt strict personal hygiene when handling sick sheep. If infection occurs in one group of sheep, then that field must be visited last at feeding times. Feeding troughs must be turned over and moved at least 10 metres across the field immediately after each feed to limit the risk of transmission by birds to others groups of sheep. Many farmers now feed cubes on a clean area of pasture each day to reduce the risk of birds contaminating the area around feed troughs.

Metaphylactic long-acting oxytetracycline injections (20 mg/kg) may reduce the number of abortions during an outbreak of salmonellosis in sheep, although there are few split-flock data to demonstrate any economic advantages of this strategy.

Economics

The economic consequences of *Salmonella* spp. abortion can be devastating, with ewe losses as high

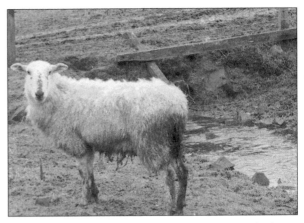

Fig. 3.82 There are many potential sources of salmonellae in a group of sheep, including contaminated feedstuffs and water courses.

as 10–20%. Unfortunately, infection is widespread throughout the group by the stage abortions/deaths are identified and confirmed. Metaphylactic long-acting oxytetracycline injections cost approximately £2–3 per ewe; therefore, ewe mortality must be reduced by around 3% to be cost effective in most situations.

Welfare implications
Prompt identification and antibiotic treatment of sick ewes should limit any welfare implications. Ewes should be euthanased for welfare reasons when autolytic lambs cannot be delivered *per vaginam*.

Campylobacteriosis
Definition/overview
Campylobacteriosis is a common cause of abortion where sheep are managed intensively, leading to heavy contamination and unhygienic environments during late gestation (**Fig. 3.83**).

Aetiology
Campylobacter fetus subspecies *fetus (intestinalis)* and *Campylobacter jejuni* infection is by the faeco-oral route, largely following introduction of carrier sheep into the flock, although wild birds have been shown to carry infection.

Clinical presentation
The common presentation is abortion during late gestation, although some lambs are carried to

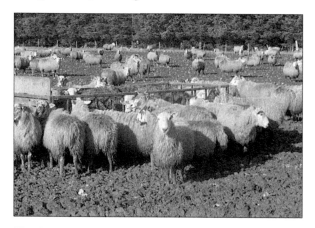

Fig. 3.83 **Campylobacteriosis is a common cause of abortion where sheep are managed intensively, leading to heavy contamination and unhygienic environments during late gestation.**

full-term and are born weakly and succumb during the neonatal period.

Differential diagnoses
Other infectious causes of abortion listed under 'Other *Salmonella* species serotypes'.

Diagnosis
The diagnosis is confirmed following culture of foetal stomach contents.

Treatment
All aborted ewes must be isolated immediately and the main flock moved to other accommodation/pasture whenever possible. Treatment options are limited because infection has already spread rapidly through the group by the time the first abortions are recognized. There are few data indicating an economic advantage from metaphylactic antibiotic injection.

Management/prevention/control measures
Sheep should be managed in clean environments and not subjected to unhygienic conditions, especially during late gestation. Particular attention should be paid to the feeding troughs/areas. Purchased sheep must be managed as a separate group until after lambing.

Following infection, ewes are immune to further challenge and should not abort. While mixing non-pregnant breeding replacement stock with aborted ewes could confer life-long protection against campylobacteriosis, this practice could also disseminate other abortion agents present within the flock (e.g. *Chlamydophila abortus*), with potentially disastrous consequences. A vaccine against campylobacteriosis is available in many countries and used routinely in some flocks.

Economics
Losses from campylobacteriosis can be high in many countries where vaccination confers affordable protection.

Welfare implications
Apart from abortion, there are no major welfare implications arising from campylobacteriosis.

Border disease

(syn. hairy-shaker disease)

Definition/overview

Border disease has a worldwide distribution. The true incidence of Border disease in the UK has not been determined. It is one of the less-commonly diagnosed causes of abortion but this statistic may not reflect its true impact upon flock reproductive performance. Losses from congenital infection are difficult to quantify because a high barren rate may be mistakenly attributed to other causes, and hairy-shaker lambs may not present in a group of neonatal lambs infected with Border disease, which has a high mortality rate.

Aetiology

Border disease is caused by a pestivirus serologically related to bovine virus diarrhoea (BVD), with cross infection between cattle and sheep.

Clinical presentation

Exposure of healthy lambs and adult sheep to Border disease virus causes nil or only mild disease. Clinical signs are only seen following infection of the foetus of susceptible ewes.

Infection during early pregnancy can cause foetal death and resorption with no outward signs other than an extended interval to return to service and/or an increased barren rate at scanning or lambing time.

Infection from mid-gestation onwards results in abortion. Infection later in gestation results in the birth at full-term of small weakly lambs that succumb during the neonatal period to adverse physical factors and/or infectious disease. It is possible that such mortality is overlooked amongst other perinatal lamb losses. Congenitally-infected lambs show symptoms ranging from few clinical signs to lambs with classical cerebellar disease, skeletal abnormalities and coat changes.

Many lambs with cerebellar hypoplasia are unable to stand or maintain sternal recumbency. They may present with seizure activity progressing to opisthotonus. Less severely affected lambs show fine muscle tremors over the head and ears which are exacerbated when the lamb is excited or stimulated (intention tremors), typically when the lamb is assisted to feed, resulting in forceful jerking movements of the head (hairy shakers). Coat changes are often difficult to appreciate in many breeds and it is important to examine some normal lambs for comparison before diagnosing a 'classical' hairy-shaker lamb on coat change alone. It is reported that affected lambs have a hairy rough fleece due to proliferation of longer guard hairs, most noticeable over the neck and back. Skeletal abnormalities include shortened long bones, which are of narrower diameter than normal. There may be evidence of hypertensive hydrocephalus with doming of the head and brachynathia.

While most lambs infected *in utero* die during the first few days of life from a combination of physical factors and infectious disease, some lambs survive but have a poor growth rate and remain susceptible to other diseases, while others survive as apparently normal but persistently infected sheep. It is this latter group which provides a source of virus for susceptible pregnant sheep.

Differential diagnoses

- The irregular and extended returns to oestrus suggest that ram infertility is unlikely to be the cause of the high barren rate.
- Toxoplasmosis would be an important differential diagnosis; the other common abortifacient agents cause abortion during the last trimester and do not cause infertility in this manner.
- Swayback must be distinguished from newborn lambs with Border disease presenting with opisthotonus.
- Bacterial meningoencephalitis rarely affects lambs less than 10 days old.
- Septicaemia is usually accompanied by depression progressing to stupor and death within 24 hours.
- Polioencephalomalacia does not occur in lambs less than 4 months old.
- There are many causes of weakly lambs with low birthweight and the reader is directed to the section on perinatal mortality, Chapter 4, Neonatal Lamb Diseases.

Diagnosis

A provisional diagnosis of Border disease can be reliably based on the clinical examination of a significant number of hairy-shaker lambs; other congenital neurological disorders are more usually sporadic in nature and tend not to occur as an outbreak. The diagnosis is confirmed following demonstration of Border disease virus in either blood samples from affected lambs before they suck colostrum or in tissues from fresh dead lambs submitted to the laboratory. In addition, serum collected from aborted ewes and those giving birth to weakly lambs show very high titres.

Treatment

There is no treatment for Border disease other than supportive therapy. Hairy-shaker lambs have a very poor prognosis and should be euthanased for welfare reasons.

Management/prevention/control measures

There are no practical preventive strategies for Border disease in commercial flocks that do not have the disease, because screening of purchased sheep is cost-prohibitive. Blood sampling to identify all antibody-negative, virus-positive purchased sheep is not economically realistic in commercial flocks (estimated cost of £3–4 for antibody detection plus a further £2–3 for virus isolation plus veterinary and labour costs). These costs represent approximately 10% of the purchase price of the sheep.

Infection could be introduced into a susceptible flock by apparently healthy rams or breeding replacements. Screening could be undertaken if only rams are introduced into an otherwise closed flock.

Virus is readily transmitted from persistently-infected BVD cattle and therefore it is essential to keep sheep separate from cattle during the breeding season and the first half of pregnancy. BVD virus is widespread in the cattle population with 1% of youngstock/growing cattle estimated to be persistently infected in the UK, although eradication programmes are progressing well.

Once Border disease is identified within a group of lambs, none of the lambs in that cohort should be kept within the breeding flock unless screened and found to be seropositive. This is likely to prove cost prohibitive in most commercial flocks.

At present there is no Border disease vaccine available in the UK, but a killed adjuvanted vaccine is available in some countries. Natural vaccination can be attempted in endemically infected flocks, whereby females to be retained for future breeding are deliberately mixed with persistently infected Border disease sheep at least 3 months before the start of the breeding season. Close confinement (i.e. essentially housing these sheep) for at least 3 weeks is considered necessary to ensure exposure to virus. This policy is by no means guaranteed and carries the risk of spread of other infectious agents, including abortifacient agents, if aborted ewes are mixed with susceptible replacements without first establishing the cause of abortion.

Economics

The true economic impact of Border disease after introduction into a susceptible flock is likely to be considerable in terms of increased barren rate, hairy-shaker lambs and increased neonatal losses, but there are few accurate data available. In endemically infected flocks, Border disease losses could be easily overlooked in the general poor performance and high losses of many commercial flocks which have little veterinary supervision.

Welfare implications

Increased perinatal mortality due to physical factors and infectious disease has obvious welfare implications.

Brucella melitensis
Definition/overview

Brucella melitensis is a sporadic cause of ovine abortion in some Mediterranean and Middle Eastern countries. It is absent from Australia, New Zealand, USA and much of Europe.

Aetiology

Brucella melitensis, and much less commonly *B. abortus*, can cause abortion in sheep. Infection of susceptible pregnant sheep may result in abortion, with excretion of the organism for many months. The mammary gland is frequently colonized, with resultant poor milk production. Sheep milk is a potential source of human infection.

Clinical presentation

Abortion close to term occurs in a percentage of susceptible ewes infected during pregnancy. Rams may occasionally develop orchitis.

Differential diagnoses

Other causes of abortion including:

- *C. abortus.*
- *Salmonella* spp. serotypes.
- *Campylobacter fetus intestinalis.*
- *Listeria monocytogenes.*
- *Pasteurella* spp.
- Border disease.

Diagnosis

Diagnosis is based upon bacteriology of aborted foetuses and placentas, and serological testing of aborted ewes.

Treatment

The intracellular nature of this organism renders it largely refractory to antibiotic therapy.

Management/prevention/control measures

Infection is transmitted to susceptible flocks by infected carrier animals, and by the products of abortion transferred between neighbouring flocks by scavenging wildlife. General approaches to biosecurity and maintenance of a closed flock strategy should prevent infection gaining entry. Strict hygiene, appropriate isolation of all aborted ewes and disposal of all aborted material will limit the spread of infection during the lambing period. *Brucella* organisms can be present in vaginal discharges for up to 2 months post abortion.

In many countries control is attempted by identification and culling of infected sheep, often in combination with a vaccination policy during the early stages of such schemes. Vaccination never affords complete protection and persistently infected vaccinated sheep can continue to disseminate infection.

Economics

B. melitensis is only a sporadic cause of ovine abortion in some Mediterranean and Middle Eastern countries. It is absent from the major sheep producing countries of Australia, New Zealand and the UK.

PART 2 MALE REPRODUCTIVE SYSTEM

MANAGEMENT OF RAMS

While the breeding period may only extend to 5 or 6 weeks on many intensive sheep farming enterprises, effective management of rams necessitates year round attention. Routine vaccination and anthelmintic treatments apply equally to rams as the ewe flock (**Fig. 3.84**). Footcare is essential to maintain ram soundness. Rams must be in good body condition prior to the mating period (typically 3.5; scale 1–5); this may necessitate a prior period of concentrate feeding. Supplementary feeding is critical during the mating period when many rams lose considerable body condition (**Figs 3.85–3.88**). Debility following such weight loss may render rams more prone to respiratory disease and other infections.

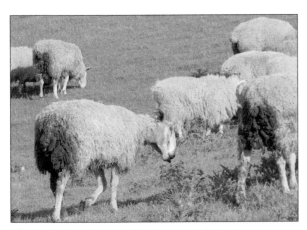

Fig. 3.84 Routine vaccination, anthelmintic treatment and footcare are essential for rams.

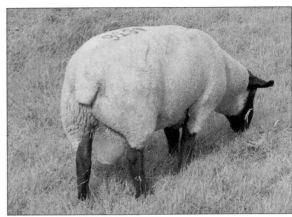

Fig. 3.85 Rams must be in good body condition prior to the mating period.

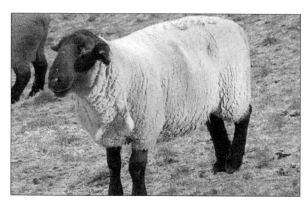

Fig. 3.86 Many rams lose considerable body condition during the mating period when not given supplementary feeding.

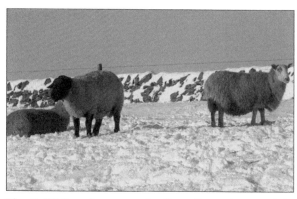

Fig. 3.87 Supplementary feeding of rams is essential during poor weather.

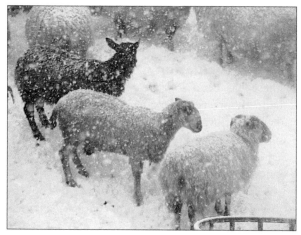

Fig. 3.88 These Leicester rams are in poor condition exacerbated by poor weather and lack of supplementary feeding.

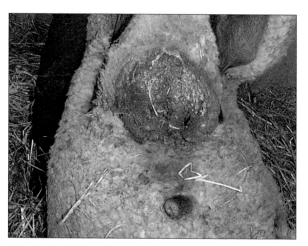

Fig. 3.89 Ill-fitted ram keel harnesses and blocks often cause large brisket sores.

IDENTIFICATION OF MATED EWES

Raddles are frequently applied to rams to determine service dates, and following colour change indicate returns to service. Knowledge of the service date and absence of return to service allow prediction of the lambing date, so that ewes can be fed more precisely during late pregnancy. Many sheep farms do not have sufficient space to house the whole flock, so ewes are housed based upon the lambing date indicated by the keel mark. In many countries, sheep are set-stocked in paddocks depending upon the expected lambing date.

Ill-fitted ram keel harnesses and blocks often cause large brisket sores (**Fig. 3.89**) which heal very slowly, if at all, and raise welfare concerns. Correct fitting of the harness is essential to avoid these sores and extra padding, usually carpet underlay material or similar, should be placed under the harness and checked daily. Some shepherds prefer to apply paint to the fleece immediately in front of the prepuce (**Fig. 3.90**) which poses no risk of brisket sores. In addition, in order to mark the ewe's tailhead, the ram must fully mount her; sometimes a harness can mark the ewe if the ram simply rests his chin on the ewe's hindquarters.

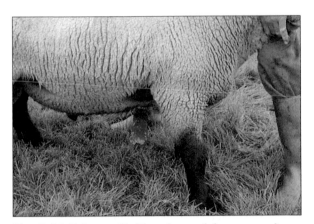

Fig. 3.90 Paint applied into front of the prepuce is a better guide to the ram's service behaviour.

Fig. 3.91 All potential ram purchases should have a maximum scrotal circumference above 36 cm for shearlings and 32 cm for ram lambs.

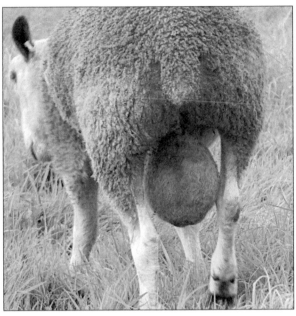

BREEDING SOUNDNESS EXAMINATION IN RAMS

Physical evaluation

Ram selection at auction sale is a lottery; therefore, farmers must undertake a basic physical examination of their potential purchases to reduce the likelihood of selecting an infertile ram. Maximum scrotal circumference has a high heritability coefficient and pedigree breeders must be alerted to this fact. Taking scrotal measurements should be seriously considered before purchase of a stud ram. Sheep breeders have made considerable progress in flock fertility management by selecting for maximal scrotal circumference.

Farmers should measure the maximum scrotal circumference of all potential ram purchases using a tape measure, with acceptable values above 36 cm for shearlings and 32 cm for ram lambs (**Fig. 3.91**). This simple measurement allows a large number of potential ram purchases to be examined prior to commencement of the sale. Rams with measurements below these threshold values must be rejected. Symmetry of the testicles and free movement in the scrotal sac can also be readily determined. Veterinary ultrasonographic examination of palpable scrotal abnormalities can provide much useful information (**Figs 3.92, 3.93**).

Semen evaluation

There has been a gradual change in the recommended practice for ram breeding soundness assessment over the past 30 years in the UK. During the 1980s it was standard practice to examine semen collected from all rams on the farm prior to commencement of the breeding season. However this practice has been largely replaced by collection of semen only from those rams that have a palpable scrotal abnormality.

Despite disadvantages with regard to assessment of rams' libido, occasional collection of an unrepresentative poor sample and animal welfare concerns, electroejaculation remains the most convenient method for checking individual suspect rams for breeding soundness on commercial farms. However, for many infertility claims, insurance companies insist upon examination of a semen sample(s) collected from an artificial vagina.

The routine semen examination should include evaluation of progressive sperm motility, the presence of white cells in the ejaculate, sperm morphology and percentage of live sperm. Volume of ejaculate is often too variable to be a useful parameter when collecting semen by electroejaculation.

Progressive motility is a more accurate assessment of forward sperm motion than the swirling action (gross motility) observed when an undiluted semen

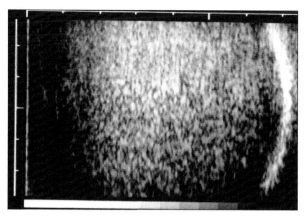

Fig. 3.92 Ultrasound scan of a normal testicle; uniform appearance of testicle measuring 7 cm in diameter.

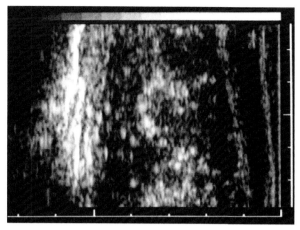

Fig. 3.93 Ultrasound scan of an atrophied testicle; multiple hyperechoic dots within the testicle which measures less than 5 cm in diameter.

sample is examined under ×10 magnification. The presence of large numbers of white cells, which can be observed in the ejaculate after the sample has been prepared and examined for progressive motility, alerts the veterinarian to the presence of an inflammatory lesion involving the urinogenital system. Sperm morphology is an integral part of all semen examinations.

Examination for the presence of white cells in the ejaculate has the disadvantage that the ejaculate must be collected from the vermiform appendage without cellular contamination from the prepuce; therefore, the penis must be extruded and held extended during the collection process.

Method for semen sample collection

The ram is positioned in lateral recumbency and the penis extruded by extending the sigmoid flexure. A gauze swab is wrapped around the penis proximal to the glans to prevent retraction into the prepuce. A warmed 7 ml plastic collection tube is held over the glans penis. A Ruakura-type electroejaculator (possibly modified to a greater diameter probe) is introduced into the rectum to a predetermined length just caudal to the pubic symphysis. The handle of the probe is gently raised positioning the stimulatory electrodes on the probe tip adjacent to the accessory sex glands. The ram is stimulated for 4 seconds, the probe is then switched off for 4 seconds. Stimulation often causes vocalization and sudden muscular spasm with resultant arching of the back and extension of

the hindlimbs. Rigid extension of one hindlimb during stimulation indicates that the tip of the probe is not positioned in the mid-line but has moved toward the side of the extended hindlimb. With the electrical current switched off, the probe is slowly moved to massage the accessory sex glands.

The ram will ejaculate during massage of the accessory sex glands while the probe is switched off. A colourless/pale yellow watery sample of 0.5 ml probably represents pre-ejaculatory fluid. A semen sample (thick creamy white, 0.7–2.0 ml) will be collected after the next cycle of electrical stimulation/accessory sex gland massage. This sequence can be repeated for a maximum of three stimulations. If no sample is collected the ram should be released and a further attempt made later.

Examination of semen sample

Progressive motility and white blood cells: One drop of semen is transferred to the centre of a warm microscope slide. A small amount of semen is then collected on the corner of a cover slip and transferred to 5 drops of warm phosphate buffered saline (PBS). After mixing, the cover slip is placed on top of the now-diluted semen sample and examined under ×100 dark ground microscopy. Vigorous forward motility of individual sperm can be readily identified in normal semen samples. White cells, whose presence is grossly abnormal, appear as round transparent cells somewhat smaller than the sperm heads.

Sperm morphology: Five drops of nigrosin/eosin stain are now added to the drop of semen in the centre of the slide and thoroughly mixed. A thin smear is then made by picking up a small amount of semen sample/stain on the corner of a microscope slide and pushing this slide at a shallow angle along the original slide.

To save time the nigrosin/eosin stained smear can be made before examining the PBS-diluted semen sample for progressive motility and white cells. By the time that examination has been performed (30–60 seconds) the stained smear will be dry and ready for examination under ×400 oil immersion.

Interpretation of results: Forward motility of 60% or greater of individual spermatozoa is expected in normal semen samples. It is important always to be aware that cold shock can dramatically reduce both swirling movement observed in undiluted ejaculates, and in samples diluted in PBS to examine progressive motility. Urine contamination of the ejaculate will also adversely affect sperm motility but this should be readily recognized by the yellow tinge to the increased volume of diluted sample collected and ammoniacal smell.

The presence of white cells is a significant finding and indicates inflammation of the urinogenital system. In rams epididymitis caused by either *Brucella ovis* or *Histophilus ovis* is the most common cause of such inflammatory changes. In countries with endemic *B. ovis* infection, detection of white cells in the ejaculate, in addition to a high percentage of detached sperm heads, may be the first indication of infection in previously uninfected flocks. Inflammatory changes in semen often occur before serological evidence of *B. ovis* infection.

Early identification of rams with epididymitis (or orchitis) caused by *B. ovis* allows these rams to be culled before transmission of infection to other rams in the male group by environmental contamination or homosexual activity. Alternatively, treatment of early *B. ovis* infections with high doses of oxytetracycline (10 mg/kg) for 10 consecutive days or longer may be effective in arresting the infection and eventual return to near-normal fertility. If palpable lesions are present in the epididymes, it is unlikely that antibiotic therapy will be effective and affected rams must be culled.

The occurrence of inflammatory lesions of the male urinogenital tract caused by bacterial infections is lower in UK flocks than in the USA, because *B. ovis* has not been reported in the UK. However, infections caused by *H. ovis* do occur in the UK, especially affecting ram lambs; the changes can be first detected at around puberty when 4–6 months old. The routine ram breeding soundness examination involving evaluation of gross motility and sperm morphology would most probably fail to detect early bacterial infections of the male genital tract. By the time palpable lesions of the tail of the epididymis are present, irreparable damage will have occurred and the ram will be infertile.

It is unlikely that veterinarians in the UK will change their routine ram breeding soundness examination until such time as infectious causes of epididymitis/orchitis become more prevalent. Nevertheless, it is important to appreciate that much additional useful information can be gained by examination of semen samples for white cells, especially in ram lambs. While a specially adapted calf crate greatly facilitates collection of semen from rams as described, the ram can be positioned to extrude the penis as usual and then transferred to lateral recumbency for electroejaculation and semen collection.

Spermatozoan abnormalities are recorded as either primary or secondary. Primary abnormalities involve the head and acrosome and are associated with serious testicular conditions. Tail abnormalities are often associated with less severe problems and disease of the epididymis. Sperm abnormalities should not total more than 30% of the 100 spermatozoa examined.

Welfare considerations

Studies have revealed that electroejaculation may be no more 'stressful' for rams than routine procedures such as shearing and handling for anthelmintic drenching. However, such examinations should be limited to those rams where there is either a history of infertility or a palpable scrotal abnormality that cannot be conclusively defined during ultrasonographic examination.

EPIDIDYMITIS

Definition/overview

Epididymitis caused by *B. ovis* and *Actinobacillus seminis/H. ovis* is a major cause of ram infertility in many countries including the USA, Australia and

New Zealand, where control measures are in operation for *B. ovis*. The condition causes reduced fertility in affected rams. While the clinical signs are similar despite the bacterial cause, the implications and control measures differ considerably. Many countries remain free of *B. ovis* infection, including much of Europe.

B. ovis infection has not been recognized in the UK. There have also been few reports of epididymitis caused by *A. seminis/H. ovis* in the UK, but the true incidence is unknown. Pedigree breeders should be encouraged to have a veterinary examination of all ram lambs and shearlings prior to sale.

Aetiology

B. ovis can enter the body via various mucous membranes, including the vagina, rectum, conjunctiva and nasal passages, localizing in the epididymis and accessory sex glands in addition to other organs. Transmission has been described from infected and non-infected rams serving the same ewe but it occurs more commonly from sodomy (**Fig. 3.94**). Significant pathological changes are largely confined to the epididymis. Infection of the ewe very rarely results in subsequent abortion under field conditions.

Epididymitis caused by *A. seminis/H. ovis* most commonly affects ram lambs and shearlings. *A. seminis/H. ovis* are also referred to as gram-negative pleomorphic organisms. In infected flocks they can be cultured from the prepuce/distal urethra in almost all rams lambs. Contamination of the prepuce may be acquired from the environment or during homosexual activity in pubertal ram lambs. Such homosexual behaviour is not uncommon even in mature rams. Infection may also be transmitted between rams mating the same ewe. It has been postulated that retrograde travel of the organism from the prepuce results in infection of the accessory sex glands and epididymis(es). Hormonal changes that effect puberty may facilitate retrograde migration of the organism from the prepuce and explain the age prevalence of males most commonly affected.

Clinical presentation

Lesions caused by *B. ovis* generally involve the tail of the epididymis, and may develop rapidly to form large palpable granulomas, which progress to abscesses. In more chronic lesions the creamy yellow pus becomes caseous then inspissated, surrounded by thick fibrous tissue. Lesions involving the head and body of the epididymis are less common.

Acute disease caused by *A. seminis/H. ovis* causes anorexia and marked lameness, progressing to recumbency. The rectal temperature may be elevated at 40.0–40.5°C. However, in most cases the disease has been present for some weeks/months and the affected ram may be in comparable body condition to others in the group, and remains bright and alert with a normal appetite. Bacteraemia involving other organs such as the lungs and heart valves is uncommon.

Infection usually affects only one side of the scrotum which is grossly enlarged and up to three times the normal size in severe cases (**Figs 3.95, 3.96**).

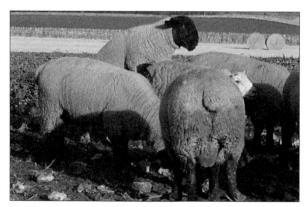

Fig. 3.94 The causal agents of epididymitis can be transmitted from an infected ram by sodomy.

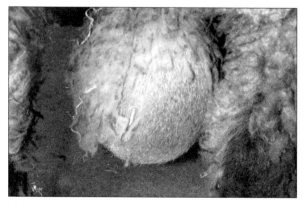

Fig. 3.95 The affected (right) side of the scrotum is grossly enlarged with loss of wool from the overlying skin.

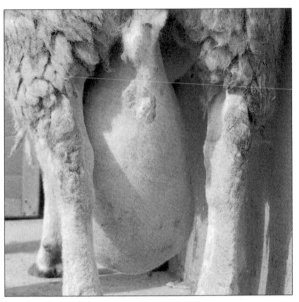

Fig. 3.96 The scrotum may be up to three times the normal size in neglected sheep.

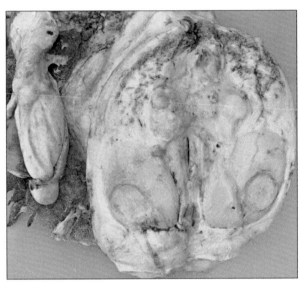

Fig. 3.97 When the lesion is unilateral, the contralateral testicle is atrophied but freely moveable within the scrotum.

If the lesion is unilateral, the contralateral testicle is atrophied but freely moveable within the scrotum (**Fig. 3.97**). Irrespective of a distal lesion, palpation reveals normal spermatic cord and neck of the scrotum. There is often increased heat in the scrotum associated with the swelling and the firm lesions may be painful, demonstrated by the ram moving away on palpation. The structures cannot readily be differentiated on palpation as the contents are firm and adherent to the scrotal skin, preventing free movement. There may be one or more discharging sinuses along the ventral border of the swelling.

Differential diagnoses

Differential diagnoses of the scrotal swelling caused by the epididymitis include:

- Orchitis.
- Sperm granuloma (several years after vasectomy).
- Inguinal hernia with omentum extending through the inguinal ring.
- Varicocoele.
- Spermatocoele.
- Puncture wound.
- Accumulation of ascitic fluid.
- Oedema of the scrotal skin.
- Haematoma.

Diagnosis

It is rarely possible to differentiate between orchitis (**Fig. 3.98**) and epididymitis (**Fig. 3.99**) on palpation alone. Ultrasonographic examination of the scrotum undertaken in the standing sheep using a 5 MHz linear scanner connected to a real-time, B-mode ultrasound machine provides the most valuable information regarding location of the lesions. If necessary, ultrasonographic examination of normal rams can be undertaken first to establish normal measurements and sonographic appearance, before progressing to those rams with scrotal swelling(s).

Sequential examination of the pampiniform plexus, testicle, and head, body and tail of the epididymis is undertaken as the transducer head is moved distally over the lateral aspect of each spermatic cord, testicle and epididymis. The pampiniform plexus reveals a matrix of hyperechoic (bright white) lines throughout the conical anechoic area. The normal testicle appears as a uniform hypoechoic area with a hyperechoic mediastinum clearly visible. The tail of the epididymis is distinct from the testicle and considerably smaller in diameter (2–3 cm compared with 6–7 cm) and with a distinct capsule. It may prove difficult to obtain good contact between the linear probe head and the smaller diameter tail of the epididymis.

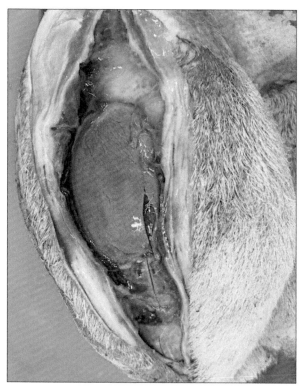

Fig. 3.98 Necropsy findings of orchitis; the scrotum is grossly swollen with the testicle adherent to the tunics by inflammatory exudate.

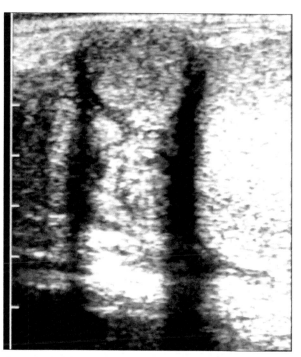

Fig. 3.99 Ultrasound examination reveals a 2 cm diameter abscess within the head of the epididymis. The pampiniform plexus is to the left (dorsal) and the atrophied 4 cm diameter testicle to the right (5 MHz linear scanner).

Ultrasonographic examination in rams with epididymitis reveals a normal pampiniform plexus. The swollen scrotal contents frequently appear as multiple 1–5 cm diameter anechoic areas containing many bright spots surrounded by broad hyperechoic lines (fibrous capsule) extending up to 1 cm in thickness, typical of thick-walled abscesses (**Figs 3.100–3.102**). Ultrasound image quality may be poor because of the large amount of fibrous tissue in the abscess capsule walls. The abscesses generally involve the tail of the epididymis (**Fig. 3.103**) but may extend to involve the body and head of the epididymis. The testicle is embedded within this fibrous tissue reaction and is much reduced in size. It appears more hypoechoic than normal and contains numerous hyperechoic spots consistent with testicular atrophy. In rams with unilateral epididymitis the contralateral testicle is much smaller than normal and appears more hypoechoic (**Fig. 3.104**). The ultrasonograms can be recorded and measurements compared with subsequent recordings at intervals after hemicastration, if such surgery is undertaken.

In countries with endemic *B. ovis* infection, detection of large numbers of white cells in the ejaculate, in addition to an increased percentage of detached sperm heads, typically greater than 20% but often much higher, may be the first indication of infection in previously uninfected flocks. Inflammatory changes in semen often occur before serological evidence of *B. ovis* infection. Similar semen changes are found in *A. seminis/H. ovis* infections. Semen collection should not be attempted in rams with palpable swellings that can readily be differentiated by ultrasound examination.

Confirmation of the cause of epididymitis follows culture of semen yielding *A. seminis/H. ovis*, or *B. ovis*. Seroconversion to *B. ovis* may occur some time after changes in semen and palpable scrotal swellings. Serological testing is based upon the complement fixation test (CFT) method, although the enzyme-linked immunosorbent assay (ELISA) test

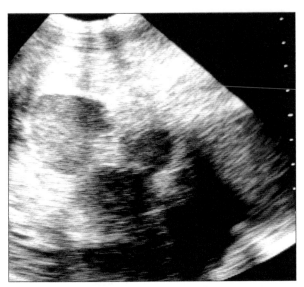

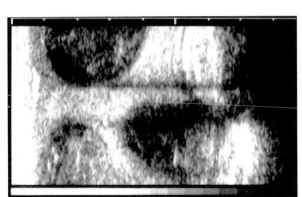

Fig. 3.101 Ultrasound examination reveals three distinct 2–4 cm abscesses within the head of the epididymis (5 MHz linear scanner).

Fig. 3.100 Multiple 2–4 cm abscesses within the epididymis (5 MHz sector scanner).

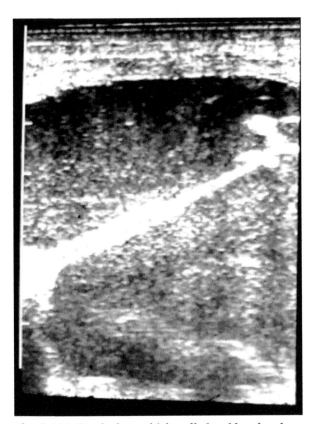

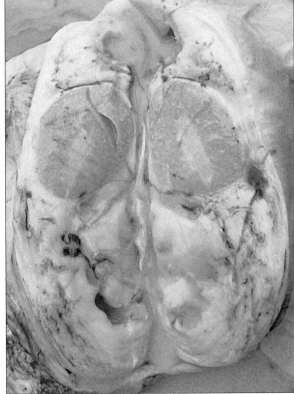

Fig. 3.102 Single, large thick-walled and loculated abscess affecting some part of the epididymis, but it is not possible to identify normal structures (5 MHz linear scanner).

Fig. 3.103 At necropsy the abscesses involve the tail of the epididymis but also extend to involve the body and head.

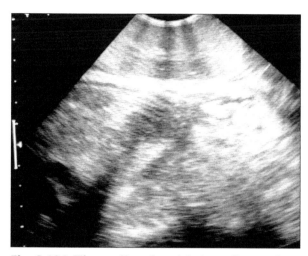

Fig. 3.104 The unaffected testicle (top of image) has atrophied to 2 cm diameter caused by inflammation in the contralateral infected epididymis (5 MHz sector scanner).

is reported to be more sensitive. There are at present no serological tests for *A. seminis/H. ovis* epididymitis.

The vendor's veterinary surgeon must be advised of all findings of disease in purchased rams, to encourage development of a control programme.

Treatment

In cases of *A. seminis/H. ovis* epididymitis, if the lesion is unilateral the owner may request hemicastration with the expectation that regeneration of the other testicle occurs over a 3–6 month period. Excellent surgical analgesia is achieved after lumbosacral extradural injection of 3 mg/kg of 2% lignocaine solution (approximately 12–15 ml of 2% lignocaine). This analgesic technique represents a cheap and readily available alternative to a protocol involving either injectable general anaesthetic drugs or sedation and local field infiltration. However, such surgery is generally ill-advised because extensive adhesions between the inflamed (and abscessed) epididymis and the vaginal tunics and skin result in debridement of a very large area of the scrotum. Wound healing and contraction draws the unaffected testicle close to the abdominal wall and may cause temperature regulation problems.

There are reports of fertile shearling rams 4–6 months after hemicastration. However, the welfare

implications of such surgery must be carefully considered and present the veterinary surgeon with a considerable moral dilemma in the situation where the ram is claimed to be especially valuable.

Management/prevention/control measures

During prebreeding ram soundness examinations, an ejaculate containing large numbers of white cells and a high percentage of dead sperm with detached heads is a significant finding, indicating marked inflammation of the testicle and/or epididymis. In rams epididymitis caused by either *B. ovis* or *A. seminis/H. ovis* is the most common cause of such inflammatory reaction and such changes in the ejaculate can be detected months before palpable enlargement of the epididymis. Antibiotic treatment can be attempted during these early stages but the best advice is to cull affected rams from the flock.

In countries with endemic *B. ovis* infection, detection of large numbers of white cells in the ejaculate in addition to a high percentage of detached sperm heads (greater than 20%) may be the first indication of infection in a previously uninfected flock. Inflammatory changes in semen often occur before serological evidence of *B. ovis* infection. These findings indicate the use of breeding soundness evaluation of rams to identify early clinical cases, allowing prompt culling. Regular serological testing and culling of positive rams will eradicate the problem. Replacement rams should be purchased from accredited flocks. If the seroprevalence is high, replacement of all rams will be the quickest method of eradicating *B. ovis* infection.

There are no recognized control measures for *A. seminis/H. ovis* epididymitis in pedigree flocks producing ram lambs and shearlings. Improved environmental hygiene may limit contamination and disease risk. Ram lambs often congregate on wet bare earth which may become contaminated; therefore, access to such areas should be prevented (**Fig. 3.105**). Regular movement through small paddocks may reduce the level of environmental exposure. Dividing the ram lambs into small groups may limit spread of infection (**Fig. 3.106**). Irrigation of the prepuce with dilute chlorhexidine solution has been recommended at regular intervals as the ram lambs

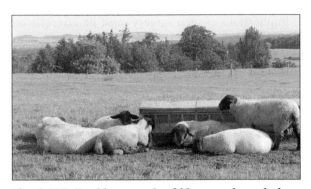

Fig. 3.105 Feed hoppers should be moved regularly and access to potentially infected areas should be fenced off.

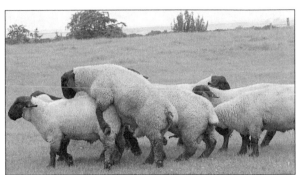

Fig. 3.106 Dividing ram lambs into small groups may limit spread of infection causing epididymitis.

reach puberty. This procedure is cheap and access to the prepuce could be achieved using a foot turning crate. Administration of parenteral antibiotics to ram lambs as they reach puberty has not proven successful but long-term inclusion of antibiotics in feed has proved beneficial. The different results achieved by these antibiotic regimens may be related to the duration of medication. These potential control measures are not exclusive and there may be good reason to adopt all of them.

Economics

Epididymitis caused by *A. seminis/H. ovis* is not a major concern to the commercial farmer purchasing rams for cross-breeding purposes, where the disease is recognized sporadically and affected rams promptly culled. Epididymitis is most problematic in pedigree flocks selling high-priced ram lambs and shearlings, where spread may occur during the pubertal period, thus rendering rams unfit for sale.

In countries with endemic *B. ovis* infection the economic effects of infection resulting from increased barren ewe rate, reduced lambing percentage and extended lambing period are considerable. Farmers must be encouraged to purchase accredited stock and maintain a *B. ovis*-free flock.

Welfare implications

Rams with palpable scrotal lesions should be culled. Hemicastration is generally ill-advised in rams with unilateral epididymal lesions.

VASECTOMY

Vasectomized rams are widely used to induce ovulation and synchronize oestrus in ewes before the introduction of fertile rams, thereby compacting the lambing period, optimizing seasonal labour and reducing the consequences of disease build-up as the lambing season progresses.

It is common practice to introduce the vasectomized ram for 1 week starting 2 weeks before the breeding season. This management practice will generally induce ovulation in ram-responsive ewes within 2–3 days, with normal behavioural oestrus around 17 days later (i.e. around 6 days after the introduction of fertile rams). The prior introduction of vasectomized rams should guarantee that the majority of ewes are mated during a 10 day period (**Fig. 3.107**) with a subsequently compacted lambing period. Before advising a client about the uses of vasectomized rams, it is essential that the veterinary surgeon checks that there are sufficient fertile rams to cope with such a compacted breeding period (approximately one ram per 30 ewes) and that there is sufficient labour to cope with the challenges of a concentrated lambing period.

Vasectomy is more easily performed in yearlings than in either 6-month-old lambs or subfertile mature rams. Crossbred sheep (e.g. Suffolk × Greyface) can grow to 120 kg and often become aggressive and unmanageable in later years; therefore, where available, it is better to vasectomize yearling

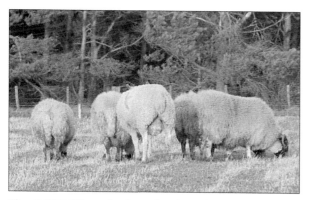

Fig. 3.107 The prior introduction of vasectomized rams should guarantee that the majority of ewes are mated during a period of 10 days.

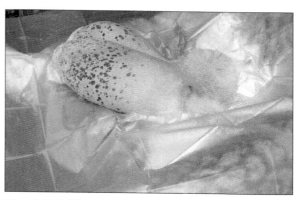

Fig. 3.108 The ram is positioned on its hindquarters for vasectomy.

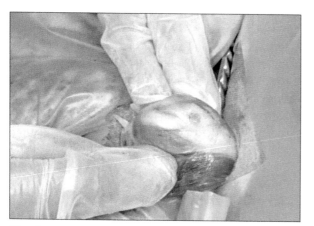

Fig. 3.109 The vas deferens is localized medially within the spermatic cord between thumb and index finger.

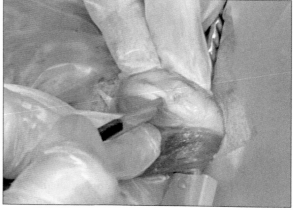

Fig. 3.110 The vaginal tunic over the vas deferens is nicked with the scalpel blade point.

Suffolk rams which have failed to make the grade for sale as breeding stock. However, with increasing awareness of biosecurity, it would be prudent to vasectomize homebred stock to reduce the number of sheep introduced onto the farm.

Surgery

Prior to vasectomy all rams should be starved for 24 hours. Shorn sheep are cleaner and easier to prepare for surgery. There is no licensed drug for general anaesthesia in sheep in many countries. Spinal analgesia using extradural lignocaine injection at the lumbosacral site is an excellent technique (see Chapter 17, Anaesthesia).

The ram is positioned on its hindquarters (**Fig. 3.108**). A 3–4 cm incision is made in the skin over the spermatic cord at the level of the accessory teats. The spermatic cord is exteriorized following blunt dissection and the vas deferens localized medially within the spermatic cord between the thumb and index finger (**Fig. 3.109**). The vaginal tunic is nicked with the scalpel blade point (**Fig. 3.110**) and a 6 cm length of vas deferens is ligated twice (**Fig. 3.111**); the 4–5 cm section between the ligatures is removed and submitted for histological confirmation in containers of formol saline correctly labelled.

During closure the ligated ends of the vas deferens are incorporated in different fascial planes to further

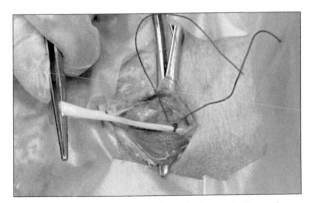

Fig. 3.111 A 6 cm length of vas deferens is ligated twice and excised.

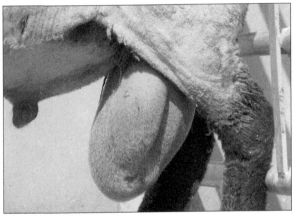

Fig. 3.112 Herniation of omentum and small intestine through the right inguinal ring; the testicle in the normal left side of the scrotum is clearly visible.

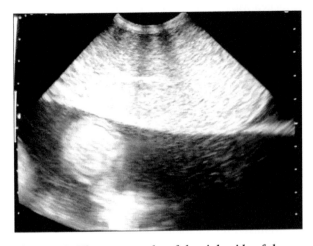

Fig. 3.113 Ultrasonography of the right side of the scrotum reveals a 4 cm diameter atrophied testicle, excess peritoneal fluid and cross-section of intestine (5 MHz sector scanner).

reduce the possibility of recanalization. The skin incision is closed with interrupted horizontal mattress or cruciate sutures and the procedure repeated for the other side.

Some veterinarians prefer to hemicastrate rams rather than remove sections of both vasa deferentes because these rams are then much more readily identifiable should a ram ever lose its ear tag and become the subject of a legal dispute.

Economic considerations/litigation

Occasionally, costly mistakes occur whereby pregnancies result from the use of 'vasectomized' rams, whether caused by errors at surgery or recanalization of one vas deferens. Effective analgesia greatly facilitates surgery and therefore may reduce the likelihood of such mistakes. Dual identification of all vasectomized rams and storage of vasa deferentes is very important in case of litigation. While some surgeons prefer to submit samples for histological examination, this can prove costly. Experienced surgeons may prefer to store specimens in formol saline and submit such specimens should a dispute arise. Electroejaculation of the 'vasectomized' ram would also be a vital part of any such investigation.

Scrotal hernia

Herniation of omentum and small intestine through the inguinal ring occurs sporadically and is readily identified by the size and fluid consistency of one side of the scrotum (**Fig. 3.112**). The scrotal contents are readily distinguished on palpation; ultrasonography (**Fig. 3.113**) can be used where there is any doubt. In most rams the hernia can be reduced when the ram is placed in dorsal recumbency. Affected rams should be culled for welfare reasons.

Sperm granuloma

Sperm granulomas are a coincidental finding in rams several years after vasectomy. The scrotal contents have a bi-lobed appearance due to testicular atrophy and abscessation/granuloma formation of the tail of the epididymis (**Fig. 3.114**). These findings are readily demonstrated by ultrasonography (**Fig. 3.115**).

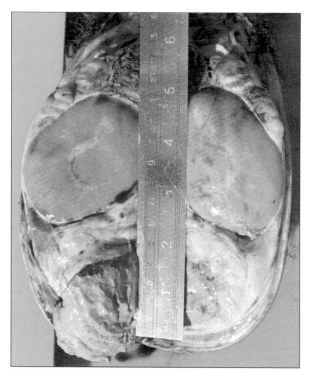

Fig. 3.114 Abscessation/granuloma formation of the tail of the epididymis in a vasectomized ram.

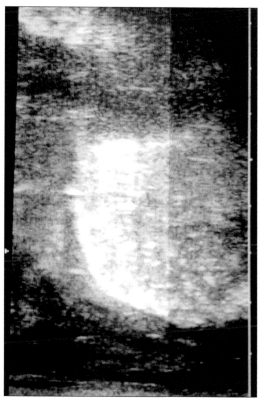

Fig. 3.115 Ultrasonography of the scrotum reveals a 4 cm diameter abscess in the tail of the epididymis; the ventral pole of the testicle is to the left of the image (5 MHz linear scanner).

PERINATAL LAMB MORTALITY

Definition/overview

Perinatal lamb mortality in the majority of UK flocks ranges from 7% to 15% with estimates as high as 25% in some flocks during adverse weather. In New Zealand the perinatal lamb mortality rate is estimated to be between 15% and 20%, with an estimated one million lambs dying each year from hypothermia alone. In the USA lamb mortality reports range from 10% to 35% of the annual lamb crop. The target perinatal lamb mortality figure should be less than 7% with 5% achievable.

Aetiology

While many factors including farm management affect perinatal mortality, lamb birthweight together with ewe body condition score and colostrum accumulation in the udder at lambing remain fundamental to ensuring a good start for the lamb during the critical first 36 hours of life. The direct influence of dam energy nutrition during late gestation on lamb birthweight and accumulation of colostrum within the udder was established more than 50 years ago. Many studies have found significantly higher lamb perinatal mortality in the progeny of underfed ewes, with the effects greater in triplet than twin lambs; singletons were largely unaffected by dam nutritional status. Perinatal lamb mortality is an area where veterinary advice can have a major impact in terms of flock production and profitability (**Fig. 4.1**) and, importantly, welfare of the flock.

Clinical presentation

Lamb birthweight: In UK lowground flocks for example, approximately 15%, 65% and 20% of ewes produce singletons, twins and triplets, respectively. However, these production statistics are influenced

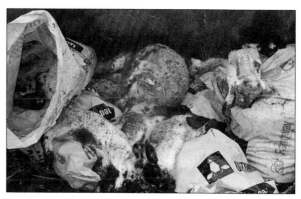

Fig. 4.1 Veterinary advice can have a major impact on perinatal lamb mortality.

by numerous factors which include breed, parity and nutrition at mating time (flushing).

Optimum lamb birthweights using a Suffolk or other terminal meat breed sire crossed onto a F1 hybrid female (e.g. Greyface, or Scottish Halfbred) are:

- Single 5.5–7.0 kg.
- Twin 5.0–6.0 kg.
- Triplet >4.0 kg.

Note that liveweights for the hybrid ewes listed above range from 70 kg to 85 kg. Hill breeds in the UK, such as the Scottish Blackface (liveweight measurements range from 45 kg to 65 kg), will have a birthweight 1–1.5 kg lighter than those stated above.

Recording birthweights: Lamb birthweight changes little within the first 24 hours of life; therefore, all lambs born within the previous 24 hours can be weighed to provide a representative sample during on-farm investigations. Lamb birthweight more than 1.0 kg lighter than those quoted above is strongly suggestive of ewe undernutrition during late gestation. Ewe body condition scores must also be checked with low values consistent with long-term poor energy supply.

Ewe body condition score: Ewe body condition scores are low (2.0 or less; scale 1–5) when late gestation nutrition has been inadequate. Where the flock is managed as one group, low body condition scores are most noticeable in multigravid ewes, especially those ewes with three or more lambs *in-utero*. Where feeding of the whole flock started on the same date, later-born lambs typically have a heavier birthweight due to a longer period of dam supplementary feeding.

Flock problems such as chronic parasitism, particularly fasciolosis, can lead to low body condition in a large percentage of ewes, but this problem is exacerbated by foetal load. In prolific flocks, it is good practice to manage pregnant ewes based upon foetal number determined by ultrasonography.

Hungry lambs within the first 24 hours of life: Hungry lambs appear dull and lethargic and spend a lot of time lying in sheltered areas. After the normal enthusiastic teat-searching behaviour immediately after birth, these lambs quickly become gaunt with a hunched-up appearance and all four limbs held close together. If neglected, the condition may progress to coma and death but this may take 2–3 days, during which time they should be detected by the shepherd and fed accordingly. Coma and death can occur more rapidly in starved lambs exposed to severe weather conditions. In many situations, lambs which have failed to ingest sufficient colostrum (protective immunoglobulins) succumb to infectious disease such as watery mouth disease or septicaemia.

Lamb starvation after 24 hours: Starvation after 24 hours occurs due to dam rejection, often after fostering a lamb; poor dam milk supply, which may be caused by mastitis; poor dam nutrition; or infectious disease (**Figs 4.2–4.4**). Hungry lambs often try to suck other ewes, especially while the ewes are at the feed trough. Hungry lambs may attempt to eat concentrates.

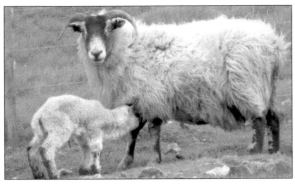

Fig. 4.2 Lamb starvation is apparent in a 24-hour-old caused by ewe mastitis.

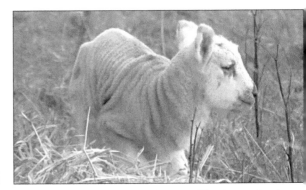

Fig. 4.3 Lamb starvation is caused by dam rejection.

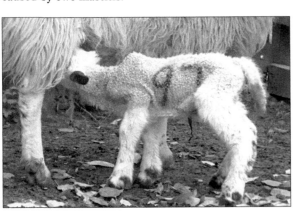

Fig. 4.4 Lamb starvation apparent in a 24-hour-old caused by poor dam milk supply.

These lambs are often found hunched up behind shelters and hedgerows. Recumbent lambs may simply be sleeping and it is therefore essential to get them to their feet for closer inspection. Diarrhoea is frequently encountered in such hungry lambs.

Differential diagnoses

Weakly lambs: There are many causes of weakly lambs at birth including the infectious causes of abortion listed below:

- Toxoplasmosis.
- Border disease.
- *Chlamydophila abortus.*
- *Salmonella* serotypes.
- *Campylobacter fetus intestinalis.*
- *Listeria monocytogenes.*
- *Pasteurella* spp.

Lack of colostrum: Lack of colostrum accumulation within the udder can arise from:

- Poor dam nutrition during late pregnancy.
- Mastitis.
- Chronic debilitating disease such as Johne's disease.
- Maedi-visna virus infection causing indurative mastitis.

Diagnosis

Birth injuries: There is considerable debate as to the relative importance of dystocia, and in particular intrapartum hypoxaemia, as a contributing factor to neonatal losses. The relative importance of dystocia as a cause of neonatal death varies between countries, and this reflects on the breed, management system and level of supervision. For example, an extensive survey in New Zealand involving 23,000 lambs suggested that dystocia was the main cause of death, with 74% of lambs showing evidence of trauma, while a survey in the UK reported only 0.5% loss due to dystocia.

It is important to define what is meant by dystocia in this respect. Postural abnormalities are very common in multigravid sheep and may affect 10–25% of all births in UK lowground flocks. Such problems are readily detected by diligent staff within 30 minutes, promptly corrected and lambs delivered with minimal traction. These lambs require close supervision but no more than any other litter.

Lambing problems that require more than 10–15 minutes of assistance may comprise another group altogether. A typical example may be anterior presentation with either unilateral or bilateral shoulder flexion. Such lambs may present with considerable oedema of the head due to reduced venous return when the head is lodged within the maternal pelvis. In these cases it is possible to envisage that intracranial haemorrhage may occur. However, practical experience indicates that with appropriate supervision these lambs have a normal survival rate. Physical injury during delivery of the lamb should not result because of the option of a caesarean operation to correct foetal oversize problems. The most common skeletal injury is fracture of a number of ribs at their costo-chondral junction along one side of the chest, when a large lamb is delivered in posterior presentation.

Meconium staining of the fleece: It has been suggested that meconium staining of the fleece is an indication of a stressful birth and that such lambs are less able to adapt quickly to extra-uterine life, although there are few supporting data. While lambs with meconium staining of the fleece may warrant special attention, in particular ensuring early colostrum ingestion, there are no convincing data which show they have a significantly higher mortality rate.

Weakly lambs at birth: The investigation of infectious causes of abortion is detailed in Chapter 3, Reproductive System. Dam dietary energy supply with respect to lamb birthweight and perinatal mortality is based upon 3-OH butyrate determination during late gestation, and is detailed in Chapter 2, Husbandry.

Determination of passive antibody transfer

Transabdominal palpation of the abomasum: Colostrum in the lamb's abomasum immediately caudal to the costal arch can readily be detected by gentle transabdominal palpation (**Fig. 4.5**). The gastrointestinal tract of the newborn lamb is empty and it is easy to detect whether the lamb has ingested up to 500 ml of colostrum (more than 10% of its bodyweight).

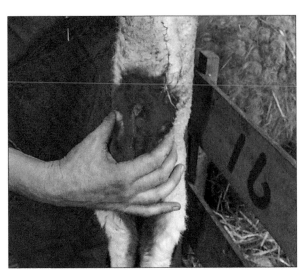

Fig. 4.5 Colostrum in the lamb's abomasum can be detected by gentle transabdominal palpation.

Abdominal distension does occur in watery mouth disease but affected lambs are usually 24 hours old and should not be confused with colostrum ingestion by lambs within the first few hours of life.

Ultrasonographic determination of abomasal diameter: Ultrasonographic examination of the abomasum of neonatal lambs provides an immediate result whether lambs have sucked or not, and may highlight an area for more detailed examination whilst the veterinary surgeon is still on the farm. The abomasal diameter is measured using a 5 MHz sector scanner. The lamb is positioned in dorsal recumbency and ultrasound gel liberally applied to the fleece immediately cranial to the umbilicus. The transducer is applied at right angles to the abdominal wall and the abomasum can be clearly identified as a hypoechoic area delineated by a hyperechoic wall. The vertical distance is measured between the probe head and the far abomasal wall. Good quality sonograms can be obtained without shaving the wool from the lambs' ventral abdomen. With experience, the ultrasonographic examination takes less than 10 seconds per lamb, with repeatable results between operators. The abomasal diameter of newborn lambs before sucking is approximately 3 cm (range = 2–4 cm) compared with 8 cm (range = 7–10 cm) recorded for lambs that have sucked normally.

Determination of total plasma protein concentration: Data from field studies consistently demonstrate that many twin and triplet lambs have failed to suck sufficient good quality colostrum. These lambs are more susceptible to neonatal disease, although the prevalence of some bacterial infections may be ameliorated by routine antibiotic administration to all lambs soon after birth, as practised on most commercial farms in the UK.

During investigations of perinatal lamb mortality, venous blood samples should be collected by the veterinarian into lithium heparin vacutainers from 10–20 randomly selected day-old lambs. Samples are then spun down in a microhaematocrit centrifuge and total plasma protein concentration determined using a hand-held refractometer. The plasma protein concentration for lambs which have not sucked sufficient colostrum is below 45g/l compared with >60 g/l for lambs which have sucked adequate colostrum within the first 12 hours. Such tests are accurate, inexpensive and very informative when the data are used in conjunction with transabdominal palpation of the abomasum and ultrasonographic determination of abomasal diameter.

Treatment
Ensuring the lamb's best start in life: There are three critically important events which must happen to ensure that newborn lambs have the best chance of survival:

1. Lambs must be born into a clean environment to an attentive dam with a good colostrum supply.
2. The lamb must ingest sufficient colostrum (200 ml/kg) during the first 24 hours of life, and 50 ml/kg within the first 2 hours, if not sooner.
3. The navel must be fully immersed in strong veterinary iodine BP within the first 15 minutes of life, and this procedure repeated at least once 2–4 hours later.

Clean environment: The importance of a clean environment cannot be over-emphasized. Poor hygiene standards increase the prevalence of watery mouth disease, infectious polyarthritis and omphalophlebitis affecting lambs, and metritis, mastitis and footrot in ewes. These diseases may not become clinically apparent for a number of days or weeks after infection but originate in the perinatal period.

These infectious diseases will be described in detail later in this chapter, but the major approach must be their prevention through good husbandry practices rather than dependence upon antibiotic prophylaxis/metaphylaxis or treatment. Antibiotics used for prophylaxis have come under increased scrutiny by regulatory authorities and consumer groups, especially where disease can largely be controlled by husbandry practices.

Colostrum accumulation in the ewe's udder: Colostrum accumulation in the ewe's udder at parturition is a direct consequence of her late gestation nutrition. The farmer's veterinary surgeon will have advised on nutritional management during regular flock visits which monitor body condition score, and based upon the metabolic profile results taken 4–6 weeks before lambing.

Maternal instinct: Maternal instinct is under hormonal control and is only adversely affected in severely debilitated or sick ewes.

Ensuring colostrum ingestion: The lamb must ingest sufficient colostrum (200 ml/kg) during the

first 24 hours of life and 50 ml/kg within the first 2 hours, if not sooner. Lambs show the strongest suck reflex within the first hour after birth.

The gastrointestinal tract of the newborn lamb is empty and it is easy to detect whether the lamb has ingested colostrum by inspection and/or digital palpation. Inexperienced farm staff can be instructed by their veterinary surgeon how to detect reliably those lambs that have not sucked colostrum.

If the lamb has not sucked colostrum then some assistance is necessary and various methods are employed:

- Restrain the ewe and gently put the teat into the lamb's mouth at the same time as gently expressing some colostrum onto the lamb's tongue to encourage sucking.
- Sit the ewe onto her hindquarters and lay the lamb on its side, then put the teat into the lamb's mouth at the same time as gently expressing some colostrum onto the lamb's tongue to encourage sucking.
- Encourage the lamb to suck colostrum stripped from either the dam or another ewe, or bovine colostrum, from a bottle and teat (**Fig. 4.6**).
- Administer colostrum stripped from either the dam or another ewe, or bovine colostrum, via a stomach tube (**Fig. 4.7**). Colostrum is very

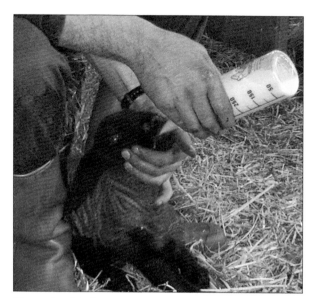

Fig. 4.6 This lamb is encouraged to suck colostrum from a bottle and teat.

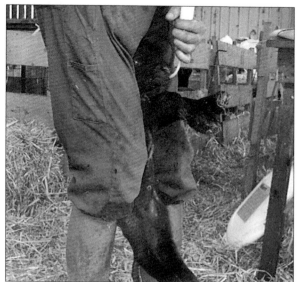

Fig. 4.7 Colostrum can be readily given to the lamb via a stomach tube.

viscous and it may prove necessary to dilute the colostrum with warm water so that it will easily flow through the stomach tube. Alternatively, a 50–60 ml syringe can be filled then discharged through the stomach tube.

Ingestion of colostrum is the single most important event in the lamb's life. Immunoglobulins in colostrum afford specific protection against clostridial and other diseases depending upon dam vaccination status, as well as non-specific immunity. Colostrum is an essential source of energy, minerals and vitamins, as well as possessing laxative properties. Despite the importance of colostrum in ensuring the health of the neonatal lamb, studies have consistently shown that many lambs, particularly triplet and small birthweight lambs, do not suck sufficient colostrum during the first few hours of life.

Teat searching behaviour: Newborn lambs should be able to stand and search for the teat within 15 minutes of birth. Normal healthy lambs nuzzle their way along the ventral abdomen until they find the udder and teat. Lambs adopt a characteristic posture when sucking with rapid tail movements and the ewe starts chewing her cud. Provided the lambs are actively searching for the teat, the ewe and lambs should be left undisturbed. In many pastoral systems, disturbance of lambing ewes may affect maternal bonding and lead to increased lamb losses through abandonment in breeds with poor mothering instincts.

In housed sheep, it is normal practice to pen the ewe with her lambs almost immediately to prevent mismothering. It is not unusual to find another ewe, which is herself within a few days of lambing, trying to 'steal' the newborn lambs. If a lamb strays from the ewe for even short periods of time within the first hour of life, it may be vigorously rejected.

Udder problems: Many shepherds gently express a small amount of colostrum from each teat when the ewe is penned to remove the small waxy plug which has sealed the teat and check that there is no mastitis.

Colostrum is uniformly thick and viscous with a yellow/white colour. Infection of the udder causes the mammary secretions to alter; mastitic milk is often straw-coloured, watery and contains white/yellow clots. The normal udder is firm but not hard, and should be neither hot nor painful. Mastitis often results in swelling of the mammary gland with accumulation of subcutaneous and interstitial fluid which will pit under pressure (oedema).

Mismothering: Mismothering occurs more commonly in housed sheep because of high stocking densities where ewes are unable to isolate themselves from the remainder of the flock during first stage labour. It is interesting to note that the ewe that is attempting to 'steal' or 'pinch' another ewe's lambs is always the more possessive sheep (**Fig. 4.8**). To differentiate which is the true mother, evidence of recent parturition including bloody vulval discharge and loss of abdominal distension should be identified. Transabdominal ballotment will also reveal if there are any foetuses *in utero*. 'Stealing' behaviour is more commonly expressed by older ewes 1–3 days before lambing, and is presumably caused by a surge of hormones as parturition approaches. This behaviour is only slightly premature and lasts for up to 12 hours although such sheep can prove a considerable nuisance during this time.

Treatment of comatose lambs: Treatment of comatose lambs is divided into two age groups; either less or more than 6 hours old.

Treatment of comatose lambs less than 6 hours old: Coma should not arise in lambs less than

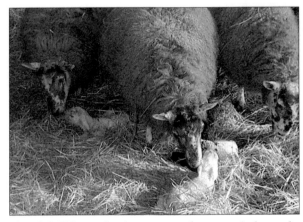

Fig. 4.8 Mis-mothering commonly occurs in housed sheep because of high stocking densities.

6 hours old unless the lambing flock has been neglected during adverse weather. This situation occurs most commonly in the UK when ewes lamb outdoors during severe weather conditions, and in hill flocks which lamb outdoors where there is no supervision during the hours of darkness.

Hypothermic lambs less than 6 hours old do not require intraperitoneal glucose injection because the lamb is born with considerable glycogen reserves, which can be mobilized to produce glucose. The lamb is placed in a warming box with the thermostat set at 45°C. Colostrum should be stomach-tubed at a rate of 50 ml/kg once the lamb has been warmed and can maintain sternal recumbency. If there is insufficient ewe colostrum, it is possible to use cow colostrum pooled in advance from more than four dairy cows previously vaccinated with a multicomponent sheep clostridial vaccine preparation 3, 6 and 10 weeks prior to calving. 'Colostrum supplements' are generally of poor quality.

The true incidence of cow colostrum-induced anaemia is very low indeed and many more lambs die of starvation than anaemia. The unlikely occurrence of cow colostrum-induced anaemia is further reduced if pooled cow colostrum is fed. Laboratory checks for anaemia factor have a low specificity and are not generally undertaken.

Artificial milk replacers should not be used for the first colostrum feed, but can be used after the first feed to save colostrum stores. Electrolyte solutions contain very little energy (as little as 15% of daily requirements) and should only be used for treating neonatal diarrhoea.

Treatment of comatose lambs more than 6 hours old: Diligent flock supervision should quickly detect all hungry lambs which can then be fed and should recover uneventfully, long before becoming comatose. Coma in lambs more than 6 hours old is a reflection of poor flock supervision, because it takes 1–2 days' starvation before the lamb finally exhausts all of its body reserves of glycogen/glucose precursors and brown fat.

Starvation of 24 to 48 hours' duration exhausts glycogen and brown reserves and the lamb becomes hypoglycaemic and hypothermic. These metabolic crises can be corrected by intraperitoneal injection of 25 ml of 20% glucose solution followed by placing the lamb in a warming box with the thermostat set at 45°C. It is essential that the intraperitoneal injection is administered before the lamb is placed in the warming box. The lamb must be regularly checked if the box does not have a thermostat to prevent overheating.

The warm 20% glucose (dextrose) solution is made up by adding 12 ml of recently-boiled water from the kettle to an equal volume of 40% glucose solution available commercially from the farmer's veterinary surgeon.

Intraperitoneal injection: The lamb is held by the forelimbs and the 19 gauge 25 mm long needle is introduced through the body wall 2–3 cm to the side of the navel and 2–3 cm caudal directed towards the lamb's tail head. The solution is slowly injected in to the body cavity once the needle has been introduced up to the hub. It is important not to inject the solution in lambs with watery mouth disease as the needle point will usually puncture the very thin wall of the hugely-distended abomasum, resulting in leakage of abomasal contents and the potential for peritonitis.

The recovery of hypothermic and hypoglycaemic lambs is dramatic within 30–60 minutes, but such neglect should not have occurred in the first instance.

Management/prevention/control measures

Veterinary monitoring and adjustment of late pregnancy ewe nutrition could have a major impact on perinatal lamb survival and prevention of disease by ensuring adequate colostrum accumulation in the ewe's udder. Such advice, incorporated into a veterinary health plan for UK flocks, could achieve increased financial returns (*Table 4.1*) and significant improvements in sheep welfare.

The data in *Table 4.1* represent a flock with moderate energy underfeeding which would require 4 MJ/head/day over the last 6 weeks of gestation to return 3-OH butyrate concentrations to target values (Russel, 1985). This increase in dietary energy supply necessitates an extra 10.5 tonnes of feed (energy value 12 MJ/kg as fed, at £200/tonne) which represents the major cost (£2100) in the total of approximately £2250.

Table 4.1 **Simplified costings for implementation of veterinary flock plan targeting late gestation ewe nutrition in a 1000 ewe lowground flock**	
	EXPENDITURE (£)
Visit farm	45
Biochemical analyses (15 ewes)	85–100
Extra feed (0.25 kg daily for 42 days)	2.10 per ewe
Total costs for 1000 ewe flock	2100
Estimated total	2250
Increased production	
5 ewes (previously died of OPT)	450
Reduction in perinatal mortality 15–17%	
110 extra lambs reared	5500
Reduced neonatal infections	1800
Increased income	£7750
Profit (income less expenditure)	£5500

The improved flock nutrition would prevent five ewes (0.5% ewes at risk) developing ovine pregnancy toxaemia. In addition, 110 extra lambs would be weaned because the perinatal lamb mortality has been reduced by 7–8% consequent to ewes lambing with adequate colostrum accumulations, thereby preventing bacteraemia in their progeny following passive antibody transfer. Perinatal mortality is inversely correlated to lamb birthweight. As well as reducing mortality due to the increasing lamb birthweight and improving immunoglobulin status, such changes would also reduce focal bacterial infections such as polyarthritis, meningitis, omphalophlebitis and hypopyon, which were estimated to cause 2% wastage in the 1800 lambs born alive.

Turnout of ewes and lambs to pasture
Ewes and their 1–2-day-old lambs should be turned out to form groups of 8–12 ewes in small 0.5 hectare paddocks with shelter provided on all sides. Ewes can be drawn to the sheltered areas by placing the feed troughs, root crops and hay in that area. The lambs (and sometimes the ewes) are numbered to allow mothering-up at regular intervals, and especially just before dusk. After 2–3 days the ewes and lambs are walked into large fields with more sheep.

Shelters: Shelters from adverse weather are very important during the first 2 weeks of the lamb's life.

WATERY MOUTH DISEASE

Definition/overview
In the UK, watery mouth disease is a colloquial expression used to describe a collection of clinical signs in neonatal lambs. This includes lethargy, unwillingness to search for the teat and suck, profuse salivation, increasing abdominal distension and retained meconium (**Figs 4.9, 4.10**). The disease process is essentially one of endotoxaemia.

Aetiology
The condition is caused by colonization of the small intestine by *Escherichia coli* with rapid multiplication, followed by cell death and release of lipopolysaccharides. The normal mean haematocrit value, high lactate and urea concentrations, leucopaenia and hypoglycaemia in naturally-occurring watery mouth disease in various field studies is consistent with data generated from an experimental model of endotoxic shock in gnotobiotic lambs. No significant relationship has been reported between serum immunoglobulin G concentrations and susceptibility to watery mouth.

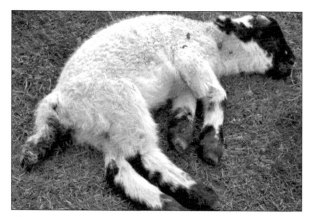

Fig. 4.9 Neonatal lambs suffering from watery mouth initially present with lethargy, increasing abdominal distension and retained meconium.

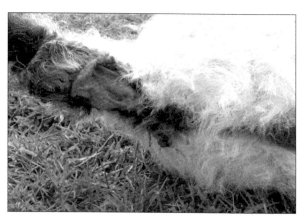

Fig. 4.10 A lamb suffering from the early stage of watery mouth presents with retained meconium.

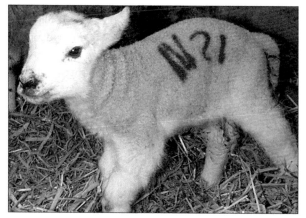

Fig. 4.11 Watery mouth disease progresses and affected lambs show profuse salivation, a wet lower jaw and increasing abdominal distension due to accumulation of fluid and gas in the abomasum.

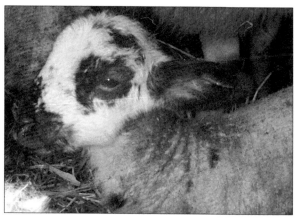

Fig. 4.12 Lambs with watery mouth disease show profuse salivation and a wet lower jaw.

Clinical presentation

Watery mouth disease is caused by colonization of the small intestine by *E. coli* with rapid multiplication and release of endotoxin following cell death. Initial contamination of the lamb's gut arises from a high environmental bacterial load in dirty wet conditions in the lambing shed and pens, and from ewes with faecal staining of the wool of the tail and perineum. Colonization of the gut and rapid bacterial proliferation is facilitated by inadequate and/or delayed colostrum ingestion, especially in small weakly triplets born to poorly-fed ewes in poor body condition with little colostrum accumulation.

Watery mouth disease is commonly encountered in twins, but especially triplet lambs aged 12–36 hours kept in unhygienic conditions. Affected lambs are dull, lethargic, depressed and reluctant to suck. Within 2–6 hours there is profuse salivation, a wet lower jaw and increasing abdominal distension although the lamb has not been sucking (**Figs 4.11, 4.12**). There is profound muscle weakness and the lamb is unable to stand. Scour is only a feature in the latter stages of disease in some lambs. Most lambs have retained meconium, which may be passed after treatment with a soapy water enema (washing-up liquid and

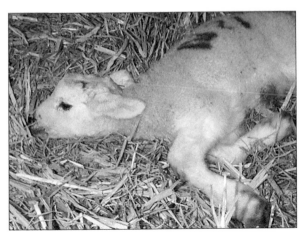

Fig. 4.13 If untreated, watery mouth quickly causes coma and death.

warm water). If untreated, the condition quickly progresses to coma (**Fig. 4.13**) and death.

Differential diagnoses
- Starvation/hypothermia/hypoglycaemia.
- Septicaemia.
- Intrapartum injury.
- Injury post partum, such as chest trauma.
- Toxoplasmosis.
- Border disease.

Diagnosis
Clinical chemistry reveals low plasma glucose concentration and leucopaenia, but elevated lactate and blood urea nitrogen (BUN) concentrations consistent with endotoxaemia.

Necropsy reveals the abomasum distended with mucin and gas. *E. coli* of varying antibiotic sensitivity patterns can be isolated from the small intestines, and agonally from heart blood, liver, spleen and lungs (agonal septicaemia).

Treatment
During the early stages soapy water enemas and mild laxatives/purgatives promote gut activity and expulsion of meconium. (Metaclopramide administered orally is also effective but is too expensive for use in commercial flocks.) These actions, in addition to supportive oral fluid therapy, are often effective in treating mild cases of watery mouth disease.

Oral antibiotics are effective during the early phase of the disease; an aminoglycoside such as spectinomycin is probably the drug of choice because it maintains high concentrations within the gut lumen. Up to 40% of advanced cases of watery mouth disease are bacteraemic; therefore, aminoglycoside antibiotics should not be used because they are not absorbed from the gut. These lambs are often treated with amoxycillin injected intramuscularly.

Despite abomasal distension in lambs with watery mouth disease, oral electrolyte therapy at a rate of 50 ml/kg qid is essential. Administration of a non-steroidal anti-inflammatory drug should be helpful based upon the endotoxic cause, but their use in farm situations is poorly documented.

Intravenous fluid therapy for watery mouth disease, whether with isotonic or hypertonic saline, has not been documented. There is no evidence that lambs with endotoxaemia are acidotic and intravenous bicarbonate administration may be contra-indicated.

Management/prevention/control measures
Problems with watery mouth disease in the UK are almost invariably encountered in housed flocks towards the end of the lambing period, caused by a build up of infection. All attempts must be made to improve hygiene standards in the lambing shed. Wherever possible, the remaining pregnant ewes should be moved to another building or, weather permitting, turned out to pasture. Whilst not the primary factor in the disease process, it is still important to ensure adequate passive antibody transfer.

The single most effective means of controlling endotoxaemia affecting neonatal lambs on commercial sheep units is the administration of an oral antibiotic preparation within the first 15 minutes after birth, to limit bacterial colonization of the gut. On most farms it should be possible to delay the prophylactic use of oral antibiotics in lambs until the second half of the lambing period.

Control measures should include (**Fig. 4.14**):

- Abundant clean, dry straw bedding.
- Use of paraformaldehyde powder on straw bedding.
- Cleaning and disinfection of individual pens between lambing ewes.

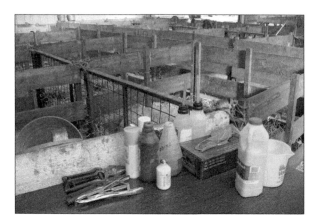

Fig. 4.14 Control measures include good management and hygienic conditions.

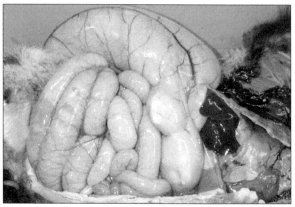

Fig. 4.15 Necropsy of watery mouth cases reveals distended abomasum and intestines containing mucin, gas and unclotted milk if recently fed by oesophageal feeder.

- Collection and disposal of placentae.
- Ensure that lambs suck colostrum as soon as possible following birth.

The role of probiotics in the prevention of watery mouth disease is uncertain although competition between the live cultures of lactobacilli and *Streptococcus faecium* in the probiotic culture may limit proliferation of *E. coli* serotypes and other potentially pathogenic bacteria. The definitive probiotics control study is still awaited.

There are anecdotal reports that oral flunixin is effective in preventing watery mouth disease but substantive on-farm controlled studies are lacking.

Necropsy: Necropsy reveals a distended abomasum containing mucin, gas and unclotted milk. Care must be taken when interpreting these findings because the lamb may have been stomach-tubed during the agonal stages of disease (**Fig. 4.15**). The intestines are gas-filled; there may be meconium in the rectum. Bacteriological culture from liver, lungs, kidneys and heart blood often reveals evidence of an agonal septicaemia.

Economics
There are no precise figures in the UK that quantify losses caused by watery mouth disease because the bacteraemia that frequently accompanies the latter stages of this disease may manifest subsequently as polyarthritis, lung, and liver abscessation some days to weeks later.

In the UK, the administration of an oral antibiotic preparation to every lamb within the first 15 minutes after birth costs 15–20 pence per head, representing a total cost of around £400 for a 1000 ewe flock.

Welfare implications
Watery mouth disease is a major welfare concern because of the associated high mortality rate.

ENTERITIS

Definition/overview
Disease caused by enterotoxigenic strains of *E. coli* (ETEC) is relatively uncommon in sheep flocks.

Aetiology
Outbreaks of neonatal diarrhoea in lambs caused by ETEC (such as K99 or F41 serotypes) are uncommon but may affect lambs less than 4 days old. There is rapid spread of disease in situations where lambs are crowded together.

ETEC possess two important properties; firstly fimbriae which attach the bacterium to the enterocytes lining the gut, and secondly the production of an enterotoxin which interferes with normal water and electrolye transport mechanisms, causing net secretion and loss resulting in rapid dehydration. There is no evidence that lambs with ETEC infections develop metabolic acidosis or bacteraemia.

Clinical presentation

ETEC enteritis affects lambs less than 4 days old with a high morbidity rate. Clinical signs include profuse yellow diarrhoea with obvious staining of the tail and perineum, rapid dehydration, weakness and death within 24 hours of onset of clinical signs. There is rapid dehydration resulting from secretion of water and electrolytes into the gastrointestinal tract which becomes distended with fluid. It is reported that death can occur before clinical signs of diarrhoea develop, but this situation is uncommon.

Differential diagnoses

- Watery mouth disease.
- Other *E. coli* infections.
- Cryptosporidiosis.
- Septicaemia.
- Salmonellosis.

Diagnosis

Diagnosis requires faecal culture and serotyping for K99 or F41 fimbrial antigens.

Treatment

The lamb(s) and the ewe should be isolated but this is rarely practical due to the high morbidity rate in the flock. Oral electrolyte therapy at a rate of 50 ml/kg qid is essential for dehydrated lambs, but this regimen presents considerable practical difficulties due to the large numbers of lambs affected.

The strains of *E. coli*, including K99 or F41 serotypes, are generally sensitive to the common oral antibiotics such as spectinomycin. ETEC do not invade the gut wall and affected lambs do not develop a bacteraemia; therefore, systemic antibiotics are unnecessary.

Administration of a NSAID should be helpful based upon its anti-endotoxic action, but its use in neonatal lambs is poorly documented.

Management/prevention/control measures

Flocks with a history of ETEC (K99, F41 etc) should be vaccinated 8 and 4 weeks prior to the expected lambing date with multivalent vaccines containing these serotypes. However, such infections rarely become endemic on sheep farms and the infection may not appear in following years even if no action is taken.

A cautious approach to vaccination is needed to avoid the overuse of gram-negative vaccines in heavily pregnant ewes because problems have been encountered with temporary malaise and inappetance post vaccination, predisposing to ovine pregnancy toxaemia in high-risk ewes. A compromise situation may be to vaccinate all introduced breeding stock and carefully monitor the disease situation.

Economics

ETEC infections can cause considerable losses in young lambs, although figures will vary depending upon the amount of supportive care provided. Losses result from mortality and the check in growth rate of those lambs which recover.

Welfare implications

While infections with ETEC only occur sporadically, they represent a major welfare concern because of the associated high mortality rate.

SALMONELLAE

Definition/overview

Salmonellae serotypes are only a problem in young lambs if there is an obvious source of infection, either from an existing abortion problem in the ewes or infection gained from cattle or pasture contamination via sewage effluent.

Aetiology

There are many *Salmonella* serotypes that can cause disease in lambs of all ages, but particularly in young lambs when intensively managed and densely stocked.

- *Salmonella typhimurium* can cause abortion in ewes leading to further environmental contamination.
- *S. typhimurium* and *S. dublin* infections can be acquired from cattle by direct contact with either aborted material or faeces, with the development of severe clinical signs.
- *S. typhimurium* and other serotypes can be contracted from sewage effluent.

In the UK, while *S. montevideo* is a common cause of abortion, neonatal enteritis is not a feature of this infection.

Clinical presentation

There is a wide range of clinical signs following infection, ranging from sudden death without pre-monitory signs to healthy carrier sheep. The clinical signs are most severe in lambs less than 1 week old.

In young lambs there is rapid onset of dysentery, rapid dehydration, toxaemia, agonal septicaemia, and death. Affected lambs appear gaunt and show signs of abdominal pain with frequent tenesmus. Initially, the rectal temperature may be raised but becomes subnormal as the severity of signs increases. Dysentery is a feature of the disease in older lambs when the faeces are malodorous and may contain mucosal casts and large blood clots.

Differential diagnoses

- Depending upon age and management, coccidiosis is an important differential diagnosis of diarrhoea, tenesmus and passage of some blood clots, although toxaemia and sudden death are uncommon.
- Lamb dysentery should also be considered in lambs that have received no specific protective immunoglobulin, for whatever reason.
- Nematodirosis can cause sudden death in lambs grazing infested pasture, while others in the group show signs of profuse diarrhoea.
- Causes of sudden death include pasteurellosis, and other septicaemic conditions.

Diagnosis

The provisional diagnosis is based upon clinical signs, and elimination of other possible causes. Confirmation requires bacteriological isolation from faecal samples and viscera of septicaemic cases.

Treatment

There is considerable debate regarding antibiotic treatment of salmonellosis in farm animals because of perceived risks of accelerated acquisition of various antibiotic resistance factors causing therapeutic problems in human infections. While many exotic *Salmonella* serotypes remain sensitive to most antibiotics, problems may arise with strains

of *S. typhimurium*. Antibiotic selection should be directed by sensitivity testing in the latter group.

Management/prevention/control measures

It is standard farm management that livestock do not have access to slurry storage areas. Overflow from septic tanks must be dealt with immediately. Sheep should not be co-grazed with cattle which have endemic salmonellosis. Feed storage areas must be vermin-proof to prevent faecal contamination. Feeding areas must be changed daily to prevent environmental contamination by vermin and birds.

Economics

Salmonellosis is not a major economic problem in young lambs.

Welfare implications

Welfare concerns are addressed by prompt treatment. Recumbent sheep with dysentery should be euthanased for welfare reasons.

OMPHALOPHLEBITIS (UMBILICAL INFECTION)

Definition/overview

Omphalophlebitis is common in young lambs born into unsanitary conditions where there is inadequate navel treatment (**Fig. 4.16**). It is more common during

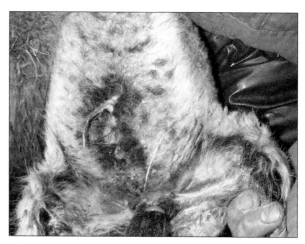

Fig. 4.16 Lambs born in unsanitary conditions without adequate navel treatment are susceptible to omphalophlebitis.

inclement weather and in male lambs, presumably because urination delays desiccation of the umbilicus and removes some of the topical astringent/antibiotic applied by the shepherd, thereby making bacterial invasion more likely.

Umbilical infections may remain localized and develop into a discrete abscess involving the body wall, or they may extend to peritonitis (**Fig. 14.17**), urachal infection (**Fig. 4.18**) and liver abscessation (**Fig. 4.19**). It is generally believed, but unproven, that omphalophlebitis may give rise to bacteraemia with subsequent localization causing polyarthritis, hypopyon and meningitis. The notable exception is umbilical infection with *Fusobacterium necrophorum* and subsequent haematogenous spread to the liver, which causes the specific condition of hepatic necrobacillosis.

It is important to consider carefully the importance of umbilical infection in newborn lambs, because sole emphasis on this potential portal of infection may overlook much more important aspects of disease prevention in neonatal lambs. While umbilical infections extend directly to the urachus, liver and peritoneum (**Figs 4.17–4.19**), it is rare to have concurrent polyarthritis lesions or other evidence of bacteraemic spread.

Polyarthritis caused by *Streptococcus dysgalactiae* can still occur on farms that immerse lambs' navels in strong iodine BP at birth and again at 2 and 6 hours old. Very few lambs with polyarthritis have macroscopic evidence of omphalophlebitis; the origin of infection is more probably via the tonsil and/or upper respiratory tract.

Bacterial meningitis is encountered in 2–3-week-old lambs. It seems unlikely that bacteraemic spread could result from chronic umbilical lesions that would be well-encapsulated after such an interval from birth and acquisition of infection.

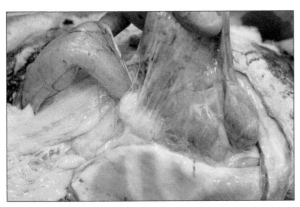

Fig. 4.17 Umbilical infection may extend to peritonitis with adhesions to small intestine and omentum in this case.

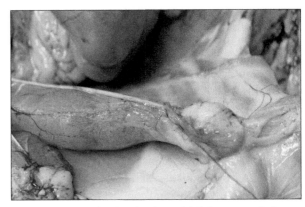

Fig. 4.18 Umbilical infection which has extended to the urachus with adherent bladder.

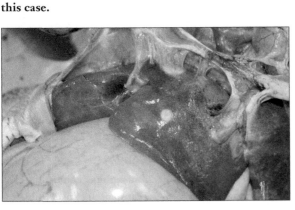

Fig. 4.19 Liver abscesses near the capsular surface with localized peritonitis arising from umbilical infection.

Aetiology

The consequences of nil/incorrect navel dressing include ascending infection to involve the body cavity, liver and urachus, and possibly more generalized infection to involve the joints, meninges, lungs, kidneys and endocardium. Navel infection can be readily prevented; prognosis is largely hopeless once adhesions develop. While infection gains entry through the undipped navel within the first few hours of life, the consequences for the lamb may not be fully appreciated until some weeks later, after a considerable period of suffering (e.g. hepatic necrobacillosis).

Clinical presentation

Septic peritonitis: The clinical signs vary with the extent and nature of the peritonitis. Lambs that develop septic peritonitis appear very dull and weak within the first 5 days of life. They stand with their back arched and their head held lowered (**Figs 4.20, 4.21**) and spend long periods lying in the corner of the pen. The rectal temperature may be subnormal. These lambs do not suck but increasing exudation in the peritoneal cavity, causing moderate distension, contrasts with the lamb's gaunt appearance and expression. The abdomen may contain up to 200 ml of turbid fluid with large fibrin clots, which may develop to pus following cellular infiltration and

bacterial multiplication. There is rapid loss of body condition with a prominent ribcage and bony prominences, which contrast markedly with the well-muscled contours of the healthy co-twin. Affected lambs rapidly become dehydrated and die within a few days of clinical signs first appearing.

Localized fibrinous peritonitis: Peritoneal lesions may often be restricted to a small number of fibrin tags, which adhere readily to intestine and may loop around intestine, causing stricture/occlusion. This presentation is not uncommon when infection has extended via the urachus. These lambs present with a distended abomasum and small intestine proximal to the constriction and often show signs of mild colic which may be mistaken for abomasal bloat. The important clinical feature in this condition is the absence of faeces over the preceding few days, but such information is rarely available to the clinician.

Hepatic necrobacillosis: The clinical presentation of hepatic necrobacillosis depends upon the number, site and size of the liver lesions. Abscesses involving the liver capsule, which stimulate localized peritonitis with adhesion formation to adjacent small intestine, are more important than deeper-seated lesions.

Typically, affected lambs are first noted from 10 to 14 days old, when they appear dull and depressed and

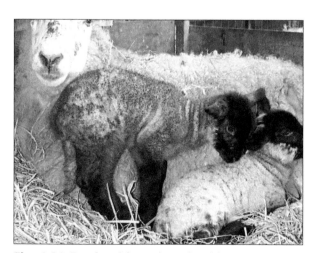

Fig. 4.20 Lambs with septic peritonitis appear very dull, weak, tucked up with four feet held together, with an arched back and do not suck.

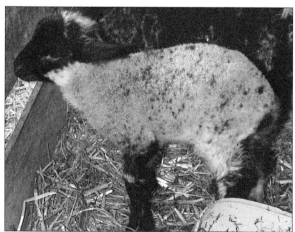

Fig. 4.21 Lambs with septic peritonitis have a gaunt appearance with evidence of abdominal pain.

in much poorer condition than their co-twin. They have an empty gaunt appearance and are too easily caught in the field. Many affected lambs may not follow the ewe and co-twin and are found sheltering behind walls and hedgerows. Affected lambs stand with an arched back and all four limbs drawn together ('like a half-closed pen knife'). In some lambs the liver can be palpated extending beyond the costal arch and digital pressure caudal to the xiphisternum may elicit a painful response. Affected lambs are much more prone to predation than healthy lambs. In extensive management systems these lambs may not be noticed as ill but are simply noted as losses at weaning.

Differential diagnoses
Septic peritonitis
- Enteric infections.
- Abomasal bloat/torsion.
- Atresia coli.

Localized fibrinous peritonitis
- Watery mouth disease.
- Pyloric outflow obstruction, e.g. wool ball.
- Abomasal bloat/torsion.
- Atresia coli.

Hepatic necrobacillosis
- Starvation.
- Pneumonia.
- Polyarthritis.
- Coccidiosis.
- Nephrosis.

Diagnosis
Septic peritonitis: Abdominocentesis of turbid fluid with a high protein concentration and large numbers of degenerative white cells confirms the clinical diagnosis of septic peritonitis. Direct smears stained with Gram's stain may identify clumps of bacteria. Care must be taken not to penetrate the abomasum during abdominocentesis, which should only be undertaken after ultrasonographic demonstration of excess peritoneal fluid.

Localized fibrinous peritonitis: Diagnosis of gut stricture caused by fibrin tags is not simple. Ultrasonography typically reveals a grossly distended

abomasum with little or no fluid within the intestines. It may be possible to visualize fibrin tags within peritoneal exudate, but large accumulations are uncommon therefore abdominocentesis would not usually be undertaken.

Hepatic necrobacillosis: Diagnosis of hepatic necrobacillosis is based upon clinical signs, and the presence of anterior abdominal pain. Ultrasonography would reveal the presence of liver abscess(es) and focal adhesions. Normal BUN concentration allows nephrosis to be excluded from the list of differential diagnoses.

Treatment
Treatment of septic peritonitis is hopeless and lambs should be euthanased as soon as the diagnosis is established. However, few sick lambs are presented to veterinarians and in most farm situations there is a standard treatment protocol for all sick lambs such that it is likely that these lambs will receive daily intramuscular penicillin injection until they either improve or are euthanased for welfare reasons/die.

Prompt recognition and antibiotic treatment of hepatic necrobacillosis may arrest growth of the infective lesions, thereafter liver regeneration may restore health although such lambs are unlikely to grow as well as their healthy co-twin. However, this is largely supposition and the extent to which the liver regenerates in hepatic necrobacillosis remains unknown.

Management/prevention/control measures
The umbilicus (navel) must be fully immersed in strong veterinary iodine BP within the first 15 minutes of life and repeated at least 2–4 hours later. Antibiotic aerosol sprays are much inferior to strong veterinary iodine BP for dressing navels and are much more expensive. All umbilical infections are a direct consequence of the farmer's neglect of sound husbandry practices.

This essential routine procedure must be undertaken when the ewe and her lambs are penned soon after birth, and again 2–4 hours later when the shepherd checks that the lambs have sucked colostrum as outlined earlier. Note that all these procedures can be fitted into a routine such that none is overlooked.

Economics

Failure to adopt sound management practices with respect to hygiene standards and routine navel dressings can lead to considerable lamb mortality.

Welfare implications

Lambs with peritonitis appear gaunt and in obvious pain. Liver abscessation leads to debility and eventual death.

POSTMORTEM EXAMINATION OF A REPRESENTATIVE NUMBER OF DEAD LAMBS

Postmortem examination of a representative number of neonatal deaths provides much useful information to the veterinary surgeon regarding lamb starvation and other causes of neonatal losses. These examinations can be undertaken very quickly on the farm, and will highlight the causes of death and allow control and prevention measures to adopted. It is vitally important that a representative sample of lambs is necropsied; this is best achieved by examining all lambs that have died 1 or 2 days previous to the veterinary visit, depending upon the number. Care should be exercised that the visit was not preceded by adverse weather conditions or other potentially unique events, which could distort the data collected. This is overcome by undertaking necropsies on serial batches of lambs.

Lamb identified by farmer

Litter size, dam parity, dystocia, any illness, treatments and age at death should be noted. Losses from starvation/exposure are greater in twins and triplets associated with lower birthweight. Losses caused by dystocia are highest in primiparous females, especially if lambed as yearlings.

Lamb weight

Depending upon breed and bodyweight of the dam, lambs <3.5 kg are more prone to starvation/exposure, while lambs with birthweights >6 kg are more likely to have caused dystocia.

Gross inspection

The presence of blood staining of fleece and sub-cutaneous oedema of head/hindlimbs may indicate dystocia. Obvious congenital abnormalities should be noted. Meconium staining causes dark yellow/brown discoloration of the whole fleece (**Fig. 4.22**) and may indicate prolonged second stage labour/dystocia.

A tapered end of the umbilicus indicates pre-partum death, a square end indicates death soon after parturition and a dry shrivelled cord indicates death after 12 hours or more, although this appearance is influenced by iodine or other topical treatments. A blood clot within the umbilical vessels indicates that death occurred after first stage labour.

Necropsy

There are a number of approaches to the necropsy examination; however, it is important that it is undertaken quickly and in a systematic manner.

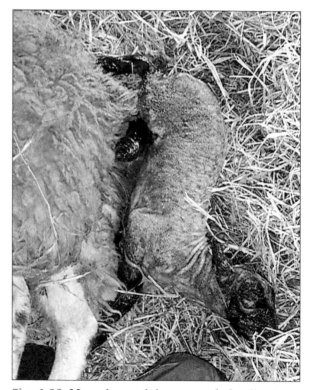

Fig. 4.22 Meconium staining causes dark yellow/brown discoloration of the whole fleece and may indicate prolonged second stage labour/dystocia.

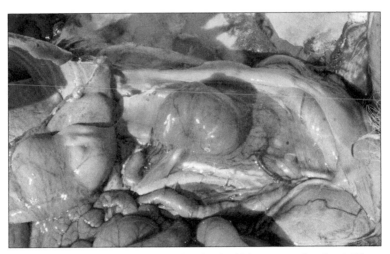

Fig. 4.23 Necropsy of a starved lamb; the kidneys are clearly visible following mobilization of perirenal fat reserves.

The lamb is positioned in dorsal recumbency and incisions made between the chest wall and scapulae. The strip of skin left covering the sternum is reflected toward the pelvis and removed, taking care not to enter the abdominal cavity. An incision can be made into each hip joint to aid stabilization but is not necessary. The skin should also be removed from the ventral neck region and extended to the jaw to allow examination of the thyroid glands.

The abdominal wall is tented and an incision made immediately caudal to the sternum and extended caudally to the pubis with scissors, thus avoiding puncturing any viscus such as distended abomasum or intestines. The sternum is then removed by cutting through the costochondral junctions using a knife (note a scalpel blade will suffice but may snap).

Often dead lambs have had their skin removed for fostering purposes. This affords ready examination of the hindlimb extremities for signs of oedema caused by dystocia. However, there is also marked oedema of the head which is obvious during inspection of the lamb such that skinning of the whole carcase is not necessary.

The size and contents of the abomasum should be noted. The abomasum of well-fed lambs contains numerous large milk clots up to 2–3 cm in diameter, as well as milk. The presence of milk suggests feeding immediately prior to death without time for clotting.

There should be evidence of chyle in the intestinal lymphatics. The presence of meconium should be noted.

The abomasum and intestines are then lifted out of the abdomen to allow inspection of the kidneys and the amount of perirenal fat deposits. In normal lambs the kidneys are embedded in 5–10 mm of fat and are not visible. Mobilization of fat reserves in starved neonatal lambs can occur within days, and the kidneys will be clearly visible (**Fig. 4.23**). Fat reserves are also mobilized from the epicardial groove. Haemorrhage into the abdomen with formation of large blood clots is uncommon but may result from liver lobe rupture.

Full expansion and aeration of lung can be checked by immersion in water: aerated lung floats, unexpanded lung sinks. The pericardium is incised to check for excess fluid and mobilization of epicardial fat.

Removal of the brain and spinal cord is rarely undertaken during on-farm investigations of perinatal lamb mortality. Intrapartum injury to the central nervous system during dystocia is reported to result in subdural, subarachnoid and extradural haemorrhages, with a prevalence of 21% in lambs that died compared with 1.4% in a control group. However, other signs of dystocia such as peripheral oedema and haemorrhages in the thymus, pleurae and epicardium are more easily observed during on-farm investigations.

Starvation/exposure

Deaths due to starvation/exposure occur 1–3 days after birth. They are much more common in multiple births and in litters of ewes in poor condition with intercurrent illness such as mastitis or metritis.

Exposure

Losses occur within the first day of life, typically within the first 6–8 hours where there is poor supervision. During winter storms and extreme weather conditions (e.g. cold driving winds and snow) lambs can die of exposure, although there will be few lesions detected at necropsy. Affected lambs may not have risen, walked or sucked. Often they are found in the morning in lateral recumbency where they were born. During adverse weather, all lambs in the litter may be found dead in addition to losses in other litters. There are fewer losses of singletons. The lamb's coat may still be covered with foetal fluids. Necropsy findings may reveal peripheral oedema, absence of colostrum and depletion of fat reserves.

Starvation

If a lamb has died from starvation, there is an absence of milk clots up to 2–3 cm in diameter and milk in the abomasum. There is no evidence of chyle in the intestinal lymphatics.

The presence of unclotted milk suggests feeding immediately prior to death. The kidneys are clearly visible (**Fig. 4.23**) with fat reserves also mobilized from the epicardial groove. There is loss of mesenteric fat. The liver may be smaller and less friable than normal.

CLINICAL EXAMINATION

History

It is important to obtain a history of the dietary management of the sheep including type and amounts of particular feeds. Sheep fed fibrous diets have a more distended rumen than those fed solely concentrates. They will have one or two full contraction cycles per minute, which is more frequent than sheep fed large quantities of concentrates.

Sheep normally pass pelleted faeces, except when grazing very lush pastures when soft stools are passed; diarrhoea is an abnormal finding under all feeding systems. The presence of dried faeces staining the tail and perineum indicates a prior episode of diarrhoea and is abnormal. Dry, mucus-coated faeces indicate an increased transport time through the gastrointestinal tract.

When presented with any sheep for examination, it is important to first inspect from a distance and compare the gross appearance (**Figs 5.1–5.3**), fleece (**Figs 5.4–5.6**), abdominal fill (**Figs 5.7, 5.8**) and body condition with sheep of the same age and production (litter size, number of lambs). Without such direct comparison, it may prove difficult to differentiate poor husbandry from disease when only affected sheep are presented (**Figs 5.8, 5.9**).

Examination of the buccal cavity

Sheep with lesions of the buccal cavity usually present in poor condition due to impaired feeding (**Fig. 5.10**). The lower jaw is wet caused by drooling of saliva. Lesions affecting the cheek result in obvious firm swellings. Infected lesions of the cheek and/or tongue may cause halitosis and swelling of the submandibular lymph node(s).

Correct dentition is of critical importance to the maintenance of body condition/weight gain in sheep. The necessity to examine the mouth fully, with particular reference to the molar teeth, cannot

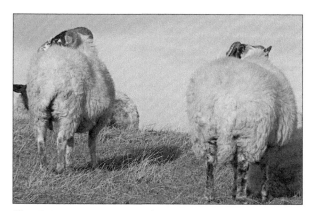

Fig. 5.1 Inspect cases and compare with normal sheep in the group. The difference in body condition score and abdominal fill contrast markedly between these two sheep, even from a distance.

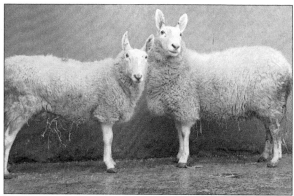

Fig. 5.2 Chronic weight loss is clearly evident in the sheep on the left.

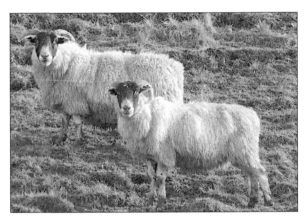

Fig. 5.3 Lower body condition score and poorer abdominal fill are readily observed in the sheep in the foreground.

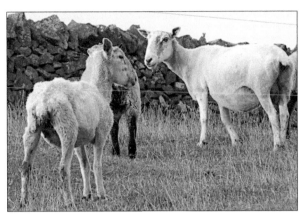

Fig. 5.4 Poorer wool growth and quality of the shearing are observed in the sheep in the foreground.

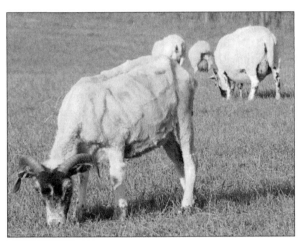

Fig. 5.5 Poor-quality shearing has occurred because there was no rise in the wool, caused by debility.

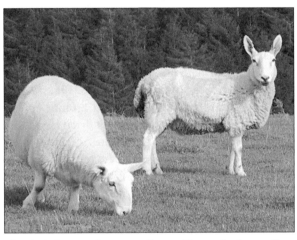

Fig. 5.6 Poorer fleece quality and lower body condition are obvious in the ewe in the background.

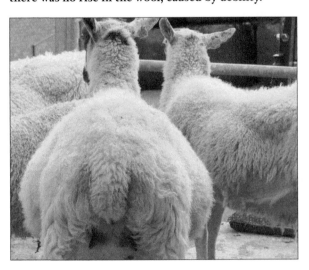

Fig. 5.7 Abdominal fill/contour can be readily compared between sheep of the same group.

Fig. 5.8 The group of sheep must be inspected otherwise it is difficult to assess only the animal(s) presented for examination.

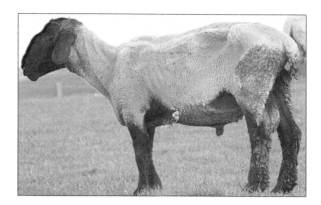

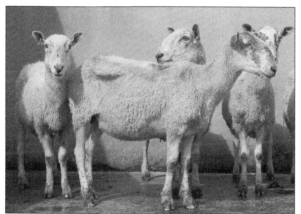

Fig. 5.9 Chronic disease or simply mismanagement; examination of the group/flock is necessary to make an informed judgement.

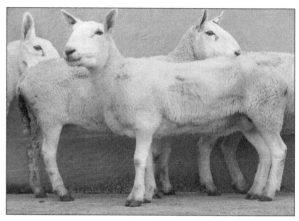

Fig. 5.10 Poor condition due to impaired feeding caused by molar dentition problems.

be over-emphasized. Overgrown, worn and absent molar teeth cause serious problems with mastication of fibrous feeds.

Sheep have 32 permanent teeth with a dental formula of 2 (incisors 0/4, premolars 3/3 and molars 3/3). Some textbooks correctly refer to the fourth (lateral or corner) incisor as the canine tooth but in essence it functions as an incisor tooth. The temporary incisor teeth erupt sequentially at approximately weekly intervals from birth. The three temporary premolars erupt within 2–6 weeks. The first permanent molar erupts at 3 and 5 months in the lower and upper jaws, respectively. The second permanent molar erupts at 9–12 months, and the third permanent molar and permanent premolars erupt between 18 and 24 months.

Incisor teeth alignment is examined by running an index finger along the dental pad and incisor teeth.

This examination will reveal any teeth projecting forward of the normal contact on the dental pad (overshot jaw or prognathia) or behind (undershot jaw or brachygnathia). This examination must be undertaken with the mouth closed and the head held in the normal resting position.

The incisor teeth can then be viewed by pulling down the lower lip, when the points should still contact with the dental pad in normal sheep. Incisor wear and loss are common in older sheep; however, such sheep can remain productive when offered appropriate supplementary feeds. Due attention must be paid to the sheep's recent nutritional management when attempting to determine the significance of missing incisor teeth, e.g. failure to bite off grass may cause loss of condition in grazing situations but prehension is of much lesser importance if the sheep are fed concentrates.

Molar tooth problems can best be identified by impaction of food in the cheeks and observing short jerky jaw movements with the mouth held slightly open. This results from excessive tooth growth or cheek lesions causing pain during mastication. The sheep will often raise its head to assist movement of the food bolus over the dorsum of the tongue and during swallowing. Affected sheep often have pieces of fibrous feed protruding from the commisures of the mouth with frequent quidding. Careful palpation of the dental arcade through the cheek reveals the sharp irregular ridges of the labial aspect of the upper cheek teeth and any lost upper cheek teeth. There is no enlargement of submandibular lymph nodes associated with molar tooth loss. Examination of the molar teeth with a gag and torch is essential, but lengthy examination is greatly resented by sheep. Radiographs can provide useful information on the jaw and cheek teeth but it proves difficult not to superimpose the cheek teeth of the contralateral jaw, even using oblique views.

Examination of the mandible

The horizontal rami of the mandible can be readily palpated through the skin. Despite the common finding of loose cheek teeth and missing teeth, tooth root abscesses with associated bone lysis and sinus formation along the ventral margin are uncommon in sheep.

Tumours involving the mandible (e.g. fibrosarcoma) appear over many months as a unilateral, firm, 3–5 cm diameter swelling of the horizontal ramus but are rare in sheep. Tissue invasion and destruction of support structures result in loosening and possible loss of associated cheek teeth.

Examination of the pharynx

Pharyngeal trauma is not uncommon following balling gun or drenching gun injury in growing lambs; however, these injuries are often not detected until infection has either extended into the cervical vertebral canal, resulting in tetraparesis, or localized abscess development has caused compression of the larynx with stertorous breathing, by which stage detailed examination of the primary route of infection is of secondary concern. Despite localized infection of the pharynx, it proves difficult to palpate the enlarged retropharyngeal lymph nodes.

Good visualization of the pharynx can be achieved under general anaesthesia (see Chapter 17, Anaesthesia). General anaesthesia is also necessary to permit complete endoscopic examination of the pharynx.

Examination of the oesophagus

Oesophageal lesions are very uncommon in sheep. While choke may occasionally occur within the proximal cervical oesophagus in sheep fed dried sugar beet or similar, this is usually relieved following retching and vigorous head tossing. The cervical oesophagus can be palpated and obstruction can be checked by careful passage of a flexible orogastric tube through a suitable mouth gag. Forcing an oesophageal obstruction using an orogastric tube is not recommended because of the likelihood of causing perforation of the oesophagus.

Examination of the forestomachs

When viewed from behind, the rumen in normal sheep pushes the lower left flank beyond the outline of the costal arch but this is usually masked by the fleece and, therefore, must be palpated. Bloat causing distension of the left sublumbar fossa is uncommon in sheep, except for those with advanced hypocalcaemia.

Auscultation of the rumen is performed in the upper left flank with the fleece parted to gain good contact between the stethoscope and the skin. The flank is then firmly pressed to contact the dorsal sac of the rumen; any gap between the rumen wall and abdominal wall will greatly reduce transmitted sounds. There are two independent reticuloruminal contraction sequences: a primary biphasic contraction cycle of the reticulum followed by rumen contractions, which occurs approximately once a minute and mixes ingesta and forces small particles into the omasum; and a secondary contraction that does not involve the reticulum but rumen activity pushes the gas cap into the cardia region, with resultant eructation. Typically, one secondary cycle follows two primary cycles such that three cycles occur every 2 minutes. Due to the fibrous nature of the ration, sheep fed fibrous diets have a more distended rumen, with more frequent contractions, than those fed solely concentrates.

Rumen fluid collection and analysis

Rumen fluid can be easily collected by aspiration through a wide-bore orogastric tube with a suitable mouth gag in place. Discarding the first few millilitres of the sample will reduce contamination with saliva. The rumen fluid can be analysed for colour, odour, pH, protozoa, sedimentation rate and methylene blue reduction time. Normal rumen fluid is green with an aromatic odour, pH 6.5–8.0, with many variably-sized motile protozoa per microscope field (×100). The methylene blue reduction time is abnormal if extended beyond 6–8 minutes.

GENERAL EXAMINATION OF THE ABDOMEN

Radiography

Radiography is rarely used to investigate abdominal disorders in sheep because lesions caused by radiodense materials such as an ingested sharp metallic object are rare; fluid accumulations are better demonstrated by ultrasonography and this also avoids the attendant health and safety restrictions.

Abdominocentesis

Abdominocentesis is undertaken when excess fluid is identified by ultrasonography. Excess peritoneal fluid associated with peritonitis is very uncommon in sheep because infections are largely confined by the omentum. Large accumulations of peritoneal fluid do occur in sheep with conditions such as subacute fasciolosis and intestinal adenocarcinoma, and in sheep with cor pulmonale. Peritoneal fluid samples can be collected from a midline site immediately caudal to the xiphisternum.

Peritoneal fluid should be collected into tubes containing EDTA. Attempts to collect peritoneal fluid by ventral midline percutaneous aspiration in sheep with no excess fluid invariably result in puncture of the rumen. In gravid ewes, careless abdominocentesis may puncture the uterine horn. Both linear and sector scanners can be used to determine the presence and extent of excess peritoneal fluid and identify the site for transabdominal fluid collection using a hypodermic needle.

Normal peritoneal fluid has a clear, slightly yellow appearance with a protein concentration of 10–30 g/l and white cell concentration <1 × 10^6/l, comprised mainly of lymphocytes. Infectious peritonitis typically results in a turbid sample with high protein and white cell concentrations comprised mainly of neutrophils.

Abdominal ultrasonography

While ultrasonography has been successfully employed in commercial flocks for the past 40 years to determine foetal number and gestation length, thus permitting more precise ewe nutrition and management during late gestation, transabdominal ultrasonographic examination can also include the peritoneal cavity (ascites, uroperitoneum, peritonitis and abscess involving the body wall), liver, rumen, reticulum, abomasum, bladder and kidney, uterus and foetus(es).

Ultrasonographic equipment

A 5 MHz linear transducer connected to a real-time, B-mode ultrasound machine can be used for all abdominal ultrasonographic examinations except examination of the right kidney and liver, where a 5.0 MHz sector transducer is necessary to ensure good contact with the concave flank of the right sublumbar fossa and between the convex intercostal spaces, respectively. The field setting of 10 cm on the linear scanner is appropriate for most abdominal examinations; occasionally the 20 cm field depth afforded by certain 5.0 MHz sector scanners more accurately determines the extent of fluid accumulation and bladder diameter but this does not significantly alter the diagnosis.

Good contact between the probe head and hair/ wool-free skin is essential to allow transmission of sound waves. The hair-free area of the abdominal wall in the inguinal region affords examination of the caudal abdomen. Ultrasonographic examination of the cranial abdomen (e.g. reticulum and abomasum in adults) is rarely undertaken in sheep but can be readily achieved after shaving the wool off with a razor or scalpel blade. The skin is then wetted with either alcohol or tap water, and ultrasound gel liberally applied. The probe head is held firmly at right angles against the abdominal wall.

Transrectal examination of the bladder and rectum has been reported in both ewes and rams but this examination has not proved necessary in practice to determine obstructive urolithiasis.

Ultrasonographic appearance of normal abdominal viscera

The abdominal wall is 1–3 cm thick depending upon the site and body condition score of the sheep. It is possible to differentiate between the various muscles forming the abdominal wall. There is scant peritoneal fluid in normal sheep and this cannot be visualized during ultrasonographic examination.

Reticular motility can readily be observed in the cranial abdomen immediately caudal to the left costal arch, but such examination is not routinely undertaken because of the rare occurrence of traumatic reticulitis.

The liver can readily be visualized from halfway down the right costal arch with the probe head angled towards the left shoulder. Alternatively, the liver can be imaged halfway down the eighth to tenth intercostal spaces with the probe head held at a right angle to the chest wall.

The intestines are clearly outlined as broad hyperechoic (white) lines/circles containing material of varying echogenicity. By maintaining the probe head in the same position for 10–20 seconds, digesta can be visualized as multiple small dots of varying echogenicity forcibly propelled within the intestines. Such movement of intestinal contents prevents confusion with other structures such as an abscess or fluid accumulation within the uterine horns (metritis/pyometra), which may present with a similar sonographic appearance but with the contents remaining static.

The bladder rarely extends beyond the pubis and therefore is not visualized in normal sheep.

Ascites

Ascites can prove difficult to quantify by ballotment, especially in sheep with fluid-distended intestines, but is readily identified during ultrasonographic examination, even in recumbent sheep. Ascites can be present without significant accumulation of fluid at other sites, such as subcutaneous tissue in the submandibular region (bottle-jaw) and brisket. Ascitic fluid appears as an anechoic (black) area with abdominal viscera displaced dorsally.

Ascites must be differentiated from urine accumulation but uroperitoneum is always accompanied by bladder distension, so permitting immediate differentiation from ascitic fluid.

Abdominal wall

The extent of subcutaneous urine accumulation along the prepuce and ventral abdominal wall can be accurately defined in male sheep with urethral rupture. Ultrasound examination of such fluid accumulation reveals multiple pockets of urine within subcutaneous tissue and clearly indicates the futility of attempted drainage using either single or multiple stab incisions in the overlying skin. Abscesses involving the body wall caused by penetration wounds, dog bites, and faulty injection/vaccination technique occur occasionally. Such abscesses appear as anechoic areas containing multiple bright hyperechoic (white) dots within a well-defined capsule.

Peritonitis

Significant peritoneal exudation is rarely seen in sheep. Reaction is limited to focal fibrinous/fibrous adhesions and localized accumulation of peritoneal fluid. When present, the hyperechoic lattice-work appearance of the fibrinous reaction within the abdomen contrasts with the anechoic peritoneal fluid.

Localized fibrinous peritonitis has been reported in severe cases of subacute fasciolosis.

Occasionally, the peritoneal reaction is limited to a few fibrinous adhesions, which cannot be visualized. In this situation the intestines are distended with fluid (anechoic appearance) rather than containing normal digesta (anechoic appearance containing multiple bright dots), and there are no propulsive intestinal contractions.

Liver

Liver abscessation caused by *Corynebacterium pseudotuberculosis*, the causal agent of caseous lymphadenitis (CLA), is common in many sheep-producing countries. In the UK visceral CLA is a rare manifestation of ovine infection. Gall bladder distension is a common finding in cachectic sheep. Hepatomegaly can be identified in sheep with subacute fasciolosis. Fibrinous adhesions between the liver and adjacent intestines have been identified ultrasonographically and confirmed at necropsy in these sheep.

Bladder, kidney and uterus

Further information on ultrasonographic examination of the bladder and right kidney is supplied in Chapter 10, Urinary System and of the uterus in Chapter 3, Reproductive System.

Abomasum in neonates

Ultrasonographic examination of the abomasum of neonatal lambs provides an immediate indication to the veterinary investigator of whether lambs have sucked or not, and may highlight an area for more detailed examination whilst the veterinarian is present on the farm. The difference in lamb abomasal diameter before and after sucking is so large (3 cm versus 8–10 cm) that minor errors in individual lamb recordings should not affect the collection of meaningful data from 20 or more lambs.

TEETH/DENTITION

Incisor loss

(syn. broken mouth)

Definition/overview

Premature loss of incisor teeth (**Fig. 5.11**) is a major problem worldwide. It leads to early culling because affected sheep are unable to bite short pasture leading to malnutrition, poor production and weight loss, particularly on marginal grazing and hill pastures. Traditionally in the UK, culling for reproductive reasons follows six crops of lambs but incisor tooth loss may affect two-crop ewes on some farms; this represents major production and financial losses.

Aetiology

Incisor loss is preceded by repeated bouts of acute gingivitis, which result in fibrosis and recession of the gingival margin with damage to the supporting periodontal ligament (**Fig. 5.11**). While this aetiology implies bacterial involvement, it may not explain the geographic prevalence of broken mouth. The incisor teeth develop an elongated appearance, become loose and are eventually lost. This process may take from 1–4 years (**Figs 5.12, 5.13**).

Clinical presentation

Incisor teeth loss is readily recognized during checks for correct dentition undertaken routinely as part of the selection procedure premating. Broken mouth can lead to chronic weight loss in situations where there is competition for grazing and grass length is short. While incisor loss is readily identified, it is preceded by slackening of the tooth support mechanism with the incisors protruding in front of the dental pad, with

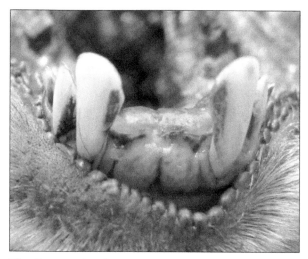

Fig. 5.11 Incisor loss is preceded by recession of the gingival margin with damage to the supporting periodontal ligament.

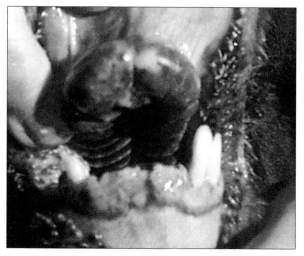

Fig. 5.12 Premature loss of permanent incisor teeth; the remaining teeth are elongated and loose.

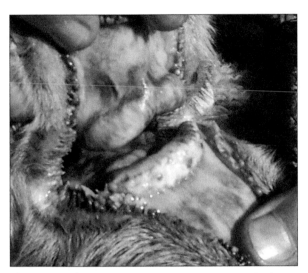

Fig. 5.13 **There are no remaining permanent incisor teeth.**

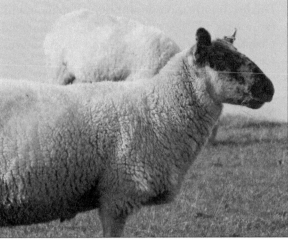

Fig. 5.14 **Undershot jaw or brachygnathia is a common hereditary defect in certain breeds.**

elongation resulting from reduced wear. Loosening of incisor teeth is readily appreciated under gentle digital pressure.

Diagnosis
Diagnosis is based upon the clinical examination.

Treatment
There is no treatment for broken mouth.

Management/prevention/control measures
There are no recognized control measures for broken mouth. Management factors in the UK include drafting broken-mouthed ewes to lowground pastures where these ewes can be as productive as full-mouthed ewes provided there is an appropriate sward height and/or supplementary concentrate feeding. Traditionally, mountain breeds are drafted off the hill onto lowground pastures after four crops of lambs. They then raise another two crops of lambs.

Shortening overgrown incisor teeth of 3–4-year-old ewes using electric grinders is ineffective and raises serious animal welfare issues such that the procedure is banned in most countries.

Economics
Broken mouth can have a serious impact on flock profitability because it necessitates supplementary feeding and premature sale, with a resultant higher replacement rate than normal. Broken-mouthed ewes command much lower prices than similar age ewes with a full mouth. Broken mouth precludes the feeding of root crops.

Welfare implications
There is discomfort and pain associated with gingivitis and periodontal disease in most species but this may be difficult to quantify in sheep. Broken mouth is a cause of emaciation whenever the grass sward has been short for a prolonged period and there has been no supplementary feeding.

Incisor teeth alignment
Examination of incisor teeth alignment is performed by running an index finger along the dental pad with the sheep's mouth closed and the head held in the normal resting position. This examination will reveal any teeth projecting forward of the normal contact on the dental pad (overshot jaw or prognathia; a very common hereditary defect in blueface Leicester) or behind (undershot jaw or brachygnathia [**Figs 5.14, 5.15**]). Sheep with such incisor teeth malalignment with the dental pad should be culled as fat lambs, but it is surprising how many sheep are kept as breeding stock despite such teeth problems.

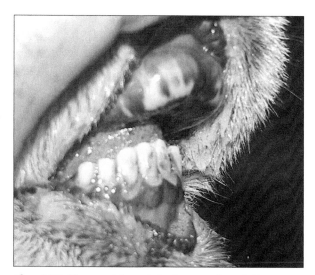

Fig. 5.15 Sheep with such incisor teeth malalignment with the dental pad should not be kept for breeding stock.

Dentigerous (odontogenic) cysts
Definition/overview
Dentigerous cysts occur very sporadically in young adult sheep. Malocclusion leads to weight loss and poor body condition.

Aetiology
The cause of these cysts remains unknown.

Clinical presentation
Affected sheep have a visible swelling of the lower jaw. Sheep aged 2–4 years are typically affected and may present in poor body condition if grazing has been sparse for some months. There is a uniform bony swelling of the mandibular symphysis measuring 5–6 cm in diameter and involving the incisor teeth roots. Some of the incisor teeth may have been lost while the remaining incisor teeth are often aligned horizontally and at unusual angles to each other. The bony swelling is not painful and there is no discharging sinus or submandibular lymph node enlargement to indicate bacterial infection.

Differential diagnoses
- Osteomyelitis of the mandible.
- Actinomycosis.
- Mandibular fracture.
- Cellulitis.
- Tumour.

Diagnosis
Diagnosis is based upon the clinical examination. Radiography reveals loss of normal bone density replaced by a uniform and poorly-mineralized matrix but it is rarely undertaken for cost reasons. The regular appearance of the swelling and absence of bone lysis suggests that these lesions are not the result of tooth root infection.

Treatment
There is no treatment.

Management/prevention/control measures
There are no recognized control measures for this sporadic condition. Affected ewes should be managed in a similar manner to broken-mouthed sheep, with preferential grazing and supplementary feeding.

Welfare implications
Sheep with dentigerous cysts require supplementary feeding when grazing is short.

Cheek teeth problems
Definition/overview
Excessive premolar and molar teeth wear leading to malocclusion and poor mastication of fibrous food is a major cause of weight loss and poor condition in older sheep. Very sharp enamel ridges develop on the labial aspect of the upper cheek teeth and the lingual aspect of the lower cheek teeth, due to lack of wear on these tooth margins. Cheek tooth loss as a consequence to gingivitis is less common than for incisor teeth but does occur, with consequent unimpaired growth of the opposite tooth into this gap leading to a step mouth.

Aetiology
Excessive wear is simply a function of the sheep's age and, possibly, diet. Tooth loss, particularly of the first and second premolar due to their shallow roots, is probably preceded by gingivitis and periodontitis, with loss of support structure similar to that recorded for incisor teeth.

Clinical presentation

Cheek teeth problems tend to be of greater significance than incisor teeth loss due to loss of masticatory function. Cheek teeth problems can best be identified by impaction of food in the cheek(s) and short jerky jaw movements with the mouth held slightly open. Prehension and initial mastication of food proves difficult. Affected sheep often have pieces of fibrous feed protruding from the commisures of the mouth (**Fig. 5.16**) and frequently drop large wads of masticated fibrous food from the mouth. Sheep with severe teeth lesions may raise their head while masticating to assist movement of food over the dorsum of the tongue and into the pharynx.

Careful palpation of the dental arcade through the cheek may reveal the sharp irregular ridges of the labial aspect of the upper cheek teeth, and any lost upper cheek teeth. Examination of the molar teeth with a gag and torch will confirm such findings but is resented by sheep. Poorly-masticated fibrous feed is typically seen impacted in the cheeks with very sharp enamel ridges on the tooth margins (**Figs 5.17–5.20**). Significant gum

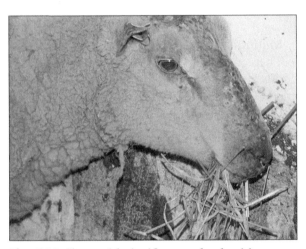

Fig. 5.16 Sheep with significant molar dentition problems often present with fibrous feed protruding from the commisures of the mouth.

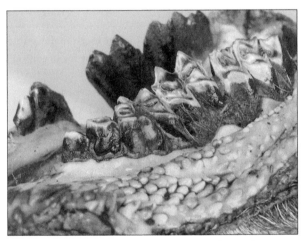

Fig. 5.17 Sharp irregular ridges of the lingual aspect of the lower cheek teeth with diastemata impacted with fibrous material.

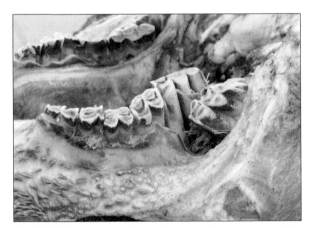

Fig. 5.18 By counting the molar teeth the presence of the temporary and permanent third molar teeth is revealed. Note the much smaller size of the premolar teeth.

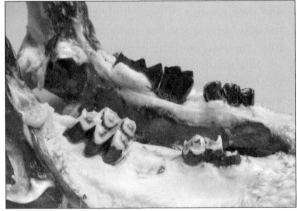

Fig. 5.19 There is loss of permanent molar teeth and considerable gum recession.

lesions are uncommon. Halitosis is not a common feature. Bony swelling of the mandible is rarely caused by tooth root infection (**Figs 5.21, 5.22, 5.23**).

Cheek teeth problems in multigravid ewes may predispose to pregnancy toxaemia due to reduced forage utilization.

Differential diagnoses

The common causes of weight loss and poor body condition have been described elsewhere (see p. 129).

- Food impaction in the cheek(s) is readily differentiated from soft tissue swellings of the face such as abscess caused by actinobacillosis, and diphtheresis.

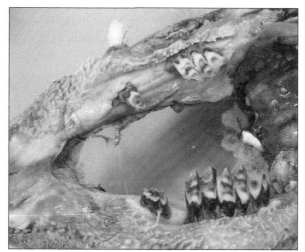

Fig. 5.20 Lost premolar and molar teeth with sharp irregular ridges on the lingual aspect of the mandibular cheek teeth, with diastemata impacted with fibrous material.

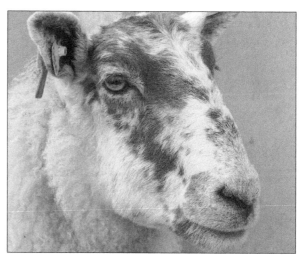

Fig. 5.21 Uniform bony swelling of one horizontal ramus of the mandible is not uncommon but is rarely caused by a tooth root abscess.

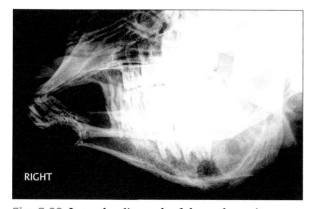

Fig. 5.22 Lateral radiograph of sheep shown in Fig. 5.21. The uniform bony swelling is not associated with tooth root infection.

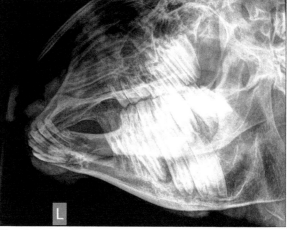

Fig. 5.23 Oblique radiograph of the skull shows little bony change despite palpable thickening of the horizontal ramus of the mandible.

- Swelling of the horizontal ramus of the mandible could be caused by osteomyelitis or tumour such as fibrosarcoma or osteosarcoma (**Figs 5.24, 5.25**); both conditions are uncommon in sheep.

Diagnosis

Diagnosis is based upon the clinical findings during examination of the mouth with a gag and torch. Radiographs are rarely needed but confirm the diagnosis (**Figs 5.26–5.29**).

Treatment

There is no treatment and affected sheep should be culled, although their body condition can be improved by generous concentrate feeding (up to 1–1.5 kg daily) over an 8–12 week period, which should command a better slaughter price.

Management/prevention/control measures

Excessive wear and molar tooth loss are largely the consequences of the sheep's age. There are no prevention measures. Problems of weight loss caused

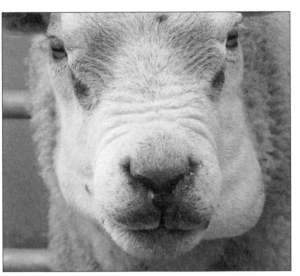

Fig. 5.24 Large uniform swelling of the left maxillary region; there is no discharging sinus (see Fig. 5.25).

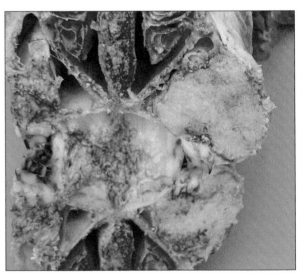

Fig. 5.25 Sagittal section through the maxillary mass shown in Fig. 5.24 reveals a fibrosarcoma.

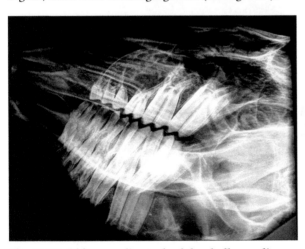

Fig. 5.26 Oblique radiograph of the skull revealing normal cheek teeth.

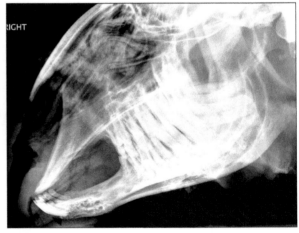

Fig. 5.27 Attempted oblique radiograph of the maxillary teeth reveals the persistence of the temporary third molar (see Fig. 5.28).

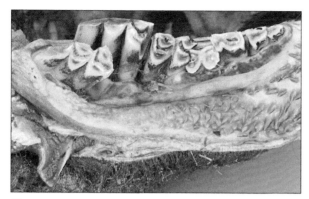

Fig. 5.28 Persistence and abnormal angulation of the temporary third molar revealed at necropsy.

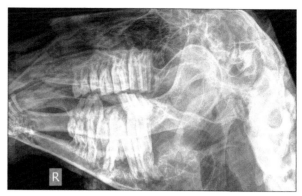

Fig. 5.29 Oblique radiograph of the skull reveals loss of the first and second molar teeth from the right mandible and abnormal angulation of the third molar tooth. There is a marked step between the premolar and molar teeth. There is considerable bone resorption surrounding the roots of the mandibular teeth.

by poor mastication of fibrous feeds (**Fig. 5.30**) can be largely offset by appropriate concentrate feeding, although care must be taken to avoid problems with acidosis when concentrates are first introduced into the ration.

Economics
Cheek teeth problems occur from 5–6 years of age in most flocks, as ewes come to the end of their productive lives. Restoration of body condition can be achieved by supplementary concentrate feeding over 2–3 months to allow sale as mutton.

Welfare implications
Sheep with cheek teeth problems managed on a forage-based ration lose weight and present in poor condition and, possibly, emaciation. Emaciated ewes should be euthanased; those ewes in poor condition should be fed concentrates and sold for slaughter when body condition has been restored.

OSTEOARTHRITIS OF THE TEMPORO-MANDIBULAR (JAW) JOINT

Definition/overview
The nature and incidence of osteoarthritis (OA) of the temporo-mandibular joint (TMJ) have recently been reported in Soay sheep but have not been studied in other breeds.

Aetiology
Sheep spend up to 10 hours per day ruminating, placing considerable wear and tear on the TMJ. Osteoarthritis is a degenerative disease of joints characterized by the destruction of articular cartilage and osteophyte formation causing pain.

Clinical presentation
Examination of skulls collected since 1984 from the Soay sheep flock on St Kilda in the Outer Hebrides revealed unilateral OA of the TMJ in 15 adult sheep (10 right side; five left side) and involving both TMJs in 19 sheep, with overall prevalence at 2.3% for females and 0.2% in males. There was a striking age-dependence in TMJ OA incidence among age classes: 30 of the 35 cases occurred in geriatric sheep (aged 7 years or more, 11% prevalence within age class), four in adults (2–6 years old, 1% prevalence), one in yearlings (0.3% prevalence) and none in lambs.

In sheep with unilateral OA, erosion of cartilage from the articular surfaces causes a significant increase in width of the articular space (**Fig. 5.31**) compared with the normal contralateral joint (**Fig. 5.32**). Erosion and remodelling of subchondral bone and osteophytosis is more severe affecting the articular condyle of the mandible (**Fig. 5.33**) than the zygomatic process of the temporal bone (**Fig. 5.34**).

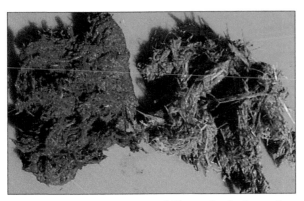

Fig. 5.30 Poor mastication of fibrous feeds shown by examining the rumen contents of an affected sheep (right) and a normal sheep (left).

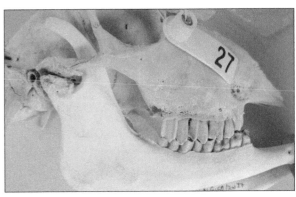

Fig. 5.31 Examination of a sheep's skull reveals a significant increase in width of the temporo-mandibular joint (TMJ) caused by erosion of cartilage from the articular surfaces (see Fig. 5.32).

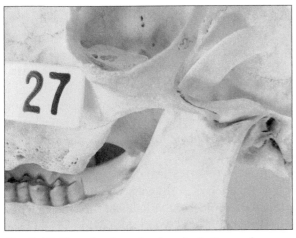

Fig. 5.32 Examination of a sheep's skull reveals a normal TMJ.

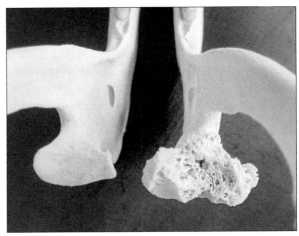

Fig. 5.33 Examination of a sheep's skull reveals erosion and remodelling of subchondral bone and osteophytosis of the articular condyle of the mandible.

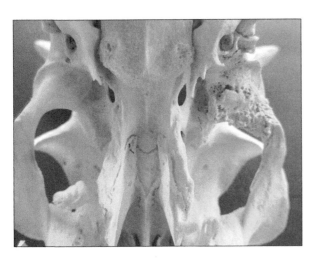

Fig. 5.34 Examination of a sheep's skull reveals erosion of articular cartilage and osteophytosis affecting the zygomatic process of the temporal bone.

These results have stimulated investigations into the prevalence of TMJ pathology in cull sheep on commercial farms in Scotland, especially in those sheep breeds with jaw malalignment, a surprisingly common hereditary condition.

Diagnosis

Diagnosis is based upon radiographic examination of the TMJ, but this is rarely undertaken in practice. A slaughterhouse survey of cull sheep is required to assess the incidence of this disease in sheep breeds other than the Soay and its significance in weight loss.

Treatment

There is no treatment and affected sheep should be culled.

Management/prevention/control measures

The potential link between brachy- and prognathia with an increased incidence of OA of the TMJ requires further investigation; however, sheep with such jaw abnormalities should not be kept for breeding replacements.

Welfare implications

OA will cause chronic pain and affected sheep should be culled.

BUCCAL CAVITY

Fusobacterium necrophorum infection of the buccal cavity
Definition/overview

Fusobacterium necrophorum causes a necrotic stomatitis in growing lambs. It may be seen as an outbreak in orphan lambs reared on milk replacer and kept in unhygienic conditions with dirty feeding equipment. Lesions may also follow trauma to the buccal cavity caused by dosing gun injuries.

Aetiology

F. necrophorum infects cuts in the buccal cavity.

Clinical presentation

Affected lambs present in poor condition due to impaired feeding. The lower jaw is wet caused by drooling of saliva. Lesions affecting the cheek result in obvious firm swellings. There is halitosis and swelling of the submandibular lymph node(s). The rectal temperature may be elevated.

Inhalation of infection is not uncommon, resulting in the formation of numerous large abscesses filled with viscous green pus which may extend to the pleural surface causing an associated pleuritis. Rupture of one of these abscesses may cause death but more commonly results in pyothorax. These lambs fail to respond to antibiotic therapy and remain in poor condition with a poor appetite.

Differential diagnoses
- Cheek lesions may result from actinobacillosis.
- Orf virus infection rarely extends from the lips and gingiva of the incisor teeth to involve the tongue.

Diagnosis

Diagnosis is based upon the clinical examination.

Treatment

Procaine penicillin by intramuscular injection for at least 7 consecutive days.

Management/prevention/control measures

The disease is prevented by high standards of hygiene when rearing orphan lambs, and taking care when drenching young lambs.

Economics

The disease occurs sporadically and is not a major cause of mortality.

Welfare implications

The oral lesions cause obvious pain and must be treated appropriately. Lambs that fail to thrive after antibiotic therapy should be euthanased for welfare reasons.

Actinobacillosis
Definition/overview

Actinobacillosis is an uncommon cause of multiple abscesses affecting the subcutaneous areas of the cheeks. The abscesses fistulate to the skin surface discharging viscous yellow/green pus.

Enlargement of the drainage retropharyngeal lymph nodes may compress the larynx causing stertor.

Aetiology

Actinobacillosis is caused by the gram-negative rod *Actinobacillus lignieresi*. A number of sheep with abscesses affecting the face may be encountered in sheep grazing pastures containing gorse or similar spiky plants.

Clinical presentation

There are numerous 1–3 cm diameter abscesses in the subcutis of the cheeks (**Fig. 5.35**), which discharge viscous yellow/green pus. Unlike caseous lymphadenitis, the lesions are in the skin rather than parotid or submandibular lymph nodes. It may prove difficult to palpate enlargement of the drainage retropharyngeal lymph nodes, which may compress the larynx and cause stertor.

Differential diagnoses

From an economic standpoint, the important differential diagnosis of actinobacillosis is caseous lymphadenitis. Stertor could result from laryngeal chondritis.

Diagnosis

Diagnosis is based upon clinical findings, and confirmed following culture.

Treatment

When confined to the subcutaneous tissue of the face, the abscesses cause few problems. Antibiotic therapy is not necessary, nor would antibiotics penetrate the fibrous capsule of these abscesses. Lancing such abscesses is not necessary as they will eventually discharge themselves, and is contraindicated in countries with endemic caseous lymphadenitis, in case the skin lesions are CLA as this might lead to contamination of the environment.

Sheep with stertor caused by compression of the larynx associated with enlargement of the drainage retropharyngeal lymph nodes should be treated with a soluble corticosteroid to reduce associated swelling and procaine penicillin daily for at least 10 consecutive days.

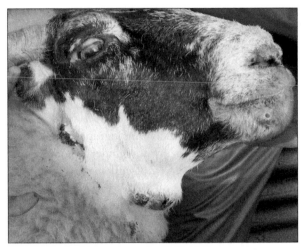

Fig. 5.35 Numerous raised 1–3 cm diameter abscesses in the subcutis of the cheeks; note the loss of overlying hair.

Management/prevention/control measures

The condition occurs sporadically often associated with grazing pastures with spiky plants. There are no specific control measures.

Economics

Actinobacillosis presents no real economic concerns.

Welfare implications

There are no real welfare concerns unless the swellings prevent prehension and mastication.

Actinomycosis

Definition/overview

Unlike cattle, actinomycosis is a rare disease of sheep.

Aetiology

Actinomycosis is caused by *Actinomyces bovis*.

Clinical presentation

There is marked enlargement of the horizontal ramus of the mandible. One or more sinuses may discharge from the bony swelling. There is enlargement of the ipsilateral submandibular lymph node. Associated pain and physical deformity result in reduced feeding and mastication, with consequent loss of body condition. The swelling is irregular and comprises fibrous tissue with considerable bone remodelling.

Differential diagnoses
- Fracture of the horizontal ramus of the mandible.
- Osteosarcoma.
- Fibrosarcoma.
- Severe orf infection.
- Tooth root abscess.

Diagnosis
The diagnosis is based upon clinical findings. Radiography reveals the extent of bone lysis and remodelling.

Treatment
The prognosis even after daily antibiotic injections with penicillin or trimethoprim/sulpha for 4–6 weeks is poor. Treatment is usually cost prohibitive unless the sheep is especially valuable but the animal's welfare must be carefully considered.

Management/prevention/control measures
The condition occurs rarely and there are no specific control measures.

Economics
Actinomycosis presents no real economic concerns.

Welfare implications
Sheep with advanced lesions should be culled for welfare reasons.

Pharyngeal abscess
Definition/overview
Pharyngeal abscesses in growing lambs, and occasionally adult sheep, result most commonly from trauma caused by incorrect drenching technique (e.g. due to inappropriate equipment or unskilled administration).

Aetiology
Penetration of the pharyngeal wall by the tip of the drenching gun frequently introduces the contents of the drenching gun (e.g. anthelmintic suspension or trace element capsule/bolus) into fascial planes. Secondary bacterial infection of the penetration site leads to cellulitis, with infection tracking to the cervical spinal canal in some cases.

Clinical presentation
There is rapid loss of body condition in growing lambs. Affected lambs appear dull and depressed and do not suck. There is continuous salivation with staining of the lower jaw. The lambs appear gaunt after 3–4 days' illness, with little abdominal fill. Closer examination of the mouth reveals halitosis and pain on palpation of the pharyngeal region. There may be oedema of the ventral neck, associated with the cellulitis lesion. It is not always possible to distinguish the retropharyngeal lymph nodes even when they are grossly enlarged. Pressure from the abscess/retropharyngeal lymph nodes onto the larynx may cause stertor.

Tetraparesis may result from compression of the cervical spinal cord following extension of the cellulitis lesion into the vertebral canal. There are many reports that describe the typical history of sudden onset tetraparesis in a number of growing lambs 5–10 days after drenching, which rapidly progresses to paralysis and lateral recumbency over 2–4 days.

Differential diagnoses
- Cellulitis:
  - Puncture wound such as dog bite.
  - Infection of vaccination site due to poor hygiene standards.
  - Oral lesions caused by *F. necrophorum*.
  - Laryngeal chondritis.
  - Caseous lymphadenitis rarely affects growing lambs.
- Weakness:
  - Vertebral empyema is a common condition of growing lambs.
  - Sarcocystosis can present with weakness affecting the pelvic limbs.
  - White muscle disease.
  - Delayed swayback.

Diagnosis

Diagnosis is not simple, especially when the infection has tracked along fascial planes and may erupt distant to the entry site in the pharynx. Recent history of drenching 10–14 days previously with numerous lambs affected provides strong circumstantial evidence of pharyngeal trauma.

Treatment

The response of cellulitis lesions to 10–14 consecutive days' penicillin treatment is poor and severely affected lambs should be euthanased for welfare reasons. Recumbent lambs must be euthanased for welfare reasons.

Management/prevention/control measures

All drenching equipment must be carefully maintained. Shepherds must work patiently amongst small groups of lambs in a confined area, with appropriate restraint to prevent lambs jumping forward when the drench nozzle is introduced into the mouth.

Economics

Pharyngeal abscesses are an avoidable problem indicating poor husbandry practice. Lamb losses totalling 2–5% have been reported on occasion from injuries caused by incorrect drenching technique.

Welfare implications

Affected sheep suffer from these painful lesions and should be euthanased for welfare reasons.

ABDOMEN

Acidosis

(syn. grain overload)

Definition/overview

Acidosis results from the sudden unaccustomed ingestion of large quantities of carbohydrate-rich feeds (**Fig. 5.36**), typically grain or concentrates, less commonly potatoes and by-products such as bread and bakery waste.

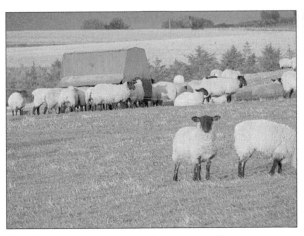

Fig. 5.36 **Acidosis results from the sudden unaccustomed ingestion of large quantities of carbohydrate-rich feeds, often associated with hopper feeding.**

Aetiology

Acidosis often results when weaned lambs are turned onto grain stubbles with quantities of spilled grain; sheep are particularly susceptible to acidosis caused by wheat and barley. Too rapid introduction onto a diet of *ad libitum* concentrates may result in acidosis. While the ration may be calculated to supply only 100 g per head per day, if the majority of weaned lambs are slow to start eating the ration, some lambs may eat in excess of 500 g.

The smaller the particle size, for example following milling, the more quickly fermentation occurs, and the more severe the clinical signs for given amount ingested by the sheep. Hill breeds, such as the Scottish Blackface, are more susceptible to acidosis than other breeds.

Pathophysiology

The sudden and unaccustomed ingestion of large quantities of carbohydrate-rich feeds results in a fall in rumen pH which kills many resident bacteria and protozoa. *Lactobacillus* spp. multiply rapidly with the production of large amounts of lactic acid, which further reduces rumen pH. There is a marked increased in rumen liquor osmolality, with fluid being drawn in from the extracellular space causing dehydration. Lactate is absorbed into the circulation leading to the development of metabolic acidosis. This metabolic crisis is further compounded by toxin absorption through the compromised rumen mucosa.

Chronic sequelae of rumen acidosis include fungal rumenitis and, occasionally, liver abscessation but the latter is less common in sheep than in cattle.

Clinical presentation

The severity of clinical signs depends upon the amount of grain ingested, whether the grain was rolled or whole, the rate of introduction of the dietary change and breed of sheep. Weaned Scottish Blackface lambs have been found *in extremis* or dead within 24 hours of sudden introduction of barley feeding. It is reported that colic signs may be observed soon after grain engorgement, and that the sheep appear restless. More usually, affected lambs are very dull and depressed and are reluctant to move. When walking, affected sheep appear ataxic; they may fall and experience difficulty rising due to weakness. They are anorexic and stand with the head held lowered. Bruxism (tooth grinding) is frequently heard. The lambs have a distended abdomen due to an enlarged static rumen. Auscultation reveals no rumen motility, and succussion reveals tinkling sounds due to the accumulation of fluid and gas within the rumen. Initially, the rectal temperature may be increased but falls to subnormal values as the condition progresses. The mucous membranes are congested and there may be enophthalmos and an increased skin tent-up duration due to moderate dehydration. There may be no diarrhoea for the first 12–24 hours after carbohydrate ingestion; thereafter, there is profuse, very fluid, foetid diarrhoea, which may contain whole grains. The most severely affected sheep become recumbent and have an increased respiratory rate from the developing metabolic acidosis. The heart rate is increased and the degree of dehydration worsens. Death may follow within 24–48 hours despite treatment. Sheep that recover have a protracted convalescence.

Differential diagnoses

- Differential diagnoses for profound toxaemia include systemic pasteurellosis, clostridial disease, especially pulpy kidney and black disease, and abdominal catastrophes such as torsion of the small intestine or caecum.
- Redgut should also be considered but is less commonly associated with grain feeding. Polioencephalomalacia may cause initial depression and isolation.
- Subacute fasciolosis can present with recumbency, weakness, anterior abdominal pain and abdominal distension associated with peritonitis and an inflammatory exudate.

Diagnosis

Diagnosis is based upon the history and clinical findings, particularly once foetid diarrhoea is evident. Rumen fluid samples can be collected by percutaneous ruminocentesis or, preferably, by orogastric tube. The rumen pH falls below 5.5. There are no live protozoa observed under microscopic examination of rumen liquor, only large numbers of gram-positive rods.

At necropsy the rumen contents are milky-grey, porridge-like and have a rancid odour. The rumen epithelium strips off readily but care is necessary to differentiate this phenomenon from normal autolytic change.

Treatment

Intravenous fluid therapy is usually cost prohibitive, and large numbers of sheep are often affected. Recumbent sheep could be 7–10% dehydrated and would require isotonic saline over 4 hours or so (3 litres for a 30–40 kg fattening lamb; 5 litres for a mature ewe or ram).

Intravenous fluids should contain bicarbonate but there are few data for treating acidosis in sheep under field situations. In emergency situations, it would be safe to administer 10 mmol/l of bicarbonate over 2–3 hours and monitor progress. In practical situations, 16 g of sodium bicarbonate = 200 mmol of bicarbonate. Therefore, an 80 kg pedigree Suffolk sheep estimated to be 7% dehydrated would require:

$$\text{Estimated base deficit} \times \text{dehydrated body weight} \times \text{extracellular fluid volume}$$

$$(\text{i.e. } 10 \times 74 \times 0.3) = 222 \text{ mmol of bicarbonate.}$$

Thus 16 g of sodium bicarbonate would approximate a 10 mmol/l base deficit of a mature Suffolk sheep (8 g for a 40 kg fattening lamb).

Severe metabolic acidosis may cause a base deficit up to 20 mmol/l, thereby necessitating further intravenous bicarbonate. The response to intravenous fluid therapy should be carefully monitored.

A rumenotomy to remove the rumen contents can be attempted but considerable care is needed to prevent leakage into the abdominal cavity during surgery, because it is not possible to exteriorize much of the rumen wall due to the large fluid contents. Unlike cattle, attempts to siphon off rumen contents are not as successful in sheep.

In most practical situations, therapy is restricted to oral fluids, intravenous multivitamin preparations and antibiotic therapy to counter bacteraemia across the compromised gut wall. Diluted oral rehydration solutions can be given by orogastric tube, which is easily achieved in sheep. Sodium bicarbonate can be added to the rehydration solution but this may result in bloat. Some authors have recommended drenching with 15 ml of milk of magnesia every few hours to counter acidosis. Some clinicians elect to inject thiamine (vitamin B1) intravenously rather than a multivitamin injection. Penicillin injections are given daily for up to 10 days to counter potential bacteraemia.

The concentrate feed must be reduced or removed from the remainder of the group although many farmers reason that as most of the sheep have already adapted to the diet, new cases may occur after reintroduction of the grain ration. Good quality hay should be provided to stimulate rumen function.

Management/prevention/control measures

Grain/concentrate feeding must be gradually introduced over a minimum of 2 weeks. If not all sheep are coming to the feed troughs the total allocated amount must be reduced accordingly. The grain can be diluted using sugar beet shreds or similar feed during this acclimatization period. As a rule of thumb, the grain ration can be increased by 50 g per head every 2–3 days provided all sheep are eating well and that all concentrate feed is eaten within 5 minutes. Good quality roughage must be available at all times. If roughage is restricted, it must be available to all sheep at the same time and not restricted to a small bunk/rack.

Economics

Mortality can be high if sheep are suddenly introduced to rations containing high levels of carbohydrates, especially rolled grain. Convalescence is protracted in those sheep which develop diarrhoea because of disturbances to the rumen microflora.

Welfare implications

Acidosis is a common problem when concentrates are introduced too quickly. Affected sheep are in obvious pain. Those sheep that survive have a protracted convalescence. Comatose sheep, and those unable to stand within 2–3 days of treatment, should be euthanased for welfare reasons.

Bloat
Definition/overview

Bloat is the sudden accumulation of free gas within the rumen causing abdominal distension. If untreated, pressure on the diaphragm causes respiratory embarrassment, reduced venous return and, eventually, death. Unlike cattle, bloat in sheep is very uncommon unless secondary to an oesophageal obstruction.

Aetiology

The sudden intake of readily fermented material such as grain can cause bloat. Oesophageal obstruction (choke) occurs sporadically when sheep are fed root crops. Ingestion of legumes may result in the formation of a stable froth in the rumen preventing presentation of free gas at the cardia for eructation, with consequent bloat.

Clinical presentation

Affected sheep with abdominal distension may simply be found dead following a sudden change in the ration. Other sheep present with predominantly high left-sided abdominal distension; some sheep may become dyspnoeic with mouth breathing.

Differential diagnoses

- Hypocalcaemia results in recumbency followed by bloat.
- Abdominal catastrophes, such as volvulus and redgut, present with abdominal distension.
- Chronic causes of abdominal distension may include peritonitis, ascites, and uroperitoneum associated with urolithiasis.

Diagnosis

Diagnosis is based upon clinical findings and confirmed by release of gas by orogastric tube or rumen trocharization.

Treatment

Free gas should be released with an orogastric tube. The administration of dimeticone may assist relief of frothy bloat. Trocharization can be undertaken as an emergency procedure but may not be successful in cases of frothy bloat.

Management/prevention/control measures

Gradual introduction onto legume or root crops and subsequent restricted grazing should reduce the likelihood of frothy bloat. Choke occurs sporadically.

Economics

Bloat is a significant economic consideration only under specific grazing conditions.

Welfare implications

There are no major welfare concerns provided sheep are treated quickly. Attempted relief of bloat using water piping by farmers has caused oesophageal rupture.

Redgut
Definition/overview

A very sporadic condition associated with torsion of the intestine/caecum of weaned lambs and adult sheep. It causes sudden death due to endotoxaemia/circulatory failure.

Aetiology

Redgut has typically been encountered in sheep grazing legumes or similar crops. This diet results in rapid transit times, reduced rumen volume and secondary fermentation in the lower gut and caecum. The altered proportions of the major abdominal viscera and increased production of gas in the lower gut lead to instability and torsion around the root of the mesentery. This causes sudden death.

Clinical presentation

Affected sheep are usually found without premonitory signs. Those that are found alive are very depressed, recumbent, have abdominal distension with dehydration and toxic mucous membranes.

Differential diagnoses

- Clostridial disease, typically pulpy kidney, black disease or struck.
- Bloat.
- Acute/subacute fasciolosis.
- Acute copper toxicity.

Diagnosis

The diagnosis is confirmed at necropsy.

Treatment

There is no treatment; those sheep found alive should be destroyed for welfare reasons.

Management/prevention/control measures

Sheep should be introduced gradually onto lush pastures or legume crops. Restricted grazing and provision of good quality fibre should reduce the likelihood of redgut.

Economics

Redgut is a significant economic consideration only under specific grazing conditions.

Welfare implications

Sheep with intestinal torsion are usually found dead, but those sheep found alive must be euthanased for welfare reasons.

Abomasal bloat
Definition/overview

Abomasal bloat occurs commonly in orphan lambs fed restricted amounts of milk replacer at variable temperatures with irregular intervals during the first 4 weeks of life.

Aetiology

Abomasal bloat is caused by the sudden fermentation of large amounts of carbohydrate with gas production that cannot escape from the abomasum.

Clinical presentation

Signs of abdominal distension and colic appear within 1 hour of feeding. Affected lambs alternate between a wide-base stance and lateral recumbency. There is frequent vocalization, tail swishing and kicking at the abdomen. Lambs have a painful expression and a wet lower jaw due to drooling saliva. In some cases, abomasal bloat may lead to volvulus.

Differential diagnoses

Differential diagnoses include lamb dysentery, abomasal foreign body such as a wool ball blocking the pylorus and abomasal volvulus.

Diagnosis

Diagnosis is based upon clinical findings and history of irregular milk feeding.

Treatment

Attempts to relieve bloat by orogastric tube are rarely successful and offer only temporary remission. Percutaneous needle decompression offers little better success because the needle often becomes blocked with milk clot and/or the abomasal wall moves and the needle comes out of the abomasum. If the lamb survives the initial bloat, leakage of abomasal contents through the needle puncture site(s) in the abomasal wall leads to localized peritonitis. Metaclopramide is unlikely to have any significant affect in advanced cases.

Management/prevention/control measures

Excellent results for rearing orphan lambs can be achieved using automated systems which regulate the amounts and frequency of milk replacer. The early introduction of high-quality concentrates will promote rumen function and lessen the risk of abomasal bloat/torsion.

Welfare implications

Many diseases can affect orphan lambs unless they are well-managed; abomasal bloat/torsion is a common cause of loss. Farmers should invest in automated feeding systems or sell excess lambs at a few days old.

Abomasal emptying defect
Definition/overview

An uncommon, yet probably underdiagnosed, disorder reported most frequently in pedigree Suffolk sheep. It also occurs in other breeds and crossbreeds.

Aetiology

The cause remains unknown but its recognition primarily in Suffolk sheep may suggest a hereditary component.

Clinical presentation

Signs develop over some months with gradual weight loss to the extent of emaciation. There is increasing abdominal distension, especially on the lower right side when the sheep is viewed from behind. Affected sheep have a poor appetite and pass firm pelleted faeces frequently coated with thick mucus. They are afebrile and appear somewhat dull and apathetic. There may be moderate dehydration. Rumen sounds are frequently increased.

Differential diagnoses

- Scrapie sheep present in poor condition/emaciation; some animals present with marked abomasal impaction.
- Abomasal impaction should be distinguished from peritonitis and adenocarcinoma, which may result in accumulations of excess peritoneal fluid.
- Poor cheek teeth with inadequate mastication of fibrous foods may result in rumen distension.
- Vagal indigestion, resulting in rumen distension with a characteristic 'papple' abdominal silhouette, is very uncommon in sheep.

Diagnosis

Determination of rumen chloride concentration gives an indication of reflux of chloride-rich secretions from the abomasum into the rumen. Values in excess of 30 mmol/l are suggestive of this condition (normal values = <15 mmol/l). The diagnosis is confirmed at necropsy with massive abomasal distension (**Fig. 5.37**).

Treatment
There is no recognized treatment and affected sheep should be euthanased when all other treatable alternative conditions have been excluded.

Management/prevention/control measures
There are presently no control measures. While it would be prudent to cull progeny from sheep which developed this condition, this is unlikely to happen because of financial losses in a pedigree flock selling breeding stock.

Economics
The true incidence of this condition has not been determined and its diagnosis is likely to be overlooked in commercial flocks that purchase individual rams.

Welfare implications
There is no recognized treatment and affected sheep should be euthanased when all other treatable alternative conditions have been excluded.

Intestinal adenocarcinoma
Definition/overview
Intestinal adenocarcinoma is a sporadic tumour of the small intestine causing weight loss, ascites and emaciation in adult sheep (**Fig. 5.38**).

Aetiology
There may be an association between the occurrence of intestinal adenocarcinoma and grazing bracken-infested pasture, but such tumours also occur in areas where there is no bracken.

Clinical presentation
The affected adult sheep presents in much poorer condition than other sheep in the group. In sheep with intestinal adenocarcinoma, ascites results from transcoelomic spread and blockage of lymphatic drainage (**Figs 5.39, 5.40**). While ascites is present in most cases, it may prove difficult to assess the extent of the transudate on clinical examination alone. Ultrasound examination provides a quick and reliable assessment of the amount of peritoneal fluid (**Fig. 5.40**).

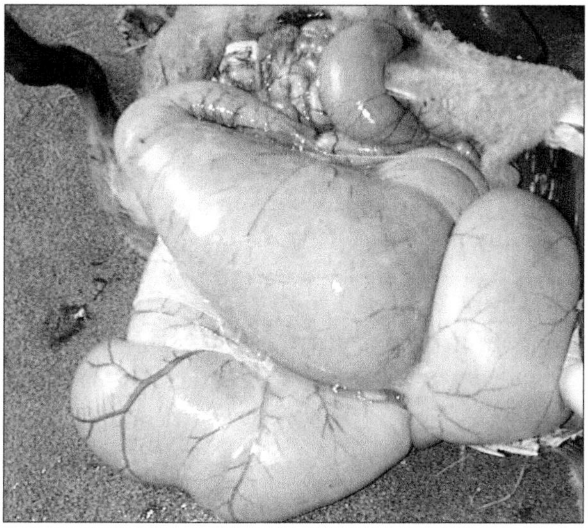

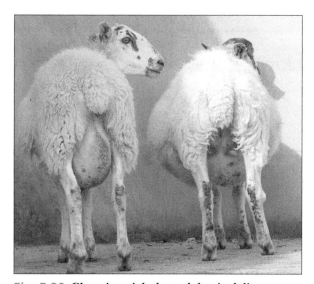

Fig. 5.37 Necropsy reveals a massively distended abomasum in a sheep with abomasal emptying defect.

Fig. 5.38 Chronic weight loss, abdominal distension caused by ascites and emaciation in an adult ewe, resulting from an intestinal adenocarcinoma.

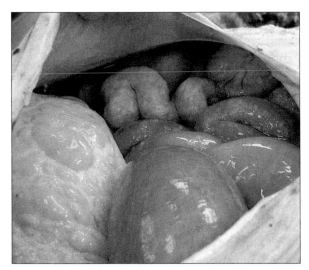

Fig. 5.39 Ascites caused by transcoelomic spread of an intestinal adenocarcinoma.

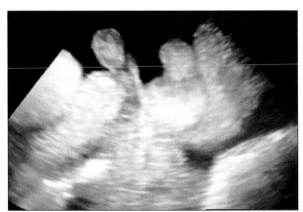

Fig. 5.40 Ultrasound examination of the ventral abdomen (5 MHz sector scanner) reveals fluid accumulation (ascites) caused by transcoelomic spread of an intestinal adenocarcinoma with dorsal displacement of small intestine.

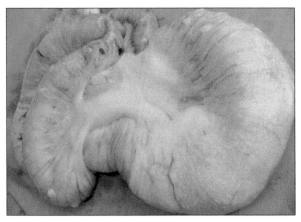

Fig. 5.41 An intestinal adenocarcinoma with localized spread to adjacent serosal surfaces revealed at necropsy.

Differential diagnoses
- Other conditions that cause weight loss in adult sheep.
- Subacute fasciolosis may cause accumulations of peritoneal exudate.
- Ascites is relatively uncommon in sheep despite the common occurrence of protein-losing conditions such as chronic fasciolosis and paratuberculosis, which can result in serum albumin concentrations below 15 g/l, and occasionally less than 8 g/l.

Diagnosis
Abdominocentesis, cytospin preparation and staining may yield exfoliated tumour cells but most cases are diagnosed at necropsy (**Fig. 5.41**) with confirmatory histopathological examination.

Treatment
There is no recognized treatment and affected sheep should be euthanased when all other treatable alternative conditions have been excluded.

Management/prevention/control measures
There are no recognized control measures.

Economics
Weight loss and poor condition occur in all sheep flocks but few cases are examined in detail. Intestinal adenocarcinoma occurs very sporadically in flocks and is unlikely to exceed 0.2 cases per annum.

Welfare implications
Sheep in poor condition despite adequate nutrition should be promptly culled for welfare reasons.

Peritonitis
Definition/overview
Infection of the peritoneal lining of the abdominal cavity may result in focal peritonitis with spread of infection limited by the omentum, or extend to septic peritonitis.

Aetiology

Uterine tears following attempted correction of dystocia are the most common cause of diffuse septic peritonitis in the UK.

Clinical presentation

The clinical signs depend upon the spread of infection within the peritoneal cavity. Focal infections with localized adhesion formation may prove difficult to diagnose with non-specific signs of poor appetite, weight loss and abdominal distension, caused by reduced gut transport (**Fig. 5.42**). Infection is often confined by the omentum and there is scant peritoneal fluid (**Fig. 5.43**). Affected sheep are rarely febrile.

Sheep with diffuse septic peritonitis are dull, depressed and anorexic. Initially, there may be abdominal distension due to gut stasis, but inappetance quickly results in a gaunt, drawn-up appearance. Affected sheep may stand with an arched back but this is much less a feature than in cattle with traumatic reticulo-peritonitis. The rectal temperature is rarely elevated but the mucous membranes are congested. There is variable dehydration. The respiratory and heart rates are elevated; there are no rumen contractions. Scant mucus-coated faeces are passed. Affected sheep often stand with their head held over the water trough but drink little. Death follows within 3–7 days.

Occasionally, adhesions may form between the rumen and abdominal incision site following caesarean operations but there are few sequelae.

Differential diagnoses

- Septic peritonitis frequently follows dystocia/ uterine tears; therefore, the most common differential diagnosis is metritis.
- Retained foetus could present with similar signs to peritonitis.
- Hypocalcaemia presents as a dull, recumbent sheep with bloat which could be confused with peritonitis at initial presentation.
- Subacute fasciolosis may result in large accumulations of inflammatory exudates within the abdominal cavity.

Diagnosis

Diagnosis of peritonitis is not simple because the infection has often been confined by the omentum and therefore cannot be identified by either abdominocentesis or ultrasonography (**Fig. 5.43**). In chronic cases of peritonitis, fibrous adhesions are the most prominent feature, with scant peritoneal fluid which cannot always be visualized by ultrasonography.

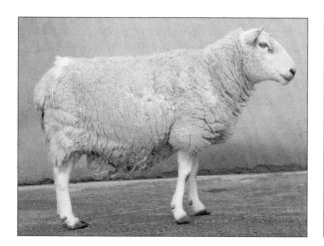

Fig. 5.42 Sheep with chronic (focal) peritonitis present with non-specific signs of poor-appetite weight loss, and abdominal distension caused by reduced gut transport.

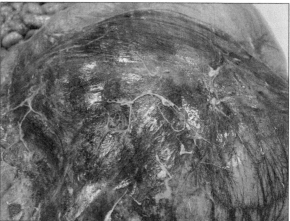

Fig. 5.43 Peritoneal infection is often confined by the omentum and there is scant exudate accumulation.

Careful ultrasonographic examination may reveal fluid accumulations within static intestines caused by the localized adhesions.

Treatment

Antibiotic therapy is hopeless and is only undertaken in case the diagnosis is incorrect and the sheep is suffering from metritis or another infectious disease.

Management/prevention/control measures

With the exception of a correct approach to dystocia management, there are no specific preventive measures. Client education with respect to careful correction of dystocia is indicated in some situations.

Economics

Peritonitis occurs uncommonly in sheep and is not a major economic concern.

Intestinal atresia

Definition/overview

Atresia ani is relatively common in lambs occurring around one case per 500 lambs. Atresia coli is diagnosed much less commonly.

Aetiology

Atresia ani occurs sporadically in newborn lambs; there is no recognized hereditary component.

Clinical presentation

Lambs with atresia ani are perfectly healthy for the first 24–36 hours after birth. Thereafter, there is increasing abdominal distension, reluctance to suck, salivation, depression and long periods spent in sternal recumbency. Examination usually reveals a bulge beneath the skin where the anus should be (**Fig. 5.44**). The clinical presentation is largely similar for atresia coli but the diagnosis is much more difficult because there is no swelling under the tail.

Differential diagnoses

Casual inspection by the shepherd often results in treatment for watery mouth disease, although the rate of deterioration in the lamb's condition is slower for atresia ani.

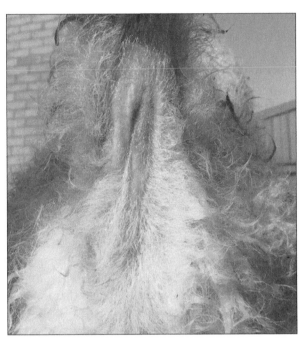

Fig. 5.44 Atresia ani – there is a bulge beneath the skin where the anus should be.

Diagnosis

Atresia ani is readily recognized upon lifting the lamb's tail, which reveals skin covering the site of the anus. Diagnosis of atresia coli is much more problematic and is based upon the clinical findings listed above plus lack of faeces produced since birth, although such detailed history may not be available.

Treatment

Correction of atresia ani is most easily achieved by an X-shaped incision in the skin bulge using a scalpel blade. This is a painful procedure and must only be undertaken after sacrococcygeal lignocaine injection (0.2 ml), which is a simple technique using a 21 gauge 12 mm needle. On incision, up to 100 ml of mucus containing meconium is passed under variable pressure (**Fig. 5.45**). The stab incision in the skin may heal over; therefore, the farmer should be advised to make sure the incision site remains patent by carefully inserting a thermometer coated with liquid paraffin into the rectum twice daily for 3–4 days. The recovery rate is good.

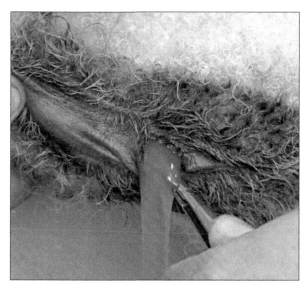

Fig. 5.45 An X-shaped incision is made in the skin bulge using a scalpel blade after sacrococcygeal lignocaine injection to correct atresia ani.

There is no cost-effective surgical correction of atresia coli for commercial value lambs and these lambs should be euthanased for welfare reasons.

Management/prevention/control measures

There is no recognized hereditary component to atresia ani, but it would be prudent not to keep these lambs for future breeding replacements.

Cryptosporidiosis

Definition/overview

Cryptosporidium parvum is a coccidian parasite that has been recognized as a significant cause of diarrhoea in young ruminants only over the past 30 years or so. Cryptosporidiosis is a zoonotic disease and has been frequently reported in children visiting open farms and 'petting' zoos. Faecal contamination of human water supplies after pastures grazed by sheep have flooded has led to numerous health scares in the UK.

C. parvum is not host specific and severe outbreaks can occur on mixed farming enterprises where there is a build-up of infection towards the end of the lambing or calving period, especially if the same fields or buildings are used for autumn/ winter calving then spring lambing, as the protozoan parasite can remain dormant on pasture for months and is very resistant to environmental stresses. In some instances no clinical disease results from *Cryptosporidium* spp. infection and these protozoa are commonly isolated from clinically healthy animals.

Aetiology

Infection is by the faecal–oral route. Adult sheep may become asymptomatic carriers and shed small numbers of oocysts during stressful periods such as around parturition. Diarrhoea is caused by the physical loss of villous absorptive area and exacerbates concurrent gut infections such as rotavirus. Cryptosporidia do not require faecal excretion for sporulation to infective stages and can invade other cells without leaving the intestine. This autoinfection can cause severe disease.

Clinical presentation

Most cases of cryptosporidiosis occur during the second half of the lambing period under intensive management systems. Lambs aged 3–7 days are most commonly affected. There is a profuse yellow/ green diarrhoea with some mucus present. Flecks of fresh blood are seen occasionally. Initially, lambs have a distended appearance but quickly become dull with a tucked-up abdomen, are reluctant to follow their dam and are often found hunched up, sheltering behind walls and hedgerows. There is rapid weight loss and lambs develop a gaunt appearance. There is gradual recovery in most lambs over 5–7 days.

A severe challenge of *C. parvum* can cause rapid dehydration with recumbency and eventual death if supportive therapy is not administered. Losses are particularly high during adverse weather conditions. Convalescence of surviving lambs is protracted.

Differential diagnoses

In lambs diagnosis of cryptosporidiosis is difficult because the clinical signs and epidemiological findings also fit *E. coli* infection in lambs aged 3–5 days. Starvation should also be considered in many advanced cases.

Diagnosis

Diagnosis is based upon the clinical findings with demonstration of *Cryptosporidium* spp. oocysts on faecal smear after modified Ziehl–Neelsen (ZN) or Giemsa stain; however, other enteropathogens may also be isolated and it may prove difficult to ascertain their relative importance. Identification of *C. parvum* on stained ileal sections of postmortem material is the preferred laboratory method for confirmation.

Treatment

There are no licensed antiprotozoal or antibiotics for the treatment of cryptosporidiosis in lambs. Anecdotal reports suggest that long-acting sulphonamides are useful in reducing clinical severity. There are also reports that halofuginone is effective in the prevention and treatment of cryptosporidiosis in lambs, but this drug is only licensed for calves.

Lambs are commonly affected at 3–7 days old when *E. coli* of varying antibiotic resistance patterns can be isolated. When morbidity and mortality rates are high it is considered helpful to use antibiotics to control *E. coli* infections and amoxycillin injections are commonly used as the first approach. Isolation and antibiotic sensitivity testing of bacterial isolates should be undertaken if losses continue.

Oral fluid therapy is essential for the treatment of dehydrated neonatal lambs and 150–200 ml of a diluted calf oral rehydration solution should be administered four to six times daily, although this regimen involves a great deal of labour. Lambs should be left with their dam as they often suck, thus preventing the energy starvation that results from prolonged feeding of oral rehydration solutions, which contain a maximum of 30% of the lamb's daily energy requirements.

Management/prevention/control measures

Three factors are critical when considering control measures for cryptosporidiosis:

1. Lack of host specificity.
2. Very short life cycle (4–7 days).
3. Persists for months on pasture.

Therefore:

1. The same fields should not be used for calving/lambing.
2. Fields should be changed every year or when clinical cases occur in that season.
3. Newborn animals should be moved immediately on to clean pasture.

Clinical cases should be isolated wherever possible but this proves difficult at lambing time. The overall standard of hygiene must be improved for housed sheep, with extra bedding to limit oocyst challenge.

Economics

Losses from cryptosporidiosis can be high during adverse weather and with concurrent bacterial infections of the gut. The lack of adequate farm staff during the lambing period limits effective fluid therapy regimens, contributing to protracted convalescence and death of lambs. Poor subsequent growth rates lead to delays in marketing and reduced sale price.

Coccidiosis
Definition/overview

Coccidiosis is a problem worldwide whenever growing lambs are intensively stocked under poor hygiene standards. With increased intensification for lamb production on many farms, coccidiosis has become a major problem in the UK.

In the UK coccidiosis is a problem of intensively-reared lambs occurring primarily indoors where stocking densities are high. It may also occur in lambs at pasture where there is heavy contamination around feed troughs in creep areas during warm wet weather. Loss of gut absorptive capacity often results in profuse diarrhoea.

Aetiology

Coccidiosis is caused by infection by the protozoan *Eimeria* spp. which parasitize the epithelium lining of the alimentary tract. Infection causes a loss of epithelial cells and villous atrophy. There are two pathogenic species in lambs, *E. crandallis* and *E. ovinoidalis*. The ewe is the probable source of the infection, which is then multiplied in young lambs, with a much greater challenge presented to later born lambs. Coccidia must sporulate outside the host to become infective, hence the importance of environmental contamination.

Clinical presentation

In lambs, infection is originally picked up from the ewes and then, following the short life cycle in the lambs, rapidly builds up in densely-stocked, dirty environments. Lambs 4–6 weeks old are most commonly affected. The common presenting signs are a rapid loss of weight combined with a tucked-up appearance (**Fig. 5.46**). In severe clinical coccidiosis there is a sudden onset of profuse foetid diarrhoea containing mucus and flecks of fresh blood. There is considerable faecal staining of the perineum and tail (**Fig. 5.47**). Tenesmus, with partial eversion of the rectum, is occasionally seen in severe infections, which may result in prolapse. Straining is often accompanied by painful vocalization. Clinical disease is often precipitated by a stressful event such as adverse weather, weaning or dietary change.

More usually, the clinical signs are less marked with weight loss and poor appetite. Small clots of fresh blood and mucus are passed but the diarrhoea is not so marked. Anaemia is an uncommon sequel. The rectal temperature is often normal. Morbidity is high but mortality, even in severe cases, is low. Convalescence is protracted in all cases. There appears to be a synergistic effect between *Nematodirus battus* and *Eimeria* spp., with relatively low levels of coccidia associated with clinical disease.

Differential diagnoses

- Group problem of scouring lambs:
  - The major differential for scouring lambs grazing contaminated pasture in many countries is nematodirosis; in the UK this typically affects 6–8-week-old lambs during May.
  - *Strongyloides westeri* infestation can cause diarrhoea in housed lambs kept in unhygienic conditions, but this is uncommon.
- Problem of poor growth in individual lambs:
  - There are many causes of poor growth in individual young lambs including poor nutrition of the dam, mastitis or other infectious disease.
  - Liver abscessation, chronic pneumonia and infectious polyarthritis cause poor growth in individual lambs.

Diagnosis

Diagnosis is based on epidemiological and clinical findings plus the demonstration of large numbers of oocysts in faecal samples (often >100,000 oocysts per gram) in which *E. crandallis* or *E. ovinoidalis* predominate. In severe infestations, disease may occur before oocysts are shed in faeces.

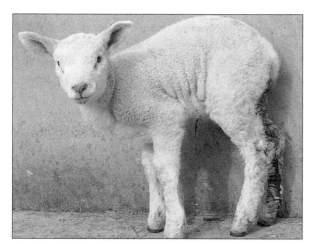

Fig. 5.46 Coccidiosis causes rapid weight loss and a resultant gaunt appearance.

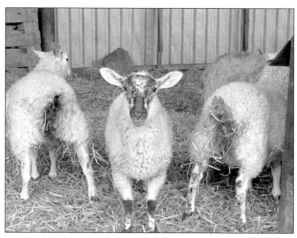

Fig. 5.47 Faecal staining of the perineum and tail caused by coccidiosis; the lambs also show tenesmus.

At necropsy the caecum is inflamed, empty and contracted with the wall thickened with a hyperaemic mucosa. The ileum and colon may also be affected. Examination of gut sections from clinical cases reveals large numbers of oocysts.

Treatment

Sulpha drugs were commonly used to treat coccidiosis but have been replaced by decoquinate, toltrazuril and diclazuril. Sheep must be moved from infected pastures/premises as soon as disease becomes apparent.

Management/prevention/control measures

Control involves avoidance of contamination around feed troughs (**Fig. 5.48**). Adequate bedding must be provided when sheep are kept indoors. Creep areas at pasture can become heavily contaminated especially during wet weather; therefore, the troughs should be moved regularly and not only when the area has become heavily contaminated.

Medication of the ewe ration with decoquinate will suppress but not totally eliminate oocyst production; therefore, this regimen is operated in conjunction with medication of the lamb creep feed. Occasionally, disease may occur because there is a problem with ration palatability; the farmer elects to medicate only the lamb ration and the lambs choose to eat the non-medicated ewe concentrate. Recent developments have suggested that suppressing oocyst production by ewes may be counterproductive because this only results in a delayed challenge to the lambs, with an increased likelihood of clinical disease in lambs.

Clinical coccidiosis may also result in growing lambs once decoquinate-medicated feed has been withdrawn, because active immunity is induced by contact with developing stages in the gut. In this situation, lambs should be moved to clean pasture once the in-feed medication has been discontinued.

Diclazuril and toltrazuril can be used for the prophylaxis and treatment of coccidiosis in lambs. For prophylaxis, the whole group is drenched as soon as clinical signs are suspected in several lambs. Treated lambs should then be moved to a clean area to prevent reinfection before they have time to develop protective immunity.

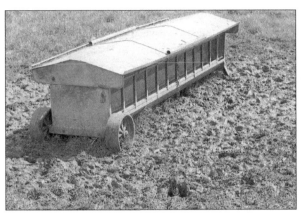

Fig. 5.48 Avoid contamination around feed troughs by regular movement to reduce the risk of coccidiosis.

In situations where lambs are moved onto suspected heavily-contaminated fields, either diclazuril or toltrazuril should be given 10–14 days later to enable some active immunity to develop during this intervening period.

Economics

In-feed medication with decoquinate is expensive, adding to the cost of rearing lambs under intensive conditions. Prophylaxis of 1-month-old lambs using diclazuril or toltrazuril is cheaper.

Paratuberculosis

(syn. Johne's disease)

Definition/overview

Paratuberculosis is a very common disease of sheep in the UK and many countries worldwide but is frequently under-diagnosed because of the vague clinical sign of weight loss over several months. The disease in sheep is characterized by emaciation (**Figs 5.49–5.52**) but not, as in cattle, chronic severe diarrhoea (**Fig. 5.53**). Disease is encountered in all sheep husbandry systems including extensively-managed Blackface hill flocks in the UK that are rarely housed and are usually confined only to small grass fields during the short lambing period (**Fig. 5.51**). Paratuberculosis is a notifiable disease in certain countries including Australia. The annual ewe mortality rate is estimated at between 2–5% in infected flocks but there are few reliable data and an underestimation of losses is likely (**Fig. 5.54**).

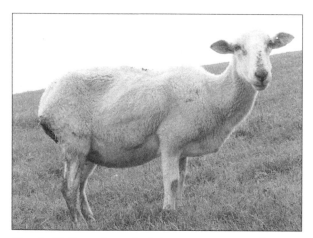

Fig. 5.49 Paratuberculosis is a very common disease of sheep in the UK.

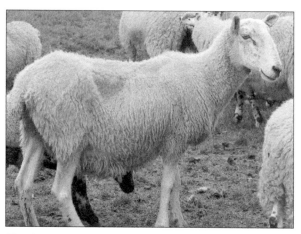

Fig. 5.50 Paratuberculosis is characterized by emaciation but not, as in cattle, chronic severe diarrhoea.

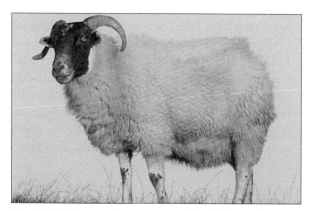

Fig. 5.51 Disease is encountered in all sheep husbandry systems including extensively-managed Blackface flocks in the UK.

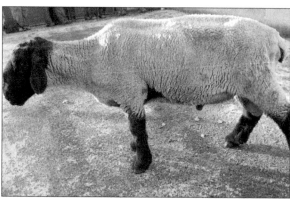

Fig. 5.52 Paratuberculosis can affect all breeds of sheep.

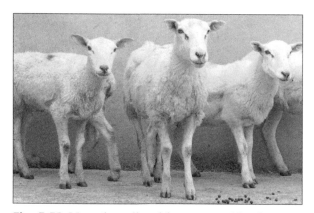

Fig. 5.53 Note the pelleted faeces passed by these sheep with paratuberculosis.

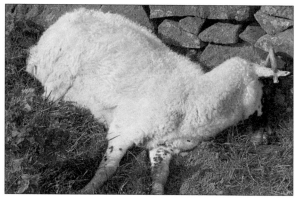

Fig. 5.54 The annual ewe mortality rate from paratuberculosis is estimated at between 2–5% in infected flocks but there are few reliable data.

In Australia annual losses as high 15–20% have been reported in heavily infected flocks.

Aetiology

The aetiological agent of paratuberculosis, *Mycobacterium avium* subspecies *paratuberculosis*, is very resistant to desiccation and can survive on pasture for many months. There are a number of strains of this organism including a pigmented strain. Sheep that develop clinical disease are infected early in life via the faecal–oral route, although infection can also be acquired in colostrum and *in utero* during the advanced stages of disease in the ewe. Infection ingested by adult sheep is unlikely to cause clinical disease. Goats can be an important source of infection when co-grazed with sheep, and this practice has led to very high levels of clinical disease in some sheep flocks. The role of cattle and various wildlife species in the epidemiology of ovine paratuberculosis is currently under investigation. Strict biocontainment measures should be undertaken to reduce the risk of spread between ruminant species on the farm. Whether rabbits are an end-stage host or act as a reservoir of infection without showing clinical signs remains unclear.

Clinical presentation

Paratuberculosis presents as chronic weight loss/low body condition score and poor fleece in individual middle-aged (typically 3–4-year-old) sheep with normal dentition and fed an appropriate plane of nutrition. Unusually, disease has been described in yearling sheep. Emaciated sheep are typically detected during routine flock handling procedures, such as premating checks, when their body condition score of 1.5 or below (scale 1–5) compares unfavourably with other sheep managed in a similar way (scores of 3.0 or greater) (**Fig. 5.55**). Unlike in cattle, chronic diarrhoea is not a feature in the majority of sheep affected by paratuberculosis; sheep often void pelleted faeces until the terminal stages. Where diarrhoea occurs (**Fig. 5.56**) it is due to concurrent parasitic gastroenteritis (PGE); affected sheep can have very high faecal worm egg counts and patent lungworm infestation with larvae visible on the McMaster slide preparation. Affected sheep appear bright and alert but are weak due to their emaciated state. They have a normal appetite but rumen fill is reduced with sunken sublumbar fossae (**Fig. 5.57**). The wool is of poor quality and the fleece appears more open than usual, and is easily detached by

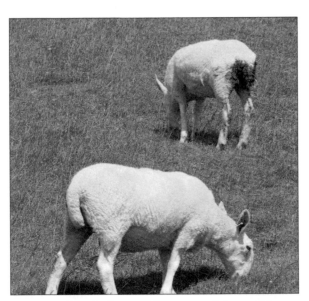

Fig. 5.55 The body condition score of sheep with paratuberculosis (background) compares unfavourably to other sheep in the group (foreground), despite similar management.

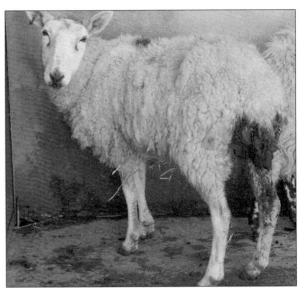

Fig. 5.56 Where diarrhoea occurs it is usually due to concurrent PGE and affected sheep can have very high faecal worm egg counts.

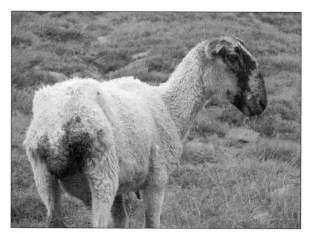

Fig. 5.57 Sheep with paratuberculosis appear to have a normal appetite but rumen fill is reduced with sunken sublumbar fossae.

rough handling. The fleece changes are best appreciated by comparing an emaciated ewe with paratuberculosis with a sheep in good bodily condition.

During the agonal stages affected sheep may become recumbent and progress to a stuporous state, which further complicates the clinical diagnosis. The emaciated state, detached poor-quality fleece and vacant expression during the agonal stages have led to a misdiagnosis of scrapie in some cases. Hypoalbuminaemia during the later stages of disease may result in accumulations of fluid within the peritoneal and pleural cavities and the pericardium, although these are not usually noted during clinical examination. Submandibular oedema presents only in extreme cases. The severity of paratuberculosis is compounded by concurrent parasitism, especially fasciolosis.

Lambs born to ewes in the terminal stages of disease have very low birthweights (often as low as 2–3 kg) due to chronic intrauterine growth retardation but they are viable. These lambs must not be kept as breeding replacement stock because of the likelihood of transplacental infection. Affected ewes should be culled for welfare reasons as they will be unable to support even one lamb.

Differential diagnoses

In order of decreasing incidence, the common causes of weight loss and ill-thrift in sheep in the UK are:

- Group problem:
  - Poor flock nutrition.
  - Fasciolosis.
  - Chronic parasitism due to poor pasture management and erroneous control strategies.
  - Chronic parasitism caused by anthelmintic-resistant strains of nematodes.
- Individual sheep:
  - Paratuberculosis.
  - Poor dentition especially molar teeth.
  - Chronic suppurative pneumonia, mastitis, septic joint, endocarditis or other septic focus.
  - Ovine pulmonary adenocarcinoma.
  - Chronic severe lameness, e.g. septic pedal arthritis, footrot.
  - Visceral form of caseous lymphadenitis.
  - Intestinal adenocarcinoma/lymphosarcoma and other tumours.
  - Scrapie.
  - Visna.

Diagnosis

While on-farm postmortem examination of individual ewes will identify gross lesions of many diseases, the intestinal changes caused by paratuberculosis can be easily overlooked. More importantly, a single necropsy provides little information regarding the prevalence of certain disease conditions on the farm. In most situations it will prove more useful to investigate weight loss in 10 or more ewes than send a single ewe for detailed postmortem examination. In general practice with a limited budget of only £2–4 per ewe for laboratory tests, serum albumin and globulin determinations could provide the most useful screening tests for the investigation of chronic weight loss in a number of adult sheep.

Serum protein analysis in the investigation of weight loss: Albumin reflects the balance between hepatic synthesis from dietary nitrogenous intake and endogenous demands/losses. Serum globulin is a long-term indicator of the body's response to bacterial infections. Other proteins, such as haptoglobin and fibrinogen, are more useful as indicators of acute disease, with significant increases within 1–3 days and 4–7 days respectively.

Sheep with paratuberculosis have profound hypoalbuminaemia (serum concentration <15 g/l but as low as 6–10 g/l in advanced disease; normal range = >30 g/l), resulting from loss of albumin across the damaged intestinal mucosa (protein-losing enteropathy) and a normal globulin concentration. These serum protein concentrations may also be encountered in cases of severe chronic intestinal parasitism such as haemonchosis, but such infestations are generally group problems. Fasciolosis may result in hypoalbuminaemia but these sheep usually show additional clinical signs, such as anaemia and submandibular oedema. In addition, many sheep with subacute and chronic fasciolosis have greatly increased serum globulin concentrations often exceeding 70 g/l (normal value = <45 g/l).

In the absence of recent anthelmintic treatment, it must be appreciated that adult sheep with paratuberculosis often have very high faecal egg counts (>5000–10,000 epg) due to immunosuppression of the host. Detailed necropsy examination typically fails to reveal significant populations of adult nematodes; the high egg output is the result of increased fecundity of a small population of adult parasites. It is not uncommon to find *Nematodirus battus* eggs and lungworm larvae (*Dictyocaulus filaria*) on the McMaster slide in these adult sheep; these parasitological findings should alert the clinician to the likelihood of paratuberculosis. Caution is needed when interpreting pooled faecal samples from 10–12 adult sheep because a single paratuberculosis case can cause a significant mean worm egg count leading to misdiagnosis of parasitism.

Chronic bacterial infections causing weight loss result in significant increases in serum globulin concentration (often >55 g/l) and low serum albumin concentration (often 18–25 g/l but rarely below 15 g/l). Low albumin/high globulin concentrations indicate a probable chronic suppurative disease process/focus (e.g. chronic suppurative pneumonia, endocarditis, liver abscessation, mastitis, infectious polyarthritis, cellulitis). Once the possibility of a chronic suppurative focus has been highlighted, the sheep should be re-examined. Further specific tests can then be selected based upon the organ system suspected of being involved, e.g. serum gamma glutamyl transferase (GGT) concentrations and faecal fluke egg count for chronic fasciolosis, chest ultrasonography if chronic suppurative pneumonia is suspected, and abdominocentesis/ultrasonography for peritonitis.

Low serum albumin/normal globulin concentrations (<25 g/l and <45 g/l, respectively) suggest that chronic bacterial infection is unlikely. A dietary effect such as low protein intake is one possible explanation. A lowered serum albumin concentration is also often encountered in ewes during late pregnancy fed poor-quality rations at a time when protein metabolism is geared toward immunoglobulin production and transfer into the colostrum in the udder.

Significant serological titres (either agar gel immunodiffusion test [AGID] or enzyme-linked immunosorbent assay [ELISA]) are detected in approximately 60% of clinical paratuberculosis cases, resulting in a high false-negative rate (low sensitivity) although the specificity is high (>95%).

Direct faecal examination will not detect the paucibacillary form of ovine paratuberculosis and thereby provides unreliable results. Cultural isolation takes at least 8 weeks, and possibly up to 6 months, and has very limited practical application. A high-throughput polymerase chain reaction (PCR) test assay has been approved for use in paratuberculosis control programmes in Australia and New Zealand. While theoretically possible, and undertaken in cattle in some situations, biopsy of the ileo-caecal lymph node or terminal ileum in live sheep is not undertaken in general practice.

Postmortem examination

There is an emaciated carcase with gelatinous atrophy of fat depots (**Figs 5.58, 5.59**) and visible lymphatics within the mesentery. However, gross changes of paratuberculosis can easily be overlooked during a cursory on-farm postmortem examination and great care must be taken not to miss potential lesions. Thickening of the ileum, with prominent ridging, is not always obvious in paratuberculosis (**Figs 5.60, 5.61**) but the mesenteric lymph nodes are visibly enlarged (**Figs 5.58, 5.62**). The diagnosis is confirmed by demonstrating clumps of acid-fast bacteria after ZN staining of ileal sections and ileo-caecal lymph nodes.

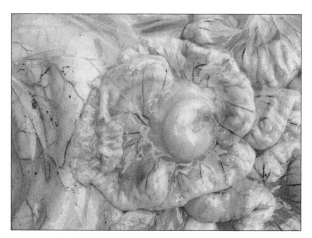

Fig. 5.58 Necropsy reveals gelatinous atrophy of fat depots with visible lymphatics within the mesentery and enlarged mesenteric lymph nodes.

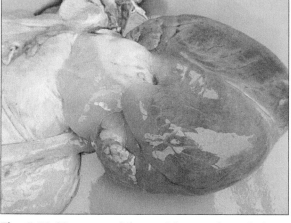

Fig. 5.59 Necropsy of sheep with paratuberculosis reveals gelatinous atrophy of fat depots around the heart.

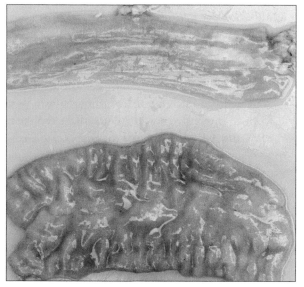

Fig. 5.60 In paratuberculosis thickening of the ileum, with prominent ridging, is not always as obvious as in the lower specimen (normal ileum upper specimen).

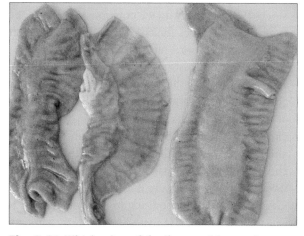

Fig. 5.61 Thickening of the ileum, with prominent ridging, is not always obvious in paratuberculosis (normal ileum in centre).

Fig. 5.62 The mesenteric lymph nodes are visibly enlarged in paratuberculosis. Note also gelatinous atrophy of fat depots.

Depending upon geographic area and strain distribution, some sheep may present with the yellow/orange pigmented strain.

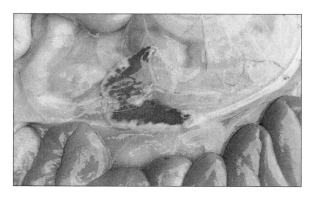

Management/prevention/control measures

The true paratuberculosis incidence in UK sheep flocks remains unknown (**Fig. 5.63**). Control measures presently operating on some commercial sheep farms in the UK are limited to culling suspected clinical cases and, where records permit, their progeny. This measure is unlikely to have a significant impact on paratuberculosis prevalence.

The wide host range of *M. a. paratuberculosis*, including cattle, goat, and wildlife reservoirs, poses many opportunities for disease transmission and may render sheep de-stocking policies useless.

Very encouraging results with much reduced disease prevalence have been reported following adoption of a vaccination programme in several countries including the UK. Vaccination against paratuberculosis has been practised in flocks in New Zealand since 1987. Currently, vaccination offers the best long-term prospect for control and is administered to sheep more than 1 month old.

Vaccine administration may cause several problems. There may be considerable localized reaction with development of a 5 cm diameter nodule at the subcutaneous injection site just behind the ear. Around 5% of sheep may develop an injection site abscess which will rupture and discharge with the potential for myiasis. Vaccinated sheep are also likely to react positively if tested for tuberculosis. Care must be exercised not to self-inject with the oil-adjuvant live attenuated vaccine as this may result in serious local reaction. These potential vaccination problems should not outweigh the benefits to be gained from effective paratuberculosis control.

Economics

Difficulties with confirmation of the provisional diagnosis of paratuberculosis, coupled with very few ewes culled for poor condition/emaciation submitted to the veterinary surgeon, lead to a gross underestimation of the prevalence and financial impact of this disease in the UK, and probably worldwide. In the author's experience of some lowground flocks in Scotland, losses and increased culling due to poor body condition in sheep with paratuberculosis can approach 5–8% of

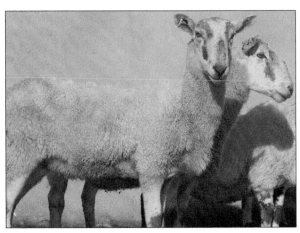

Fig. 5.63 The true paratuberculosis incidence in UK sheep flocks remains unknown because involuntary culls are rarely examined.

adult stock per annum. This figure compares with the UK average ewe mortality rate of 5–7% per annum. Their debilitated state may also render affected ewes more susceptible to infectious disease, parasitic infestations and predation.

The culling rate due to paratuberculosis in the UK must currently exceed 2% to offset the cost of vaccinating ewe lambs. The unit cost of vaccination may decrease as more vaccine is used, and as new vaccines are developed. Problems with bovine paratuberculosis worldwide, and fears surrounding zoonotic risk, may accelerate vaccine development and its use in sheep.

Welfare implications

Suspected/confirmed paratuberculosis cases during the early stages of disease (poorer body condition compared to peers) should be culled immediately to reduce environmental contamination (**Fig. 5.64**). Emaciated sheep must be destroyed immediately on the farm for welfare reasons (**Fig. 5.65**).

CLOSTRIDIAL DISEASES

Definition/overview

Clostridial diseases remain a serious threat to unvaccinated sheep in all countries worldwide. Typically, death occurs within hours of rapid bacterial multiplication and exotoxin production (**Figs 5.66, 5.67**)

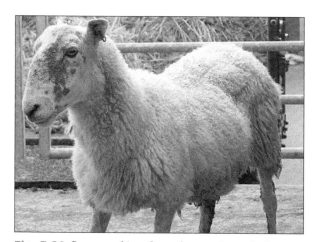

Fig. 5.64 Suspected/confirmed paratuberculosis cases during the early stages of disease should be culled immediately to reduce environmental contamination.

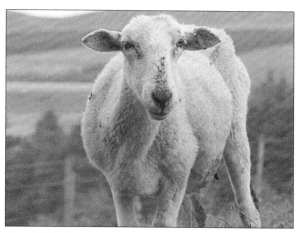

Fig. 5.65 Emaciated sheep must be destroyed immediately on the farm for welfare reasons.

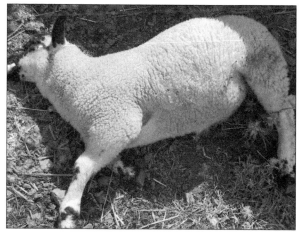

Fig. 5.66 Clostridial diseases cause death within hours due to rapid bacterial multiplication and exotoxin production.

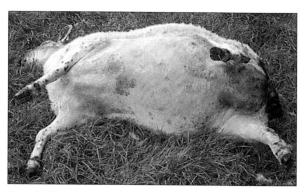

Fig. 5.67 Clostridial diseases cause rapid carcase autolysis.

although lambs with tetanus can survive for several days. Despite effective control from timely vaccination and the protection afforded lambs by passive antibody transfer, clostridial diseases still occur all too frequently because of management errors. Surprisingly, a UK survey revealed that almost 20% of sheep farmers did not vaccinate their adult sheep on an annual basis. The growth of certain organic food schemes in some countries,

including the UK, is a concern when membership can restrict clostridial vaccination until these diseases occur on the farm.

This chapter will not deal with the clostridial diseases in detail because they do not occur in well-managed sheep flocks. Furthermore, such details can be readily accessed from standard bacteriology references. More importantly, it is the veterinarian's duty to ensure that all sheep clients operate an effective clostridial vaccination programme for both economic and welfare reasons. With this point in mind, the reader is directed to the sections detailing late gestation ewe nutrition (Chapter 2, Husbandry) and neonatal lamb management (Chapter 4, Neonatal Lamb Diseases) because clostridial disease in young growing lambs is readily prevented by ensuring adequate specific antibody accumulation in colostrum and timely transfer to lambs within the first 6 hours of life. Farmers and veterinarians must not overlook such basic husbandry measures.

Aetiology

Clostridia are generally considered to be ubiquitous in the environment, particularly in organic material, with disease triggered by various factors including changes in feeding and parasite damage to tissues. Such microenvironments within the body permit extremely rapid clostridial multiplication and exotoxin production, characteristically leading to death within hours. In general, there is excessive blood-stained fluid within body cavities and pericardium at necropsy (**Figs 5.68–5.71**).

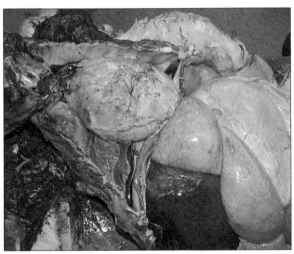

Fig. 5.68 Necropsy reveals excessive blood-stained fluid within body cavities and the pericardium caused by clostridial disease.

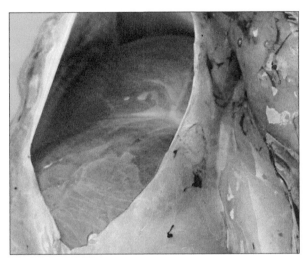

Fig. 5.69 Necropsy reveals excessive fluid in the pericardial sac caused by clostridial disease.

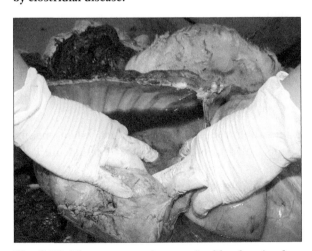

Fig. 5.70 Necropsy reveals excessive blood-stained fluid within the chest caused by clostridial disease.

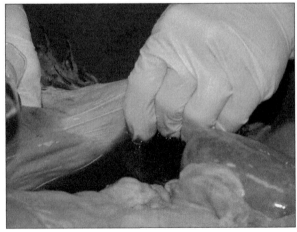

Fig. 5.71 Necropsy reveals excessive blood-stained fluid within the abdominal cavity caused by clostridial disease.

Lamb dysentery

Aetiology

Clostridium perfringens type B.

Clinical presentation

Sporadic cases may occur in the flock in those lambs that have received nil or inadequate specific antibody in colostrum, This may be due to various factors including: individual ewe not vaccinated; lack of colostrum accumulation in the ewe's udder due to poor feeding/mastitis; large litter; or feeding colostrum supplements/bovine colostrum from unvaccinated donors.

Lamb dysentery is more typically identified as a disease outbreak in lambs born to unvaccinated ewes, with losses approaching 20–30% of susceptible lambs. Lambs less than 1 week old are affected at the beginning of the outbreak; thereafter losses occur in older lambs. Initially, lambs are found dead without any observed clinical signs; in intensive systems these lambs have been turned out to pasture with their dams at 2 days old and are then less closely supervised. Thereafter, careful observation reveals lambs that are lethargic, do not suck, have a gaunt appearance, show frequent tenesmus with painful bleating and develop dysentery during the agonal stages, which is accompanied by rapid dehydration, recumbency and death within 2–12 hours.

Differential diagnoses

Differential diagnosis of sudden death in young lambs includes:

- Pasteurellosis, colisepticaemia, and other acute bacterial conditions.
- Salmonellosis rarely causes disease in young lambs.
- Starvation, exposure, hepatic necrobacillosis, cryptosporidiosis and bacterial enteric infections cause lethargy and a gaunt appearance, often with evidence of diarrhoea, but these signs should be detected before death ensues some days later.

Diagnosis

The provisional diagnosis of lamb dysentery is based upon history of ineffective vaccination/failure of passive antibody transfer, clinical findings and postmortem examination. Necropsy findings include a haemorrhagic enteritis (**Fig. 5.72**) with excessive blood-stained fluid within body cavities and pericardium. The demonstration of specific toxins by ELISA may give a number of false-positive results and such laboratory tests must be interpreted in conjunction with clinical and epidemiological findings.

Treatment

With the exceptions of blackleg and bighead, there are no effective treatments for the clostridial diseases. (Please refer to the particular sections on blackleg and bighead for specific treatments.)

Management/prevention/control measures

There are well-established vaccination protocols using toxoid vaccines which prevent all common clostridial diseases; protection against botulism and *C. sordellii* is not provided by some polyvalent clostridial vaccines. Clostridial disease invariably results from failure to adhere to vaccination instructions and good management practices. Clostridial diseases are not encountered in well-managed sheep flocks.

Prevention of pulpy kidney and the other clostridial diseases that can affect weaned lambs is achieved by two vaccinations 4–6 weeks apart, administered before weaning at around 4 months

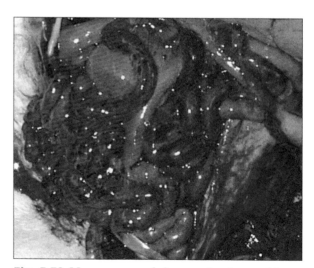

Fig. 5.72 Necropsy reveals haemorrhagic enteritis caused by lamb dysentery.

old (**Fig. 5.73**). All purchased lambs must be assumed to be unvaccinated unless there is written confirmation from the vendor that this has indeed been correctly undertaken.

A gradual change in diet, such as the step-wise introduction of concentrate feeding may reduce the incidence of clostridial disease, and is in any case sound practice to reduce the risk of acidosis and polioencephalomalacia (PEM). Prophylactic antibiotic injections following unskilled correction of dystocia may reduce the likelihood of blackleg, but there is no reason why all sheep should not have been correctly vaccinated.

In some countries, vaccination against pasteurellosis is combined with clostridial vaccination.

Economics
Clostridial vaccination is cheap (15–20 pence per dose) and very effective indeed. Initially, two vaccinations are given 4–6 weeks apart followed by annual vaccination of ewes 4–6 weeks before the expected lambing date (**Fig. 5.74**) to ensure adequate accumulation of protective immunoglobulins in colostrum. Lambs are vaccinated from 3–4 months old, with the programme complete before weaning unless sold for slaughter before waning of maternal antibody,

at around 4–5 months old. Rams are commonly forgotten in vaccination programmes and veterinarians must remind their clients of this oversight.

Welfare implications
Illness from clostridial disease has serious welfare implications, especially when there is an effective vaccination strategy to prevent such losses.

Pulpy kidney
Aetiology
C. perfringens type B.

Clinical presentation
Pulpy kidney occurs in 4–10-week-old lambs born to unvaccinated dams, and in weaned lambs from around 6 months old when passively derived antibody has waned and the lambs themselves have not been vaccinated. Losses in weaned lambs often follow dietary improvements such as the introduction of concentrate feeding or movement to lush pastures (**Fig. 5.75**).

The major clinical feature is sudden death. Affected sheep are initially very dull, almost stuporous but progress rapidly to seizure activity and opisthotonus, followed rapidly by death.

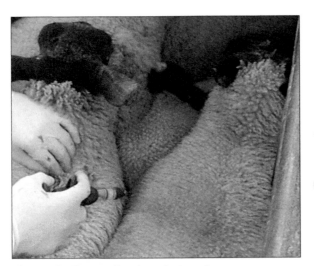

Fig. 5.73 Two vaccinations 4–6 weeks apart are administered to lambs before weaning at around 4–5 months old to prevent clostridial disease.

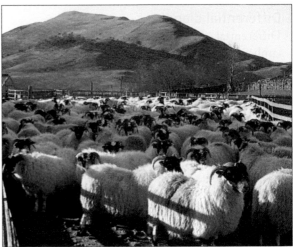

Fig. 5.74 Vaccination of ewes 4–6 weeks before the expected lambing date protects lambs from clostridial disease.

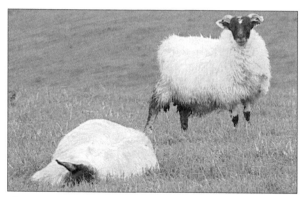

Fig. 5.75 **Deaths from clostridial disease in weaned unvaccinated lambs often follow dietary improvements, such as the introduction of concentrate feeding or movement to lush pastures.**

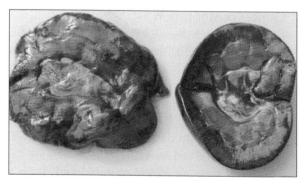

Fig. 5.76 **Necropsy revealing a very friable kidney on cut section (left) compared to a normal kidney (right) supports a diagnosis of pulpy kidney.**

Differential diagnoses

Sudden death in growing lambs includes nematodirosis and pneumonic pasteurellosis. The main differential diagnosis in weaned lambs is septicaemic pasteurellosis. In certain geographic areas acute fasciolosis and black disease must also be considered. Sheep recently introduced onto a concentrate ration/ access to stubbles are susceptible to acidosis.

Diagnosis

The diagnosis is based upon epidemiology, lack of vaccination history (although this may be uncertain in purchased sheep) and necropsy findings.

There is rapid autolysis of the carcase with excess serosanguinous fluid in the body cavities, more especially the abdomen. The kidneys are very friable (**Fig. 5.76**). A glycosuria, consequent to hepatic glycolysis, is present which is readily detectable on urinary dipstick and is a useful field test. Characteristic lesions of focal symmetrical encephalomalacia can be demonstrated by histopathological examination of brain tissue.

Treatment

There is no treatment for pulpy kidney.

Braxy
Aetiology

Braxy is caused by *C. septicum* and is characteristically seen in unvaccinated weaned lambs during the winter months, associated with ingestion of frosted root crops.

Clinical presentation

Affected sheep are almost invariably found dead. Those that are observed alive are profoundly depressed and may show abdominal pain, but this is difficult to appreciate. There is rapid carcase decomposition despite the prevailing low environmental temperatures.

Differential diagnoses

The main differential diagnoses include other clostridial diseases such as pulpy kidney and black disease. Other causes of sudden death include systemic pasteurellosis and subacute fasciolosis. Sheep recently introduced onto a concentrate ration are susceptible to acidosis. Ingestion of root crops may lead to frothy bloat/choke.

Diagnosis

The diagnosis is based upon epidemiology, including recent frost, and lack of vaccination history.

Treatment

There is no treatment for braxy.

Black disease
(syn. infectious necrotic hepatitis)

Aetiology

C. novyi type B.

Clinical presentation

In the UK black disease is typically associated with migration of immature liver flukes during late summer/early autumn and can affect unvaccinated sheep of all ages. In the absence of rapid intervention and appropriate action, losses can be very high in unvaccinated sheep. Sudden death in 2–4-year-old unvaccinated sheep due to black disease is reported in New Zealand and Australia.

Clinical signs are rarely observed and sheep are simply found dead. There is rapid carcase decomposition and accumulation of blood-tinged fluid within body cavities and widespread petechial haemorrhages. The liver is congested and very dark, with areas of necrosis visible on cut section. There is evidence of fluke tracks throughout the liver in those geographical areas where disease is associated with acute fasciolosis.

Differential diagnoses

The main differential diagnosis is acute fasciolosis but also includes other clostridial diseases and systemic pasteurellosis. Louping-ill should be considered in tick-infested areas in certain countries. Sheep recently introduced onto a concentrate ration are susceptible to acidosis.

Diagnosis

The diagnosis is based upon necropsy findings, and lack of vaccination history. Laboratory tests, such as FAT, may yield false-positive results and should not be interpreted in isolation.

Treatment

There is no treatment. An appropriate fluke control plan, combined with an appropriate clostridial vaccination programme, will effectively control black disease, although very occasional deaths may still occur.

Bacillary haemoglobinuria
(syn. redwater)

Aetiology

Bacillary haemoglobinuria occurs sporadically in many countries worldwide. It is caused by *C. haemolyticum*.

Clinical presentation

Affected sheep are dull, depressed, inappetent with pyrexia and have dark red urine. Jaundice is present during the agonal stages and affected sheep die in 2–3 days.

Differential diagnoses

Differential diagnoses include copper toxicity and nitrate poisoning. Acute fasciolosis can also result in anaemia and death within days from severe infestation.

Diagnosis

Necropsy reveals large infarcts in the liver and haemorrhage into the renal cortex, with red urine in the renal pelvis and bladder. Laboratory tests, such as FAT, may yield false-positive results and should not be interpreted in isolation.

Treatment

There is no treatment for bacillary haemoglobinuria.

Blackleg
(syn. postparturient gangrene)

Aetiology

Blackleg occurs in all countries worldwide. Blackleg is caused by *C. chauvoei* which, in common with the other clostridial organisms causing disease in sheep, can survive in soil for many years. Entry of clostridia occurs through skin wounds, dog bites, shearing cuts, via contaminated needles/injection equipment, untreated umbilicus and trauma to the posterior reproductive tract during attempted dystocia correction.

Clinical presentation

Blackleg usually occurs sporadically within a flock due to individual factors such as dystocia or dog bite, but outbreaks of disease have been reported after tail docking in unhygienic and contaminated handling facilities, and via contaminated needles.

Involvement of one limb results in sudden onset severe lameness with the limb often dragged along. Once recumbent, the sheep has great difficulty raising itself. There is marked swelling of the limb with oedema, subcutaneous emphysema and purple discolouration of overlying skin (**Figs 5.77, 5.78**). The limb often has a crepitant feel due to gas accumulation. The drainage lymph node is markedly enlarged.

Invasion and infection of traumatized tissues of the posterior reproductive tract result from excessive unskilled interference in dystocia cases without appropriate hygienic precautions. The ewe is extremely dull, depressed and inappetent, often spending long periods in sternal recumbency. The rectal temperature is increased (>41.0°C) and the mucous membranes have a toxic appearance. The ewe has no milk and the lambs are very hungry and gaunt. There may be considerable swelling and oedema of the vulva with a scant sero-sanguinous discharge. Further clinical signs depend upon the site of bacterial entry.

Infection of the umbilicus in neonatal lambs leads to rapid death.

Differential diagnoses

The important differential diagnoses for sudden onset severe lameness include cellulitis from dog bites, long bone fractures and joint infection. Foot abscess and septic pedal arthritis can cause severe lameness but are not so acute in presentation.

The important differential diagnoses for postparturient gangrene are uterine rupture and metritis, which occur under similar conditions of unskilled interference and poor hygiene. Severe metritis is common in some cases of infectious abortion, particularly *Salmonella typhimurium* and, less commonly, *Chlamydophila abortus*.

Other differential diagnoses include failure to detect foetal malpresentation (commonly breech presentation), which results in prolonged first stage labour with foetal death and emphysema, with toxin absorption across the compromised endometrium causing illness. Failure to deliver all foetuses and retention of a foetus causes severe toxaemia 36–48 hours after foetal death. Obvious infectious diseases such as gangrenous mastitis will be detected during the clinical examination.

While much less common after lambing, hypocalcaemia causes recumbency and depression, leading to bloat and stupor, although there is no pyrexia.

Diagnosis

The diagnosis of blackleg is based upon typical clinical findings in unvaccinated sheep. Death results in very rapid carcase autolysis and bloat. There is obvious muscle necrosis with associated blood-tinged oedema, although these lesions may be deep-seated within a muscle mass, necessitating methodical sectioning.

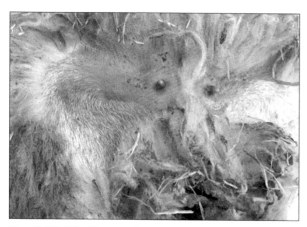

Fig. 5.77 Blackleg, with marked swelling of the limb with oedema, subcutaneous emphysema, and purple discoloration of overlying skin (see Fig. 5.78).

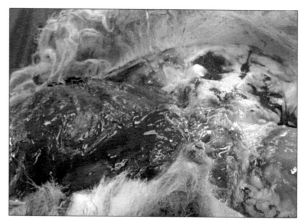

Fig. 5.78 Necropsy reveals marked oedema and discolouration of hindlimb muscles consistent with a diagnosis of blackleg.

Treatment

It may prove difficult to be certain of the blackleg diagnosis during the early stages based upon clinical examination alone. Penicillin is the drug of choice for clostridial disease, with the first dose given intravenously wherever possible. A non-steroidal anti-inflammatory drug such as flunixin or ketoprofen is unlicensed for sheep in many countries but they have anti-endotoxic action. Corticosteroids, such as dexamethasone, assist reduction of oedema and localized swelling.

Malignant oedema

(syn. bighead)

Aetiology

Various clostridia, including *C. chauvoei, C. perfringens* type A, *C. septicum, C. novyi* type A and *C. sordellii*, are associated with malignant oedema.

Clinical presentation

Malignant oedema is typically seen in rams during late summer/early autumn when headbutting is a common behaviour in establishing a hierarchy prior to, and during, the breeding season. Cases often occur within days of introducing purchased rams into an established group. Malignant oedema has been reported after contaminated intramuscular injection and following injection of substances that cause local tissue necrosis.

Affected sheep are dull and depressed and stand isolated from others in the group. The most obvious clinical sign is marked swelling of the head, particularly surrounding the eyes, which forces the eyelids closed. There may be skin abrasions to the poll and blood streaked along the wool of the flanks, but such indications of fighting are common in groups of rams. There is obvious subcutaneous oedema of the face which may extend onto the neck but this is unusual. The mucous membranes are congested. It may prove difficult to palpate the submandibular lymph nodes because of the oedema. Affected sheep are febrile (41.0–42.0°C). Occasionally, narrowing of the upper airways may cause inspiratory dyspnoea.

Differential diagnoses

The main differential diagnosis is cellulitis following infection of head wounds caused by fighting injuries. Myiasis of such head wounds is common. Periorbital eczema causes marked swelling and oedema with closure of the palpebral fissure but these sheep are not sick.

Diagnosis

The diagnosis is based on the clinical findings.

Treatment

Malignant oedema is the only clostridial disease that responds well to antibiotic therapy. Penicillin is the drug of choice, with the first dose given intravenously. Corticosteroids, such as dexamethasone, assist reduction of oedema and localized swelling.

Management/prevention/control measures

Management factors to control malignant oedema are centred round reducing fighting injuries in rams. Care must be exercised when introducing rams to a group; mixing is best achieved by keeping rams confined together in handling pens for several hours. Such confinement aids spread of odours amongst the rams whilst preventing charging each other and head butting. Many farmers coincide mixing groups of rams with plunge dipping as this is claimed to reduce fighting, presumably due to a 'common odour'. Antibiotic treatment of head wounds will prevent clostridial multiplication but not all wounds are detected promptly. Collecting areas with large accumulations of organic matter should be avoided but rams actively search out such areas whilst avoiding clean pasture.

Tetanus
Definition/overview

Tetanus is caused by production of a powerful neurotoxin with clinical signs most frequently seen in young lambs. The neurotoxin progressively causes spasticity, recumbency, opisthotonus (**Fig. 5.79**) and death. Tetanus has a worldwide distribution but its occurrence depends upon failure of well-established

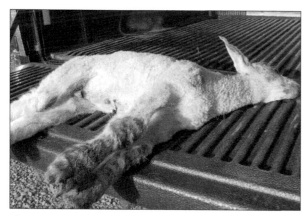

Fig. 5.79 There is marked spasticity and opisthotonus in this lamb suffering from tetanus.

vaccination regimens. All animals, including man, are susceptible to tetanus.

Aetiology

Production of a neurotoxin by *C. tetani*.

Clinical presentation

Tetanus is rarely encountered where clostridial vaccination forms an integral part of management practice. However, errors occur and vaccination is forgotten and this can lead to the appearance of clostridial diseases, including tetanus.

Historically, tetanus was observed approximately 1 week after surgical castration and tail docking. Traditionally, these procedures were carried out when lambs were 4–6 weeks old. The handling pens rapidly became contaminated with clostridial spores leading to infection of skin wounds.

Lambs show hindlimb stiffness and difficulty following their dam. Difficulty walking leads to long periods spent in sternal recumbency. Affected lambs are hungry and have a gaunt appearance. The condition progresses over 24–48 hours to lateral recumbency, seizure activity progressing to opisthotonus and death from respiratory failure.

Differential diagnoses

The initial period of hindlimb stiffness can be differentiated from bacterial polyarthritis on clinical examination, although it is likely both conditions could occur synchronously in the lamb crop. Lateral recumbency with extensor tone is observed in lambs with a cervical spinal lesion, typically vertebral empyema affecting C1–C6 in 1–4-month-old lambs. Pelvic limb ataxia occurs during the early stages of delayed swayback when lambs are 2–3 months old. Louping-ill is uncommon in lambs because of protection afforded by maternally-derived antibody.

Seizure activity and opisthotonus are observed during the agonal stages of bacterial meningoencephalitis, which most commonly affects 2–3-week-old lambs. Bacterial meningoencephalitis occurs only sporadically in lambs and never as an outbreak. PEM is not seen in lambs less than 4 months old.

Diagnosis

Diagnosis is based upon the clinical signs and history of recent castration/tail docking in lambs from unvaccinated ewes.

Treatment

There is no effective treatment and all affected lambs should be euthanased for welfare reasons. Treatment with high doses of penicillin and tetanus anti-toxin accompanied by wound debridement has been described in textbooks. Theoretically, large doses of tetanus anti-toxin is given slowly intravenously (lambs 12,500 IU daily) until a treatment response is observed. Injection at the site of suspected infection has also been recommended. While intrathecal tetanus anti-toxin injection has been described in cattle and horses, and could be achieved in lambs, there is no conclusive evidence of its greater efficacy by this route.

Focal symmetrical encephalomalacia
Definition/overview

Focal symmetrical encephalomalacia (FSE) occurs sporadically in unvaccinated sheep, more commonly in young lambs and in lambs after weaning. It is reported that disease more commonly affects sheep in poor condition, and may occur following dietary change and/or anthelmintic treatment.

Aetiology
C. perfringens type D.

Clinical presentation
The clinical signs are poorly defined but include depression, lethargy, separation from other sheep in the group with progression to ataxia, recumbency, opisthotonus and death after a few days.

Differential diagnoses
- Louping-ill could occur in sheep introduced onto hill pasture with autumn tick activity. Polioencephalomalacia is common in weaned lambs more than 4 months old, often occurring following pasture change.
- Hepatic encephalopathy has been described in severely cobalt-deficient lambs. Nephrosis is uncommon in lambs more than 3 months old but presents with many of the early clinical signs of FSE.

Diagnosis
Diagnosis is based upon clinical signs in sheep from unvaccinated flocks, with confirmation following histological examination of brain tissue.

Treatment
There is no treatment for FSE.

Botulism
Definition/overview
Botulism is much less frequently diagnosed in sheep than in horses and cattle, despite the recent upsurge in feeding big-bale silage to sheep in the UK. The feeding of ensiled poultry manure has caused serious losses in cattle on individual properties but this practice is never undertaken on sheep farms. Sporadic cases of botulism in cattle have been associated with poultry litter spread onto pasture and neighbouring properties. There are rare reported flock outbreaks of botulism in sheep, with very high mortality (150 of 500 ewes) occurring over 2 weeks after access to poultry manure.

The epidemiology of botulism differs in countries other than the UK; outbreaks, particularly in cattle, in other countries are associated with either pica in phosphorus-deficient animals on extensive grazings or prolonged starvation due to drought.

Aetiology
Botulism is caused by the ingestion of preformed toxins of *C. botulinum*.

Clinical presentation
Depending upon the amount of toxin ingested, affected sheep may simply be found dead. Clinical signs are confined to the central nervous system with ataxia and hyperaesthesia, and characteristic head-bobbing action. This state quickly progresses to flaccid paralysis and death.

Differential diagnoses
Diagnosis is difficult in individual sheep. Large numbers of dead sheep under extreme grazing conditions in some countries, including Australia, highlight the possibility of botulism.

Diagnosis
Botulism is uncommon in ruminants and sporadic losses may frequently be overlooked. The sudden loss of numerous animals with some of the risk factors listed above, and the lack of other plausible cause, may warrant further consideration of botulism, but sheep are rarely affected in the UK.

Treatment
There is no effective treatment. Disease can be controlled in those areas where botulism occurs by specific vaccination but it is not included in standard multivalent clostridial vaccines.

Management/prevention/control measures
There are well established vaccination protocols using toxoid vaccines which effectively prevent all common clostridial diseases; protection against botulism and *C. sordellii* is not provided by some polyvalent clostridial vaccines. Clostridial disease invariably results from failure to adhere to vaccination instructions and good management practices.

Prevention of pulpy kidney and the other clostridial diseases that can affect weaned lambs is achieved by two vaccinations 4–6 weeks apart, administered before weaning at around 4 months old. All purchased lambs must be assumed to be unvaccinated unless there is written confirmation from the vendor that this has been correctly undertaken.

A gradual change in diet, such as the step-wise introduction of concentrate feeding may reduce the incidence of clostridial disease, and is in any case sound practice to reduce the risk of acidosis, PEM and so on. Prophylactic antibiotic injections following unskilled correction of dystocia may reduce the likelihood of blackleg, but there is no reason why all sheep should not have been correctly vaccinated. Furthermore, such trauma in unhygienic conditions should not have occurred in the first place.

Economics

Clostridial vaccination is cheap and very effective. Initially two vaccinations are given 4–6 weeks apart followed by annual vaccination 4–6 weeks before the expected lambing date, to ensure adequate accumulation of protective immunoglobulins in colostrum. Lambs are vaccinated from 3–4 months old with the programme complete before weaning unless sold for slaughter before waning of maternal antibody at around 4–5 months old. Rams are commonly forgotten in vaccination programmes.

Welfare implications

Illness from clostridial disease has serious welfare implications, especially when there is no excuse not to operate an effective vaccination strategy and prevent such losses.

CHAPTER 6

CARDIOVASCULAR SYSTEM

CLINICAL EXAMINATION

The rate, rhythm and intensity of heart sounds are determined by auscultation over the chest in the region immediately beneath the elbow joints. It is essential to listen to both sides of the chest because unilateral space-occupying lesions in the cranial thorax frequently displace the heart, leading to a marked disparity in intensity and origin of heart sounds. The heart rate of neonatal lambs may approach 180 beats per minute; older lambs and adult sheep have a heart rate 65–80 beats per minute. Handling and other stresses may increase the heart rate by more than 50% but it returns to normal within 5–10 minutes. The heart can also be reassessed at the end of the clinical examination. While the heart rate is usually regular, it is not uncommon to find every fourth or fifth beat dropped in otherwise healthy adult sheep.

Peripheral pulses are not easy to find in sheep and are not usually assessed during the clinical examination; the femoral artery affords the best opportunity. Blood gas analysis, electrocardiography and echocardiography are rarely undertaken in sheep; echocardiography would be most useful in the diagnosis of vegetative endocarditis, the most common condition affecting the heart.

There are few conditions affecting the cardiovascular system in sheep; many reference textbooks do not include this body system. Congenital cardiac disorders are very uncommon in lambs. Unlike calves where ventricular septal defect is relatively common and can be diagnosed with a reasonable degree of accuracy on clinical examination, this condition is rarely reported in lambs. Septic pericarditis secondary to traumatic reticulitis, while common in cattle, is not seen in sheep. Vegetative endocarditis is encountered occasionally in adult sheep, although there are no specific reports of endocarditis detailed in the literature.

VEGETATIVE ENDOCARDITIS

Definition/overview

There are few detailed clinical reports of ovine vegetative endocarditis because, as described for cattle, vegetative endocarditis in sheep commonly presents with no audible murmur. Furthermore, unlike cattle, polyarthritis is relatively common in growing sheep, whereby this common pointer to endocarditis in cattle is often attributed to erysipelas or other infectious cause. The provisional diagnosis of vegetative endocarditis is based upon clinical findings of chronic weight loss, pyrexia and polyarthritis, with confirmation at necropsy. Such detailed necropsy is rarely undertaken in farm animal practice, leading to potential under-reporting of endocarditis. Lesions involving the tricuspid valve may result in ascites and peripheral oedema.

In this author's experience vegetative endocarditis is typically encountered in ewes 2–4 months after lambing. The occurrence of cases at this time may suggest that the uterus is one potential source of infection, but obviously does not explain endocarditis in rams where another septic focus must be the origin of the bacteraemia. There may be clinical evidence of concurrent focal infection such as mastitis in ewes with endocarditis.

Aetiology

Bacteraemia with localization in the heart valve; more commonly involves the tricuspid valve.

Pathophysiology

Vegetative growths on the tricuspid valve may be associated with dilation of the right ventricle and a thinner wall than usual. There may be evidence of bacteraemic spread to other viscera, such as the lungs. Right-sided heart failure has been described in association with vegetative lesions on the tricuspid valve.

Clinical presentation

Affected sheep typically present with depression and weight loss manifest as poorer body condition compared to other sheep in the group. The rectal temperature is elevated, typically within the range 40.0–40.5°C. The sheep spends long periods in sternal recumbency (**Fig. 6.1**) and, when standing, adopts a roached-back appearance and continually shifts weight from one limb to another (**Fig. 6.2**). The respiratory rate may be normal but the heart rate is often irregular and elevated to 100 beats per minute; no murmur is audible in most cases. There may be a marked jugular pulse/distension. Typically, there is effusion of the hock, carpal and all four fetlock joints but no thickening of the joint capsules (**Fig. 6.3**). In some cases there may be fibrin accumulation within the joint, but this is difficult to differentiate from pannus. There may be palpable enlargement of the drainage lymph nodes associated with these joints.

Differential diagnoses

Bacterial polyarthritis is the most important differential diagnosis but such infections are uncommon in adult sheep.

Diagnosis

Diagnosis is based upon clinical findings of chronic weight loss, pyrexia, and associated joint effusions, and confirmed at necropsy. Some vegetative lesions can be identified during ultrasonographic examination using a 5 MHz sector scanner (**Figs 6.4, 6.5**).

Treatment

Bacteriology of vegetative lesions is rarely undertaken although isolates have included *E. rhusiopathiae* and streptococci. Extended treatment of vegetative endocarditis with procaine penicillin for up to 28 consecutive days has been unsuccessful, with the diagnosis confirmed at necropsy (**Figs 6.6, 6.7**). As in cattle, a marked reduction in joint effusion follows dexamethasone injection in

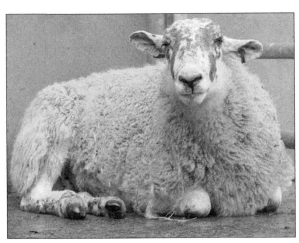

Fig. 6.1 Sheep with endocarditis present with chronic weight loss and spend long periods in sternal recumbency.

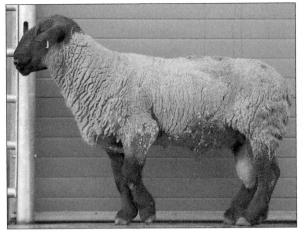

Fig. 6.2 Sheep with endocarditis are lame, caused by joint effusion.

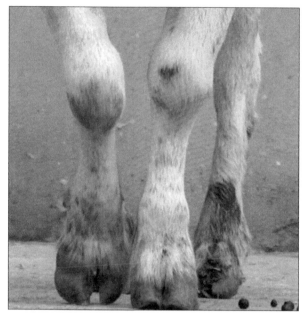

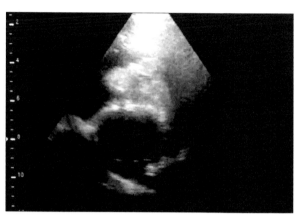

Fig. 6.4 Vegetative lesion (irregular 2 cm hyperechoic area) on the tricuspid valve identified using a 5 MHz sector scanner (see Fig. 6.5).

Fig. 6.3 Sheep with endocarditis may present with effusion of the hock, carpal and fetlock joints.

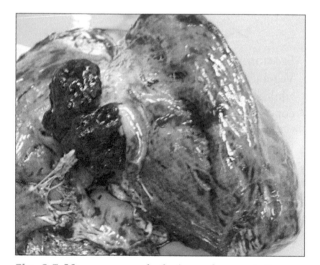

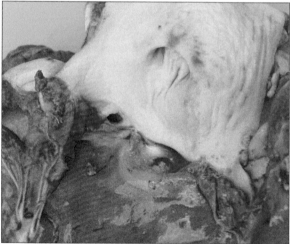

Fig. 6.5 Necropsy reveals the irregular vegetative lesion on the tricuspid valve identified using a 5 MHz sector scanner (see Fig. 6.4).

Fig. 6.6 Prolonged antibiotic treatment of the vegetative lesions affecting the aortic valve was unsuccessful in this case.

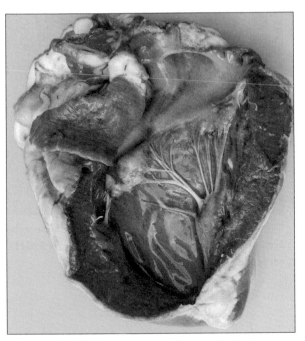

Fig. 6.7 Antibiotic treatment of vegetative lesions on the heart valves is rarely successful.

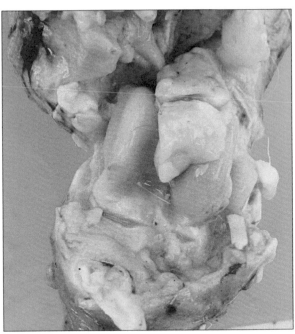

Fig. 6.8 In some cases the joint lesion comprises pannus rather than an effusion. This image shows pannus within an infected hock joint.

many cases, but the condition deteriorates after 2–3 days. In advanced cases there may be considerable fibrin/pannus within affected joint(s) (**Fig. 6.8**), which causes severe lameness.

Management/prevention/control measures

Prevention of endocarditis is based upon timely and effective treatment of focal bacterial infections, but these may, in themselves, not present with outward clinical signs (e.g. metritis, mastitis, foot abscess and bacteraemia from the gut).

Economics

Vegetative endocarditis occurs sporadically in adult sheep and is not a disease of major economic concern.

Welfare implications

The joint effusions associated with vegetative endocarditis cause marked lameness. Affected sheep should be euthanased for welfare reasons if their condition remains refractory to an extended course of penicillin therapy (at least 10 consecutive days).

CHAPTER 7

RESPIRATORY SYSTEM

INTRODUCTION

In many countries the perception of a high disease prevalence is widely held but the true incidence is not known; respiratory infections represented only 5.6% of sheep submissions to veterinary laboratories in the UK in 2008. The presumptive clinical diagnosis of acute respiratory disease caused by *Mannheimia haemolytica* and *Bibersteinia trehalosi* ('pasteurellosis') in growing lambs (**Fig. 7.1**) and adult sheep (**Fig. 7.2**) is based upon findings of sudden severe illness, inappetence, pyrexia, marked toxaemia and tachypnoea consistent with endotoxaemia. However, many other infectious diseases have a similar clinical presentation (**Fig. 7.3**). Respiratory infections often result from adverse physical and physiological stress (**Fig. 7.4**) combined with viral and bacterial infections; virus infection alone does not cause acute respiratory disease.

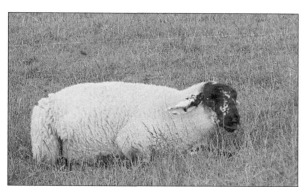

Fig. 7.1 The presumptive clinical diagnosis of acute respiratory disease in growing lambs is based upon findings of sudden severe illness and endotoxaemia.

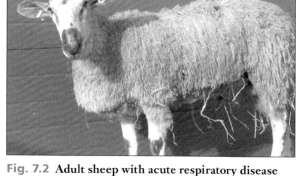

Fig. 7.2 Adult sheep with acute respiratory disease present with inappetence, pyrexia and tachypnoea, consistent with endotoxaemia.

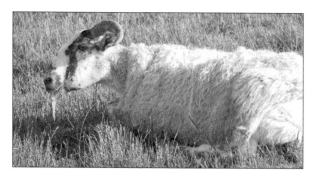

Fig. 7.3 Findings of inappetence, pyrexia, toxaemia and tachypnoea are consistent with endotoxaemia seen in many infectious diseases other than respiratory disease.

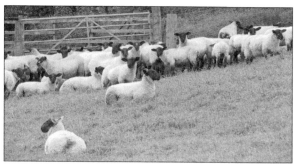

Fig. 7.4 Respiratory infections often follow physical and physiological stresses, such as dietary change and weaning, combined with viral and bacterial infections.

EXAMINATION OF THE THORAX

Respiratory disease is believed to be common in sheep but few specific conditions can be diagnosed by clinical examination alone (**Fig. 7.5**). In most veterinary practice situations the provisional diagnosis of ovine respiratory disease is based upon history, clinical examination and response to antibiotic therapy. Fortunately, many other infectious disease conditions respond to such antibiotic therapy. Occasionally, the diagnosis of respiratory disease may be supported by on-farm postmortem examination, but interpretation of necroscopy findings presents many opportunities for error and misdiagnosis (**Figs 7.6, 7.7**). For example, pasteurellosis is a common all-encompassing diagnosis in sheep practice; necropsy findings, however, require expert interpretation supported by histopathology and bacteriology, especially when several hours, possibly days, have elapsed between death and necropsy (**Fig. 7.8**).

History

Recent management events may precipitate respiratory disease including weaning, purchase, source, transport, vaccination status, housing, severe weather changes and diet (**Fig. 7.9**). The frequency of flock supervision will influence the accuracy, and thereby usefulness, of the animal's given history for the current complaint. It is also human nature to report that the sheep's illness has been shorter that its actual duration. In this respect, body condition score relative to others in the group may provide some indication of likely duration, although two conditions may co-exist. Alternatively, one disease may precede and/or predispose to another (e.g. ovine pulmonary adenocarcinoma frequently predisposes to a peracute episode of illness caused by *M. haemolytica*) (**Fig. 7.10**).

Visual inspection

It is essential to examine the sheep from a distance to observe their attitude, response to the observer, respiratory rate and effort, frequency of coughing and the presence and nature of any ocular and nasal discharges. Painful conditions, especially lameness, can have a considerable influence on observed respiratory parameters; therefore, it is essential to note the sheep's stance and gait.

During inspection of sheep under farm conditions, the respiratory rate is variably affected by gathering, handling stresses and body condition score. The presence of a full fleece in a hot environment can rapidly induce panting, which may further complicate interpretation of auscultation findings.

Clinical examination

At least 1 hour should elapse between gathering and veterinary examination and, whenever possible, the sheep should be left in shade. If doubts

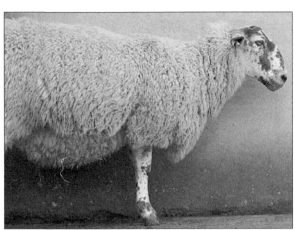

Fig. 7.5 Few specific respiratory diseases can be diagnosed by clinical examination alone.

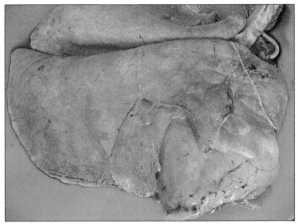

Fig. 7.6 Necropsy reveals the appearance of normal lungs.

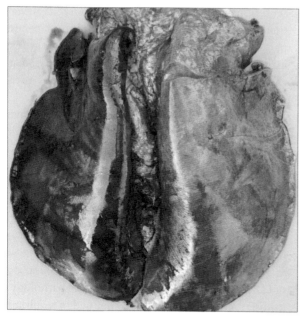

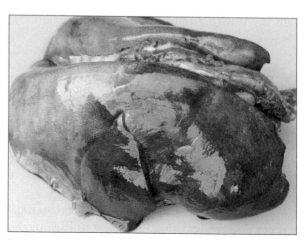

Fig. 7.8 Diagnosis of pasteurellosis requires expert interpretation often supported by histopathology and bacteriology.

Fig. 7.7 Necropsy performed quickly on-farm presents many opportunities for error and mis-interpretation; hypostatic congestion of the left lung could be mistaken for respiratory disease.

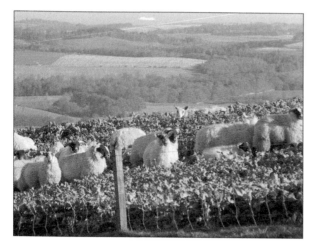

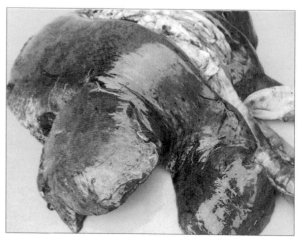

Fig. 7.9 Recent management events including a change of diet may precipitate respiratory disease in weaned lambs.

Fig. 7.10 Ovine pulmonary adenocarcinoma frequently predisposes to per-acute illness caused by *Mannheimia haemolytica*.

exist concerning the effects of recent exercise on a sheep's rectal temperature, it is essential to check some normal sheep from the same group which were gathered. Similarly, the rate and depth of respirations should always be compared with these normal sheep.

Increased audibility of normal breath sounds over the entire lung field can simply reflect tachypnoea, which increases the amplitude of breath sounds by increasing the velocity of airflow in the large airways. The common causes of tachypnoea excluding respiratory diseases are transport, pain, handling stresses in sheep with a full fleece during hot weather and endotoxaemia.

Adventitious sounds

Adventitious (abnormal) lung sounds are noises superimposed upon normal lung sounds and tend to occur consistently at the same stage of the breath cycle, over many consecutive breaths. There is a wide range of descriptors used in the literature for adventitious lung sounds in sheep, but the terms 'wheezes' and 'crackles' are used here.

Wheezes are prolonged musical sounds that usually occur during inspiration and occasionally throughout the breath cycle. They result from vibration of airway walls caused by air turbulence in narrowed airways. Wheezes are musical adventitious lung sounds, also called 'continuous' since their duration is much longer than that of 'discontinuous' crackles. They will typically last longer than 80–100 ms.

Crackles are loud, explosive, short duration (typically 10–30 ms), non-musical, 'rattling or bubbling' sounds. Crackles are possibly caused by air bubbling through, and causing vibrations of, respiratory secretions within the larger intrathoracic airways, including those that are pooling within the dependent part of the rostral thoracic trachea. Crackles are typically heard in sheep with ovine pulmonary adenocarcinoma (OPA), with fluid accumulations within the larger airways, bronchi and trachea.

Increasingly, authors of recent papers on ovine respiratory disease have not described auscultation findings but have referred to their distribution; no abnormal sounds recorded (score 0), abnormal sounds audible predominantly anteroventrally (score 1), abnormal sounds audible throughout the entire lung field (score 2), or have simply commented in a more general sense on the presence of 'loud and prolonged respiratory sounds'.

Routine interpretation of auscultated sound does not allow the presence of superficial lung pathology or its distribution to be accurately defined in respiratory disease. Focal pleural abscesses cannot be detected on auscultation alone (**Figs 7.11, 7.12**), which may explain why there are no clinical descriptions of this condition in sheep textbooks. Attenuation of lung sounds is recorded in cases of pleural effusion, pyothorax

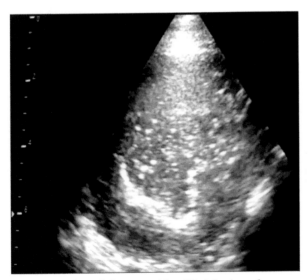

Fig. 7.11 Pleural abscesses identified during ultrasonographic examination cannot be detected by auscultation. The anechoic area containing multiple hyperechoic dots is bounded by the broad hyperechoic abscess wall 6–7 cm from the probe head (5 MHz sector scanner).

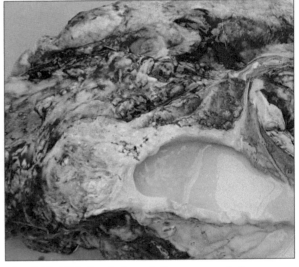

Fig. 7.12 This focal pleural abscess revealed at necropsy was not detected during auscultation of the chest.

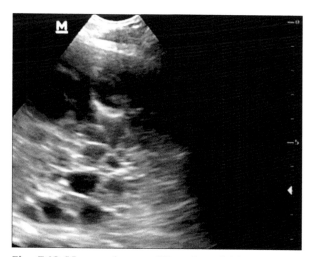

Fig. 7.13 No sounds resembling pleural friction rubs were heard in this sheep with fibrinous pleurisy. Ultrasonography shows the pleural space containing fibrinous exudate measuring 8 cm deep appearing as a hyperechoic matrix within anechoic fluid (5 MHz sector scanner).

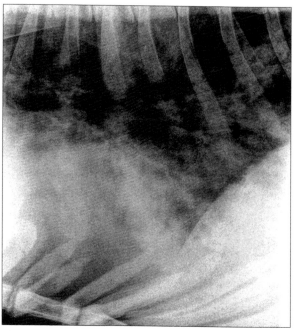

Fig. 7.14 Lateral radiography of the chest taken from a sheep suffering from ovine pulmonary adenocarcinoma (OPA). Health and safety regulations limit radiography in the investigation of respiratory disease on-farm (see Fig. 7.15).

and extensive fibrinous pleurisy. No sounds resembling the description of pleural friction rubs are heard in cases of marked fibrinous pleurisy (**Fig. 7.13**) or associated with pleural abscesses. Moderate to severe coarse crackles detected in advanced cases of OPA are audible over a larger area than lesion distribution identified during ultrasound examination.

Laboratory tests

Chronic respiratory disease is common in sheep but few specific conditions can be diagnosed by clinical examination alone. Changes in the leucogram, haptoglobin, fibrinogen and serum protein concentrations may indicate an inflammatory response to bacterial infection, but these changes are not specific for respiratory disease. Indeed, chronic suppurative pneumonia in adult sheep frequently arises following bacteraemia from another infected organ, such as the udder (mastitis).

Serological tests are available for some respiratory tract viral infections, such as maedi/ovine progressive pneumonia, but not OPA. However, sheep populations with a high seroprevalence of ovine progressive pneumonia may also suffer from another respiratory disease which may prove more important, such as OPA.

Radiography has limited application in the investigation of respiratory disease in sheep practice (**Fig. 7.14**). Ultrasonography, using both 5 MHz sector and linear scanners (**Fig. 7.15**) can yield specific information regarding the nature and extent of the lesions (**Fig. 7.16**) within 5 minutes, including skin preparation time, making this diagnostic imaging technique cost-effective.

Thoracocentesis

Pleural effusion is rare in sheep with respiratory disease. Fluid accumulation within the chest cavity may result from right-sided heart failure, but this is invariably preceded by large accumulations within the abdominal cavity (ascites). Prior recognition of pleural effusion by ultrasonographic examination is essential before ever attempting thoracocentesis.

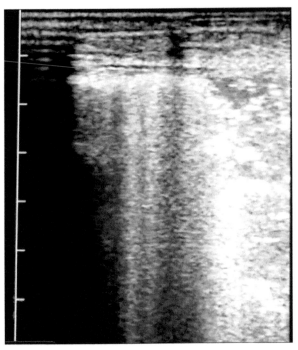

Fig. 7.15 5 MHz sector and linear ultrasound scanners yield immediate information regarding the nature and extent of the lesions, enabling specific diagnosis, in this case OPA. (See radiograph of the same case in Fig. 7.14.) Examination reveals an abrupt loss of the normal visceral pleura replaced ventrally by a hypoechoic area extending at least 6 cm into the lung.

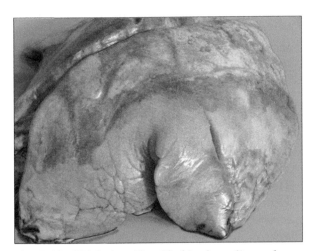

Fig. 7.16 OPA lesions identified in the radiograph in Fig. 7.14 and the sonogram in Fig. 7.15 revealed at necropsy.

This procedure can be undertaken under local anaesthesia using a narrow gauge needle; the length necessary is determined during the ultrasound examination. For example; the chest wall is typically 1.5–2 cm thick in mature sheep; a thick-walled pleural abscess may be 1 cm thick, necessitating a 4 cm needle or greater.

Broncho-alveolar lavage

Transtracheal broncho-alveolar lavage (BAL) is not routinely undertaken in ovine respiratory disease because respiratory pathogens can frequently be isolated from the major airways of healthy sheep with no respiratory disease. A recent study, however, reported that the detection of *M. haemolytica* and *Mycoplasma ovipneumoniae* and respiratory viruses was closely correlated with clinical disease. Sheep with clinical respiratory disease also had a higher mean percentage of neutrophils in the lavage fluid than did normal sheep.

Culture and antibiotic sensitivity testing are rarely indicated in ovine respiratory disease because the majority of respiratory pathogens remain susceptible to the commonly used antibiotics, such as oxytetracycline and tilmicosin. However, the major limitation arises from the fact that BAL results cannot quantify the extent of lung/pleural pathologies.

Radiographic examination of the thorax

Radiographic examination of the thorax is relatively expensive and necessitates health and safety precautions. In most situations radiographs would be taken at the veterinary surgery. Interpretation of radiographs is not as simple as for ultrasound images; nonetheless, a specific diagnosis can be reached in many cases (**Figs 7.17, 7.18**). The position of the forelimbs and associated musculature in the standing animal often restricts radiographic examinations to the caudo-dorsal thorax (**Fig. 7.19**); pathological changes associated with aerosol infection more commonly involve the cranio-ventral lung field. Physical restraint of dyspnoeic sheep in lateral recumbency to facilitate radiographic examination of the chest may exacerbate the clinical condition.

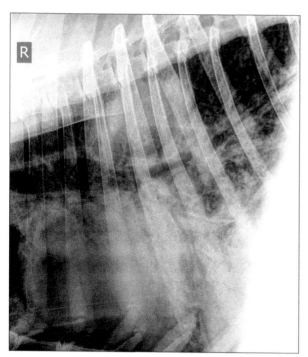

Fig. 7.17 Lateral radiograph of the chest permitting confirmation of OPA; note the tumour mass present in the dorsal lung field.

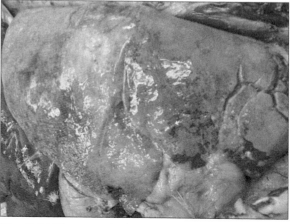

Fig. 7.18 Necropsy findings confirm the OPA lesions shown in the radiograph in Fig. 7.17.

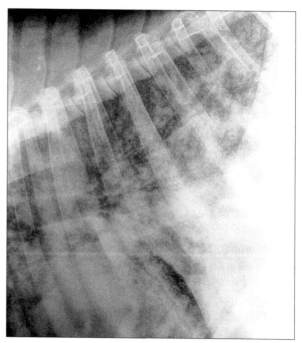

Fig. 7.19 The forelimbs and associated musculature in the standing sheep restrict radiographic examination to the caudo-dorsal thorax.

Ultrasonographic examination of the thorax

In many farm animal veterinary practices ultrasonography has been restricted to early pregnancy diagnosis in cattle, despite reports detailing the considerable information that can be obtained by ultrasonographic studies of the thorax and abdominal viscera, including reticulum, abomasum, liver, bladder and kidney.

Ultrasonographic examination of the ovine chest is inexpensive, non-invasive, takes less than 5 minutes and, unlike radiography, there are no special health and safety procedures or restrictions. Furthermore, the equipment is readily transportable, thus ultrasonographic examinations can be performed on the farm. A 5 MHz linear transducer, used for early pregnancy diagnosis in cattle, achieves sufficiently good contact to the chest wall to allow examination of the pleurae and superficial lung, although a 5 MHz sector transducer generally provides better images.

A 5 cm wide strip of fleece is carefully shaved from both sides of the thorax, extending in a vertical plane from the point of the elbow to the caudal edge of the scapula (**Fig. 7.20**). It is not necessary to use alcohol to remove natural oils/grease from the skin in order to achieve good quality sonograms. The prepared skin overlying the chest wall can be freely moved up to 5 cm, which allows examination of the caudal aspect of the dorsal lung field. The skin is soaked with warm tap water then ultrasound gel liberally applied to the wet skin to ensure good contact.

The transducer head is firmly held against the skin overlying the intercostal muscles of the 6th or 7th intercostal spaces, and the thorax examined in both longitudinal and transverse planes. The dorsal lung field is selected at the start of all ultrasound examinations in an attempt to visualize normal lung tissue, as this area is less commonly affected in the majority of ovine respiratory disease processes. The cranial thorax is scanned by advancing the transducer head from the 6th or 7th intercostal space to the next more cranial intercostal space once or twice as the transducer is moved down the chest wall. The ipsilateral forelimb can be held forward to facilitate access to the ventral aspect of the thoracic wall. The caudo-dorsal aspect of the thorax is examined by moving the transducer head two or three intercostal spaces more caudally from the 6th or 7th intercostal space to the 9th or 10th intercostal space. The ultrasonographic examinations are made with a depth setting of 6–7 cm, which includes 1–2 cm of chest wall. Good contact between the transducer head and skin overlying an intercostal space is evident by the intensity of the ultrasound image.

Interpretation of ultrasonographic findings

The sonograms are presented with the chest wall at the top of the image; dorsal is to the left and ventral to the right of the image. An air interface, created by aerated lung parenchyma, reflects sound waves and appears as a bright white (hyperechoic) linear echo (**Figs 7.21, 7.22**). The sonogram below the white linear echo may contain equidistant reverberation artefacts. The area visualized below the linear echo, including the reverberation artefacts,

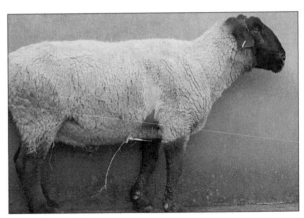

Fig. 7.20 A 5 cm wide strip of fleece has been shaved from both sides of the chest, extending in a vertical plane from the point of the elbow to the caudal edge of the scapula, to enable ultrasound examination.

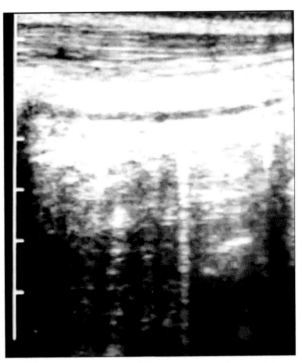

Fig. 7.21 Ultrasonographic appearance of normal lung where the aerated lung surface reflects sound waves and appears as a bright white (hyperechoic) linear echo 1.5–2 cm from the probe head (5 MHz linear scanner).

does not represent lung parenchyma. Air contained within a major airway in consolidated lung appears as a hyperechoic spot within the hypoechoic lung parenchyma.

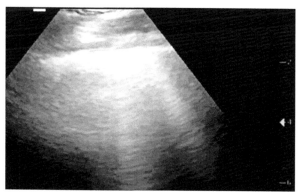

Fig. 7.22 Ultrasonographic appearance of normal lung where the normal aerated lung parenchyma reflects sound waves and appears as a bright white (hyperechoic) linear echo 1 cm from the probe head (5 MHz sector scanner).

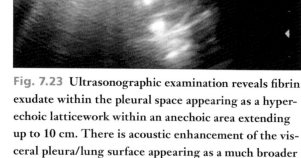

Fig. 7.23 Ultrasonographic examination reveals fibrin exudate within the pleural space appearing as a hyperechoic latticework within an anechoic area extending up to 10 cm. There is acoustic enhancement of the visceral pleura/lung surface appearing as a much broader white line than normal (compare with Fig. 7.22).

Ultrasonographic examination of fibrinous pleurisy reveals separation of the pleurae and lung lobes by a hypoechoic area with acoustic enhancement of the visceral pleura. In more severe cases the fibrin deposits have a hyperechoic latticework appearance containing hypoechoic areas extending for up to 8–10 cm (**Fig. 7.23**).

Pleural fluid transmits sound waves readily and appears as an anechoic area. Gas-filled pockets within an abscess capsule appear as bright hyperechoic spots within the anechoic area (**Fig. 7.24**).

Normal sheep

The surface of normal aerated lung (visceral or pulmonary pleura) of normal sheep is characterized by the uppermost white linear echo, with equally-spaced reverberation artefacts below this line. In normal sheep the visceral pleura is observed moving 1–3 mm in a vertical plane during respiration. No pleural fluid is visualized in normal sheep. The chest wall is approximately 1 cm thick in 20–40 kg lambs, extending to 2 cm in adult sheep in good body condition and with a reasonable amount of subcutaneous fat. The intercostal space is often too small to obtain good quality sonograms using most large animal ultrasound scanners in lambs <15 kg.

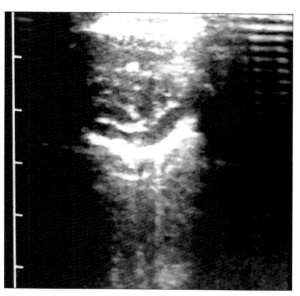

Fig. 7.24 Gas bubbles within a 2 cm abscess appear as many bright hyperechoic spots within the anechoic fluid, bordered distally by the thick hyperechoic capsule (5 MHz linear scanner).

Ovine pulmonary adenocarcinoma

The first indication of changes in the superficial lung parenchyma caused by OPA is the abrupt loss of the bright linear echo formed by normal aerated lung tissue (visceral or pulmonary pleura). This is

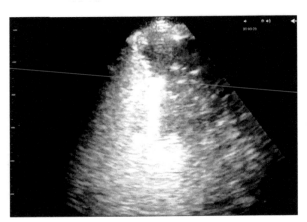

Fig. 7.25 Ultrasonography reveals a typical OPA lesion with sudden loss of the bright linear echo formed by normal aerated lung tissue (visceral or pulmonary pleura), replaced by a large hypoechoic area ventrally (5 MHz sector scanner).

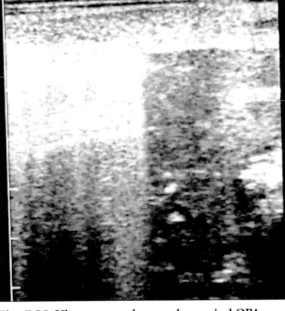

Fig. 7.26 Ultrasonography reveals a typical OPA lesion with abrupt loss of the bright linear echo formed by normal aerated lung tissue (visceral or pulmonary pleura), replaced by a large hypoechoic area ventrally (5 MHz linear scanner).

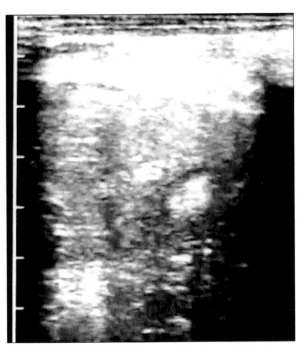

Fig. 7.27 Ultrasonography reveals a 2 cm diameter abscess within an OPA tumour appearing as a discrete hyperechoic circle with an anechoic periphery (5 MHz linear scanner).

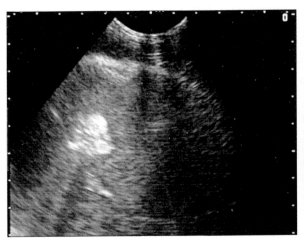

Fig. 7.28 Ultrasonography reveals either a 2 cm diameter abscess or necrotic centre within an OPA tumour; note the shadowing distal to the lesion (5 MHz sector scanner).

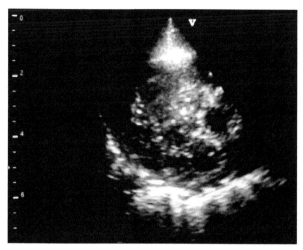

Fig. 7.29 The pleural abscess appears as an anechoic area extending to 8 cm, containing many hyperechoic spots bordered by a thick hyperechoic capsule (5 MHz sector scanner).

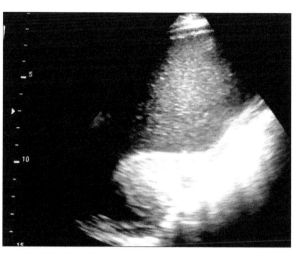

Fig. 7.30 The pleural abscess extends for 14 cm to involve one side of the chest (pyothorax) (5 MHz sector scanner).

replaced by a large hypoechoic area in the ventral margins of the lung lobes at the 5th or 6th intercostal spaces (**Figs 7.25, 7.26**). The hypoechoic areas visualized during ultrasonography correspond to lung tissue invaded by tumour cells causing consolidation, which allows the extent and distribution of the OPA lesions to be accurately defined during the ultrasonographic examination. Focal hyperechoic areas clearly identified within the more cellular-dense areas represent airways.

There are no appreciable ultrasonographic differences between lungs affected with OPA only and those with OPA and secondary septicaemia. Abscesses/necrotic centres are readily identified within the tumour mass; discrete hyperechoic circles with an anechoic periphery are typical of an inspissated abscess (**Figs 7.27, 7.28**).

Chronic suppurative pneumonia

Typically, there are large irregular hypoechoic areas extending 4–6 cm from the lung surface in the ventral margins of the lung lobes. The lung lesions are not clearly defined, as occurs in OPA cases.

Pleural abscesses

There is loss of the white linear echo formed by the visceral or pulmonary pleura and no reverberation artefacts are visualized. Individual pleural abscesses appear as uniform anechoic or hypoechoic areas extending up to 8–10 cm in depth, containing many hyperechoic spots (**Fig. 7.29**).

Pyothorax

With extensive pleural abscessation the lesion involves most of one side of the chest and may contain up to 3 litres of pus. The pleurae are separated by a uniform hypoechoic to anechoic area containing many hyperechoic spots, representing gas echoes within the abscess. The pleural abscess may extend up to 14 cm deep (**Fig. 7.30**) to involve all of one side of the chest (pyothorax), with the lung compressed to 1–2 cm thick against the mediastinum.

Fibrinous pleurisy

The visceral pleura (bright linear echo) appears thicker than normal and displaced from the parietal pleura by an area of varying hypoechogenicity, representing fibrin exudation (pleurisy) between the parietal and visceral pleurae (**Figs 7.31–7.34**). A hyperechoic matrix is present within the pleural exudate.

Ultrasound-guided thoracocentesis

Ultrasound-guided thoracocentesis can be attempted using a 5 cm 19 gauge hypodermic needle. The skin

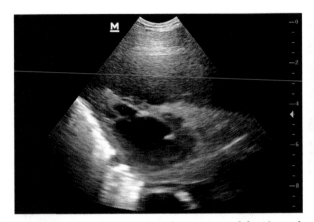

Fig. 7.31 There is acoustic enhancement of the visceral pleura (bright linear echo) of the right lung which is thicker than normal and displaced up to 10 cm from the parietal pleura by an anechoic area containing large hyperechoic strands of fibrin (5 MHz sector scanner).

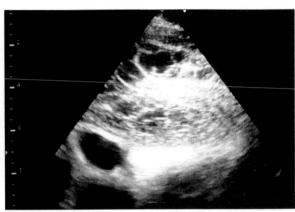

Fig. 7.32 Fibrin exudation (pleurisy) within the right pleural space presents as an anechoic area containing an extensive hyperechoic fibrin matrix; the lung surface is not imaged in this case (5 MHz sector scanner).

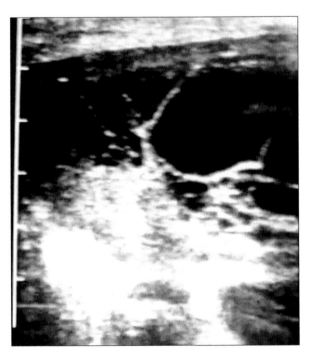

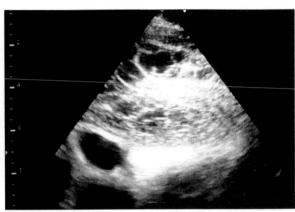

Fig. 7.34 Ultrasonographic examination of the chest shown in Fig. 7.30 3 months later; note there has been resorption of much of the exudate to leave a discrete 5 cm diameter fibrin clot (5 MHz sector scanner).

Fig. 7.33 Fibrin exudation (pleurisy) occupying the right pleural space; note the visceral pleura is not visible because of the limited field depth of the 5 MHz linear scanner.

of an intercostal space overlying the abscess, previously identified by ultrasonographic examination, is surgically prepared and along with the intercostal muscles infiltrated with 2% lignocaine solution. The transducer head is placed adjacent to the site where the hypodermic needle is introduced, but it may prove difficult to image the needle continuously. Care is also needed to avoid contamination of the prepared site and needle with ultrasound gel from the probe head.

ENZOOTIC NASAL TUMOUR

Definition/overview
Enzootic nasal tumour occurs in many countries worldwide but has not been recognized in Australia and New Zealand. Only sporadic cases have been reported in the UK.

Aetiology
The condition is caused by an exogenous retrovirus referred to as enzootic nasal tumour virus (ENTV). The condition can be transmitted experimentally by tumour homogenates, which would explain the widespread occurrence of this condition within some flocks.

Clinical presentation
Clinical signs of continuous mucopurulent nasal discharge and stridor are noted in sheep aged 2–6 years (**Fig. 7.35**). The tumour may be unilateral or bilateral. Occlusion of the nasal passage can readily be demonstrated by holding a piece of cotton wool close to the nostril. Weight loss occurs in those advanced cases with inspiratory dyspnoea. Rarely, pressure resulting from tumour proliferation from the ethmoid turbinates may cause thinning of overlying bone and deformity and, possibly, exophthalmos. Metastatic spread is uncommon.

Differential diagnoses
The differential diagnoses for nasal discharge and respiratory distress may include OPA and *Oestrus ovis* infestation. Stridor may also be caused by compression of the larynx by enlarged retropharyngeal lymph nodes associated with abscessation of the head. Laryngeal chondritis also results in inspiratory dyspnoea of varying severity.

Diagnosis
Diagnosis is based upon clinical findings and, possibly, prior occurrence in the flock. Endoscopy reveals occlusion of the caudal part of one or both nasal cavities by a greyish mass with a granular surface covered by mucus. Radiography reveals the extent of the lesion (**Fig. 7.36**). Biopsy of the mass

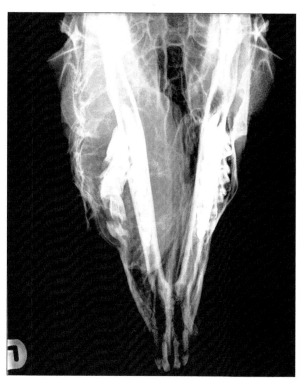

Fig. 7.36 Dorso-ventral radiograph of the anterior skull reveals the extent of the proliferative enzootic nasal tumour in the left nasal passages shown clinically in Fig. 7.35.

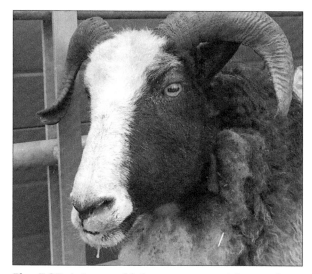

Fig. 7.35 A 6-year-old sheep presents with a continuous unilateral (left side) mucopurulent nasal discharge caused by enzootic nasal tumour.

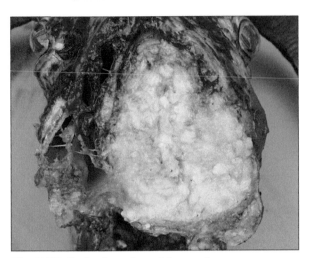

Fig. 7.37 Sagittal section of the nasal passages at necropsy reveals the extent of the enzootic nasal tumour affecting a 6-year-old sheep (see Figs 7.35, 7.36).

during endoscopic examination and subsequent histopathological examination confirms the provisional diagnosis.

Treatment
There is no effective treatment (**Fig. 7.37**) and affected sheep must be culled immediately because they act as a source of virus for other sheep in the flock, especially when closely confined. Surgical removal of the tumour is not indicated.

Management/prevention/control measures
Prevention is based upon strict biosecurity with all purchased replacement stock obtained from flocks with no known history of this condition. There is no vaccine available. In endemically infected flocks, all suspected cases must be isolated immediately and promptly culled once the diagnosis has been confirmed.

Economics
Enzootic nasal tumour is not considered a disease of major economic importance.

Welfare implications
Affected sheep must be promptly culled once the diagnosis has been confirmed.

OESTRUS OVIS INFESTATION

(syn. nasal bot)

Definition/overview
Oestrus ovis infestation has a worldwide distribution. There are only sporadic infestations in the UK restricted to the warmer south of the England and Wales.

Aetiology
Adult flies deposit L1 larvae into the nasal cavity. These migrate to the maxillary, frontal or palatine sinuses, where they develop to the third instar. Third stage larvae are sneezed onto pasture after 30–40 days where they pupate and emerge as adults 2–10 weeks later.

Clinical presentation
During the summer months, adult flies cause irritation to the sheep, demonstrated by frequent head shaking and sneezing. Larval infestation of the nasal passages may cause a mucopurulent nasal discharge and, in severe cases, stridor.

Differential diagnoses
Sporadic cases could be confused with enzootic nasal tumour.

Diagnosis
Diagnosis is based upon clinical findings affecting a large number of sheep during the summer months.

Treatment
Autumn treatment with ivermectin eliminates larval stages from the nasal cavity, thus preventing build-up of fly numbers.

Management/prevention/control measures
There are no specific control measures.

Economics
O. ovis infestation is not an economic concern in most situations.

Welfare implications

Prompt treatment removes any welfare concerns.

PASTEURELLOSIS

Despite different bacterial aetiologies, 'pasteurellosis' is the term commonly used by veterinarians and farmers to describe acute respiratory disease in both growing lambs (**Fig. 7.38**) and adult sheep (**Fig. 7.39**). *Mannheimia haemolytica* is considered to be of major economic importance to the sheep industry, causing septicaemia in young lambs and pneumonia in older sheep. *Bibersteinia trehalosi* (previously termed *Pasteurella trehalosi*) causes septicaemia in 4–9-month-old lambs (systemic pasteurellosis). *P. multocida* only rarely causes disease in the UK, but recent reports have described septicaemia in young lambs.

Diseases caused by *M. haemolytica*
Clinical presentation in adult sheep

Acute respiratory disease caused by *M. haemolytica* is uncommon in adult sheep unless there is a predisposing problem, such as OPA (**Fig. 7.40**). The clinical signs include acute onset depression, lethargy and inappetence, and are consistent with profound endotoxaemia. Affected sheep are typically separated from the remainder of the flock and are easily caught and restrained. On approach they may show an increased respiratory rate with an abdominal component. Affected sheep are typically febrile (>40.5°C), but periods of exercise before restraint may increase rectal temperature in normal sheep. There may be a scant serous nasal discharge. The mucous membranes are congested and there may be evidence of dehydration with sunken eyes and extended skin tent duration. Auscultation often fails to reveal significant changes

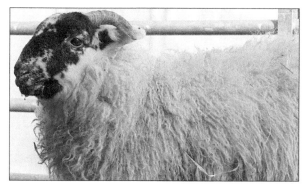

Fig. 7.38 'Pasteurellosis' is a term commonly used by veterinarians and farmers to describe all acute respiratory diseases of growing lambs.

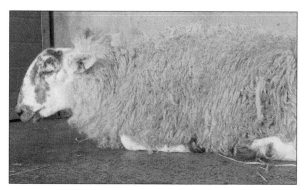

Fig. 7.39 'Pasteurellosis' is a common presumptive diagnosis of sick adult sheep, but is rarely confirmed at necropsy.

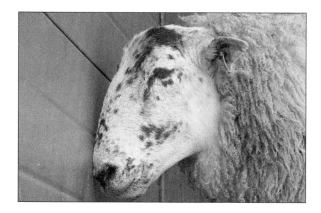

Fig. 7.40 Acute respiratory disease caused by *Mannheimia haemolytica* is uncommon in adult sheep unless there is a predisposing problem, such as OPA (see Fig. 7.41).

other than an increased respiratory rate. Rumen contractions are reduced or absent. There may be evidence of diarrhoea. Frothy fluid may be noted around the mouth during the agonal stages. In some situations, the animal is found dead. Ultrasonography fails to reveal any abnormality unless disease has been predisposed by OPA, when characteristic lesions are clearly visible.

Pathology

There are subcutaneous ecchymotic haemorrhages over the throat and ribs. The lungs are heavy, swollen and purple-red in peracute cases (**Fig. 7.41**), and the airways contain blood-stained froth. Cases of longer duration show anteroventral consolidation and fibrinous pleurisy. The lungs must be carefully examined/palpated for evidence of OPA.

Great care must be exercised when attempting to establish the cause of death in acute cases as many causes of sudden death, including clostridial disease, may cause heavy congested lungs.

Differential diagnoses

Clostridial disease must be considered in all cases of sudden death in unvaccinated sheep.

Acute bacterial infections of other organ systems such as mastitis, endocarditis or metritis present with endotoxaemia (**Figs 7.42–7.44**) manifest as acute onset pyrexia, depression and inappetence; however, these are identified during the clinical

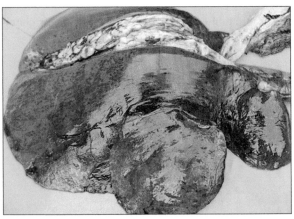

Fig. 7.41 At necropsy, the lungs are heavy, oedematous, and purple-red with ecchymotic haemorrhages following death from *Mannheimia haemolytica* infection.

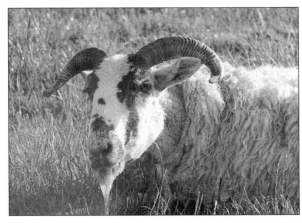

Fig. 7.42 Sheep with acute mastitis can present with clinical signs consistent with endotoxaemia.

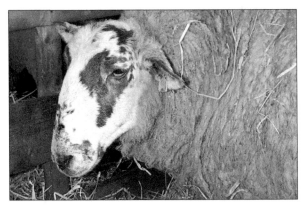

Fig. 7.43 Sheep with acute metritis can present with clinical signs consistent with endotoxaemia.

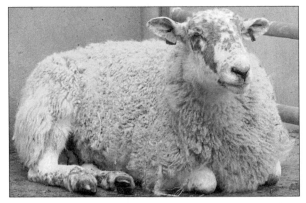

Fig. 7.44 Sheep with endocarditis can present with clinical signs consistent with endotoxaemia.

examination. Farmers frequently mistake hypocalcaemia for respiratory disease because affected sheep are apathetic, anorexic and, in the case of recumbent sheep, may have green-stained fluid (rumen contents) at the external nares. Subacute fasciolosis may present with some of the clinical signs listed above but anterior abdominal pain is usually present.

Infections of the respiratory tract include:

- Laryngeal chondritis.
- OPA.
- Pleuropneumonia/pleural abscesses.

Diagnosis

Diagnosis of respiratory disease caused by *M. haemolytica* is based upon clinical signs but there is no confirmatory test in the living sheep. At necropsy, testing whether lung tissue sinks (pneumonia) or floats (normal) remains a very useful screening test in field situations (**Fig. 7.45**). Confirmation of diagnosis is made following histopathological examination and culture of lung lesions.

Treatment

A good treatment response to antibiotic therapy necessitates rapid detection of sick sheep by shepherds. Oxytetracycline, administered intravenously, is the antibiotic of choice for pasteurellosis as there are few resistant strains in sheep, unlike in cattle. Tilmicosin could also be used by veterinary surgeons but is considerably more expensive than oxytetracycline. Extrapolation from other gram-negative diseases in ruminants suggests that injected intravenous injection of a non-steroidal anti-inflammatory drug (NSAID) should be helpful in countering endotoxaemia, but there is little published supporting evidence in ovine respiratory disease. Corticosteroids, such as dexamethasone, are used successfully in the treatment of peracute bovine respiratory syncytial virus infection because of the allergic nature of this severe presentation. Similar allergic-type reactions have not been reported in sheep and NSAIDs are the more rational treatment for endotoxaemia. A prescribing dilemma arises in those countries where corticosteroids are licensed for use in sheep but not NSAIDs.

An improvement in demeanour and appetite is expected within 24–48 hours of treatment, with a corresponding fall in rectal temperature to the normal range (e.g. from 41–42°C to 39.5°C).

Management/prevention/control measures

Following investigations to rule out OPA, prevention of pasteurellosis is best attempted using vaccines incorporating iron-regulated proteins. Since these iron-regulated proteins are antigenically similar, they confer cross protection against other serotypes.

Breeding ewes require a primary course of two injections 4–6 weeks apart, followed by an annual booster 4–6 weeks before lambing. However, this vaccination regimen only provides passive immunity to the lambs for up to 5 weeks. Lambs can be protected by two doses of vaccine administered from 10 days old, as colostral antibody does not interfere with the development of active immunity.

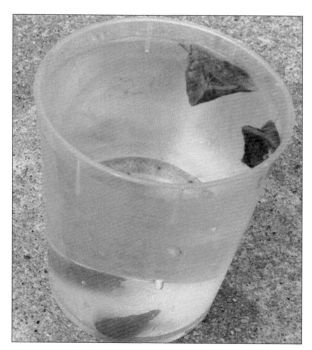

Fig. 7.45 At necropsy, testing whether lung tissue sinks (pneumonia) or floats (normal) remains a useful screening test for suspect pneumonic lesions.

Economics

The low cost of vaccine (ca. 25 pence per dose) should permit vaccination of all susceptible sheep where appropriate.

Septicaemic pasteurellosis

M. haemolytica also causes septicaemia in young lambs up to 12 weeks old.

Clinical presentation in growing lambs

This is an important cause of sudden death in lambs up to 12 weeks old. Typically, the best lambs in the group are lost over 1–2 weeks (**Fig. 7.46**) with no obvious predisposing factor(s). Some affected lambs may be found alive and are profoundly depressed and easily caught. They are pyrexic (rectal temperature often >41.0°C) with injected mucous membranes and marked dyspnoea. There is often a large amount of frothy saliva around the mouth and lower jaw.

Pathology

In peracute cases there are widespread petechiae over the myocardium, spleen, liver and kidney, with enlarged lymph nodes and congested and oedematous lungs (**Fig. 7.47**). Less acute cases are characterized by a considerable fibrinous pleurisy, which may be unilateral and extend up to 1 cm thick.

Differential diagnoses

Causes of sudden death include lamb dysentery and pulpy kidney in lambs which have not received sufficient passive antibody.

Diagnosis

Diagnosis is based on clinical signs and postmortem findings, including bacteriology from untreated cases (lung, liver, kidney, spleen, thoracic fluid and heart blood).

Treatment

Oxytetracycline is the antibiotic of choice for bacterial respiratory infections in sheep. However, the prognosis is poor because of the advanced clinical signs when animals are presented for treatment.

Management/prevention/control measures

M. haemolytica is an inhabitant of the nasopharynx of healthy sheep. It is important to limit potential predisposing factors that may trigger clinical disease such as handling stresses. Large daily temperature fluctuations and wet weather, however, cannot be controlled.

Maternal vaccination using vaccines incorporating iron-regulated proteins provides passive immunity for up to 5 weeks. Lambs can then be protected after two doses of vaccine 4 weeks apart from 10 days old.

Tests for the possible role of parainfluenza 3 virus in respiratory disease of young lambs has produced equivocal results. Good protection was reported in a UK study after intranasal administration of the

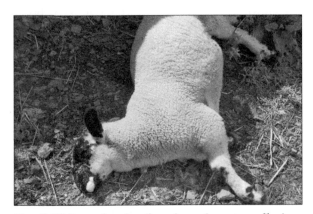

Fig. 7.46 In outbreaks of septicaemic pasteurellosis, some of the best-grown lambs in the group are lost over 1–2 weeks.

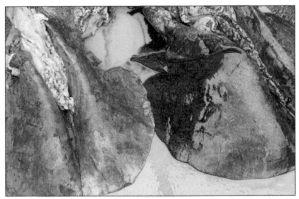

Fig. 7.47 Congested and oedematous lungs revealed at necropsy from a lamb that died of septicaemic pasteurellosis (normal lungs on left).

temperature-specific bovine intranasal PI3 vaccine to 2–3-week-old lambs.

Welfare implications

If there is no improvement within 12–24 hours, lambs in severe respiratory distress should be euthanased for welfare reasons.

Systemic pasteurellosis

Definition/overview

The disease is most common in recently-weaned lambs, occurring in the UK from August to December. Outbreaks frequently follow weaning, sale and/or movement of lambs onto rape, turnips or improved pastures. Gastrointestinal erosions and ulcers caused by dietary change may be the portal of entry for bacteria, leading to septicaemic disease. Outbreaks start with sudden deaths 7–10 days after the potential stressor(s), with the number of losses falling rapidly over the following 2 weeks. Mortality averages 2% but may reach up to 10% in severe outbreaks.

Clinical presentation

Systemic pasteurellosis caused by *B. trehalosi* is the most common cause of sudden death in lambs in the UK between August and December. Those lambs found alive are separated from the remainder of the group and profoundly depressed (**Figs 7.48, 7.49**). They stand with the neck extended and the head held lowered. The respiratory rate is increased, with frothy saliva around the lower jaw during the agonal stages. The mucous membranes are dark red/purple with injected scleral vessels. Auscultation of the chest fails to reveal any dramatic changes in lung sounds.

Pathology

There are subcutaneous haemorrhages in the neck and thorax and over the pleura, diaphragm and epicardium. The lungs are swollen (**Fig. 7.50**) with

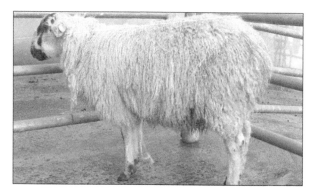

Fig. 7.48 Sudden onset disease in a weaned lamb caused by *B. trehalosi*.

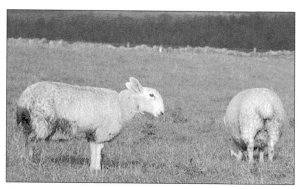

Fig. 7.49 Systemic pasteurellosis caused by *B. trehalosi* in a weaned lamb. The lamb is very dull and not grazing.

Fig. 7.50 Necropsy findings of systemic pasteurellosis caused by *B. trehalosi*; the lungs are swollen and oedematous.

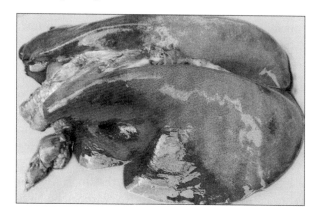

haemorrhages and blood-stained froth in the airways. There are necrotic erosions in the pharynx around tonsils, nasal mucosae and upper alimentary tract. The liver is congested and there are necrotic infarcts in liver, kidney and spleen.

Differential diagnoses

The clinical signs should be differentiated from other septicaemic, toxic or stress-induced conditions including clostridial disease (pulpy kidney, braxy, black disease), ruminal acidosis, Rhododendron poisoning, brassica poisoning and nitrite poisoning. Acute and subacute fasciolosis may present as sudden death.

Diagnosis

Confirmation involves isolation of large numbers of *B. trehalosi* from lung, liver or spleen.

Treatment

Oxytetracycline is the antibiotic of choice for systemic pasteurellosis. The prognosis is guarded because of the advanced clinical signs when animals are presented for treatment. Intravenous NSAID injection, such as flunixin, meglumine and ketoprofen, would help counter endotoxaemia but these drugs are off-label in many countries worldwide.

Management/prevention/control measures

It is important to limit potential predisposing factors which may trigger clinical disease such as handling stresses, long periods held in markets without food, mixing with other stock, repeated journeys to markets and sudden dietary changes.

Lambs can be protected by two doses of vaccine given 4 weeks apart, with the second injection 2 weeks before weaning/sale, but this has rarely been undertaken in most store lambs presented at markets.

Antibiotic metaphylaxis in the face of mounting deaths has produced equivocal results in split-flock trials in the UK, with benefit over cost in only one of 10 test flocks. Injection with either long-acting oxytetracycline or tilmicosin is often delayed until losses exceed 1%, with total losses unlikely to exceed 2%. The low financial value of many store lambs and high cost of antibiotic dictates that mortality must exceed 4% to be cost effective, without budgeting

for labour costs. It has been reasoned that stresses involved with handling and antibiotic injection may increase losses. Meat withdrawal periods must be observed after antibiotic injection; care is also necessary to avoid injection site reaction in lambs destined for slaughter within a few months.

Welfare concerns

The treatment response of severely affected lambs is very poor and these sheep should be destroyed for welfare reasons. Every effort must be made to convince farmers to vaccinate store lambs against clostridial diseases and pasteurellosis.

OVINE PULMONARY ADENOCARCINOMA

(syn. jaagsiekte, sheep pulmonary adenomatosis)

Definition/overview

Ovine pulmonary adenocarcinoma (OPA) is a contagious tumour of the lungs of sheep. It is also commonly known as jaagsiekte, ovine pulmonary carcinoma or sheep pulmonary adenomatosis. OPA is generally considered a chronic wasting disease (**Fig. 7.51**), with progressive respiratory distress leading to emaciation. However, it may be that early lung lesions predispose to secondary bacterial pneumonia causing sudden death despite antibiotic treatment (**Figs 7.52, 7.53**). OPA is common in the UK and most other countries where sheep are farmed, but the disease may be grossly under-reported because few deaths are investigated on sheep farms.

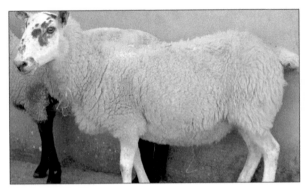

Fig. 7.51 Ovine pulmonary adenocarcinoma (OPA) is generally a chronic wasting disease with progressive respiratory signs over 3–12 months.

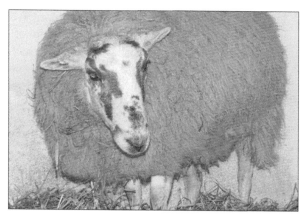

Fig. 7.52 OPA may predispose to secondary bacterial pneumonia causing sudden illness and death despite antibiotic treatment.

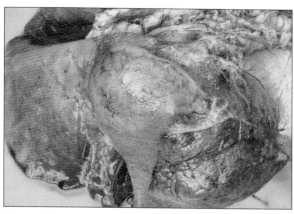

Fig. 7.53 Necropsy examination reveals that the fibrinous pleurisy is confined to areas of lung affected by OPA.

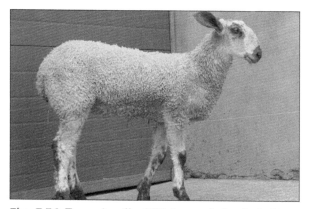

Fig. 7.54 Exceptionally, OPA is seen in lambs 8–12 months old where infection has been contracted very early in life; they are generally the progeny of infected dams.

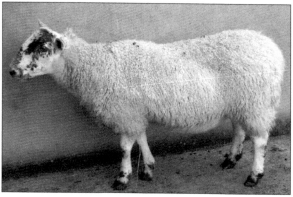

Fig. 7.55 Appetite remains good in OPA and affected sheep are bright, alert and afebrile.

Aetiology

OPA is an infectious neoplastic lung disease resulting from infection with a beta-retrovirus called jaagsiekte sheep retrovirus (JSRV). The virus replicates predominantly in the tumour cells and is released into the airways, and is found in respiratory secretions. Transmission of JSRV occurs predominantly through the aerosol route by inhalation of infected respiratory secretions, although the virus may also be transmitted via colostrum and milk.

Clinical presentation

The incubation period in naturally-infected sheep is long with clinical disease apparent in 2–4-year-old sheep. Exceptionally, disease is seen in lambs 8–12 months old (Fig. 7.54), generally the progeny of infected dams. The early clinical signs include exercise intolerance, manifest as an increased respiratory rate. Appetite remains good and affected sheep are bright, alert and afebrile (Fig. 7.55) unless there is significant secondary bacterial pneumonia. As the disease progresses, sheep become increasingly tachypnoeic with an increased abdominal component to their breathing effort. Fluid gathers in the respiratory tract, which first appears as a scant serous nasal discharge. A soft cough is often audible. Crackles may be heard over a wide area of the chest, although there is a lack of correlation between lung sounds and distribution of pathology.

Moderate to severe crackles are recorded in sheep with advanced OPA but are audible over a much larger area than the distribution of lesions determined ultrasonographically. The fluid that generates the audible crackles accumulates within the larger airways dorsal to the actual pathology, which may explain this apparent lack of correlation. During the advanced stages of clinical disease, when the tumour mass may occupy up to 50% of lung parenchyma (**Fig. 7.56**), a clear frothy fluid may flow freely from both nostrils when the head is lowered during feeding, and this quantity may exceed 50 ml if the hindquarters are raised when the head is simultaneously lowered (colloquially referred to as the 'wheelbarrow test'). This 'test' causes affected sheep considerable distress and must be discontinued as soon as some clear fluid appears at the nostrils. Euthanasia must be undertaken once this positive result is obtained (**Fig. 7.57** – note that this sheep had been euthanased before the wheelbarrow test and this image is for demonstration purposes only). It should be noted that not all cases of OPA produce this fluid in detectable amounts even in the advanced stages of disease. Therefore a negative wheelbarrow test should not be considered conclusive, although a positive wheelbarrow test is pathognomonic for OPA.

Death may follow a brief illness manifest as profound depression, inappetance and pyrexia (**Fig. 7.58**), secondary to infection of compromised lung with *M. haemolytica* (**Fig. 7.59**). Antibiotic treatment of such secondary bacterial infection often results in improvement of these clinical signs but this is only a temporary remission and affected sheep must be culled as soon as the disease is confirmed on ultrasonographic examination.

Differential diagnoses

A thorough postmortem examination must be undertaken on all ewe deaths to ascertain the significance of OPA within the flock because many losses attributed to 'pasteurellosis' may be predisposed by underlying OPA.

- Chronic suppurative pneumonia.
- Pleuropneumonia/pleural abscess.
- Mediastinal/lung abscess caused by caseous lymphadenitis (CLA) (**Fig. 7.60**).

These conditions would present with tachypneoa, possibly dyspnoea during exercise and chronic weight loss, but none show classical ultrasonographic images of OPA nor give a positive wheelbarrow test, noting the limitations of this latter test.

Diagnosis

There is presently no commercial confirmatory serological test for OPA. The polymerase chain reaction (PCR) test has been used in research on OPA for

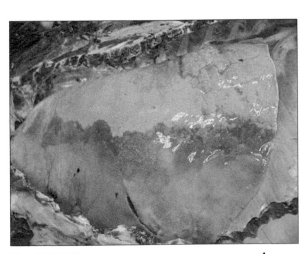

Fig. 7.56 The tumour mass may occupy more than 50% of lung parenchyma in the advanced stages of clinical disease.

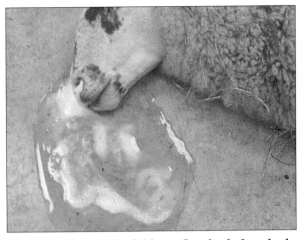

Fig. 7.57 Clear frothy fluid may flow freely from both nostrils when the head is lowered and the hindquarters raised (note this sheep has already been euthanased).

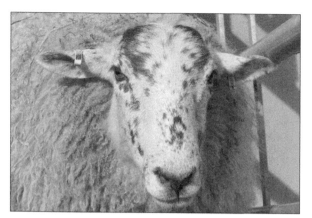

Fig. 7.58 Death may follow a brief illness manifest as profound depression, inappetence and pyrexia, due to secondary bacterial infection of OPA.

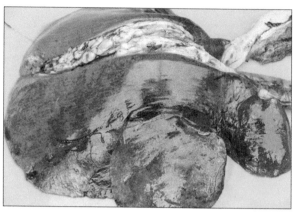

Fig. 7.59 Secondary infection of compromised lung with *M. haemolytica*.

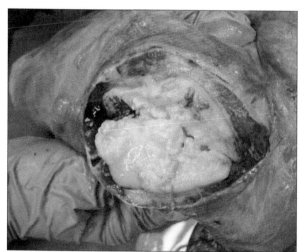

Fig. 7.60 Caseous lymphadenitis mediastinal/lung abscesses may also cause tachypneoa and chronic weight loss.

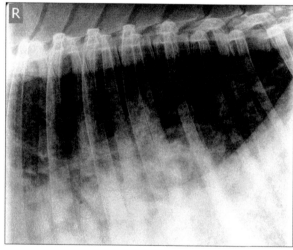

Fig. 7.61 Lateral radiograph of the chest. Radiography of the chest is limited to the caudo-dorsal lung field; this case was confirmed as OPA.

several years. However, while the test is highly sensitive in laboratory assays, it fails to detect JSRV in most infected sheep other than overt clinical cases. This is because there are few infected cells in the blood during the early stages of disease progression. BAL has been employed on sedated sheep in order to collect cells from the airways. Deoxyribonucleic acid (DNA) was extracted and the PCR detection method was used. Whilst the method appears to offer better sensitivity than the blood test, the sample collection method does not lend itself to large scale routine testing on-farm.

Radiography of the chest is limited to the caudo-dorsal lung field in the standing sheep (**Figs 7.61, 7.62**). Greater access to the lung field can be achieved by placing the sheep in lateral recumbency with the forelimbs drawn forward (**Figs 7.63–7.65**); however, such restraint may exacerbate respiratory distress. Radiography reveals the dorsal extent of the OPA lesion in advanced cases because only the caudo-dorsal lung field can be imaged, while the tumour mass is typically distributed antero-ventrally during the early stages of disease. Wider use of radiography on-farm is largely restricted by cost and health and safety regulations.

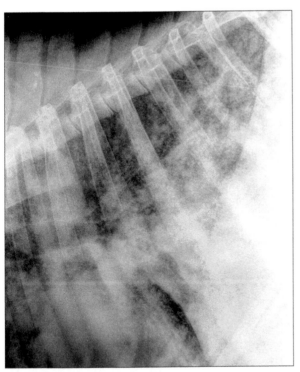

Fig. 7.62 Lateral radiograph of the chest reveals the typical appearance of OPA.

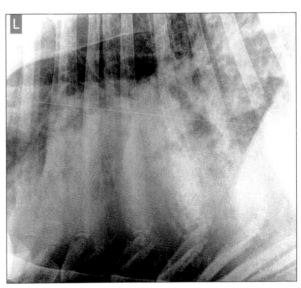

Fig. 7.63 Lateral radiograph of the chest. The sheep is placed in left lateral recumbency with the forelimbs drawn forward.

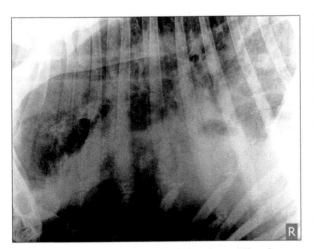

Fig. 7.64 Lateral radiograph of the chest. The sheep is placed in right lateral recumbency with the forelimbs drawn forward.

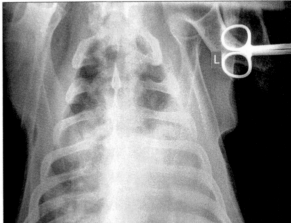

Fig. 7.65 Ventro-dorsal view of the thorax of sheep featured in Figs 7.63, 7.64.

Ultrasonography (see also below under potential control measures) can be used to differentiate most chronic lung pathologies and support a diagnosis of OPA, including superficial lung lesions as small as 1–2 cm in diameter (**Figs 7.66, 7.67**). The first indication of changes in the superficial lung parenchyma caused by OPA is the abrupt loss of the bright linear echo formed by normal aerated lung tissue (visceral or pulmonary pleura), replaced by a hypoechoic area in the ventral margins of the lung lobes at the 5th or 6th

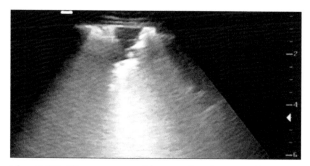

Fig. 7.66 Ultrasonographic examination can detect superficial OPA lesions as small as 1–2 cm (5 MHz sector scanner).

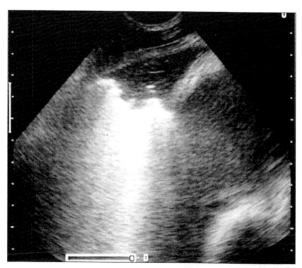

Fig. 7.67 Loss of the bright linear echo formed by normal aerated lung tissue (visceral or pulmonary pleura), replaced by a hypoechoic area bordered distally by a hyperechoic line delineating the OPA lesion (5 MHz sector scanner).

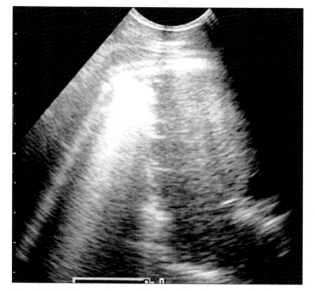

Fig. 7.68 Abrupt loss of the bright linear echo formed by normal aerated lung replaced by a large 7 cm deep hypoechoic area in the ventral margins of the lung lobes at the 5th or 6th intercostal spaces, representing OPA tumour (5 MHz sector scanner).

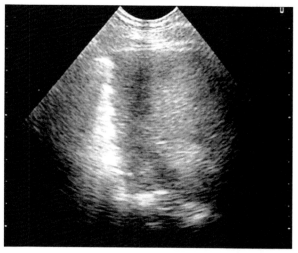

Fig. 7.69 Abrupt loss of the bright linear echo formed by normal aerated lung replaced by a large 8 cm deep hypoechoic area in the ventral margins of the lung lobes at the 5th or 6th intercostal spaces, representing OPA tumour (5 MHz sector scanner).

intercostal spaces (**Figs 7.68–7.70**). The hypoechoic areas visualized during ultrasonography correspond to lung tissue invaded by tumour cells causing consolidation. This allows the extent and distribution of the OPA lesions to be defined accurately during the ultrasonographic examination (**Figs 7.71, 7.72**). Focal hyperechoic areas clearly identified within the more cellular-dense areas represent large airways. While the

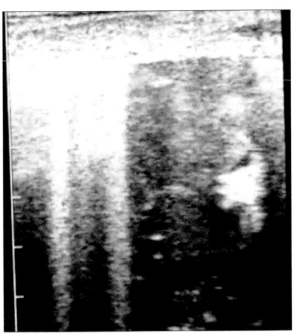

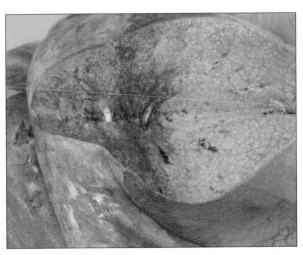

Fig. 7.71 The hypoechoic areas visualized ventrally during ultrasonography correspond to lung tissue invaded by tumour cells causing consolidation. The abrupt change from normal lung to tumour is clearly visible on cut section of lung tissue at necropsy.

Fig. 7.70 Abrupt loss of the bright linear echo formed by normal aerated lung replaced by a large 6 cm deep hypoechoic area ventrally, representing OPA tumour (5 MHz linear scanner).

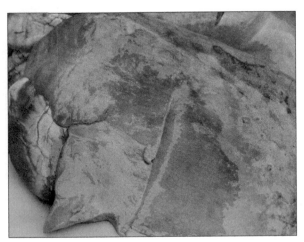

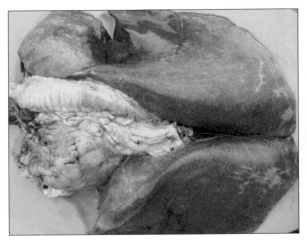

Fig. 7.72 The sharply demarcated OPA lesions evident at necropsy permit accurate definition during ultrasonographic examination.

Fig. 7.73 It is important to examine both sides of the chest ultrasonographically because the OPA lesions can vary considerably between lungs.

tumour usually affects both lungs, it is important to examine both sides of the chest as the extent of lesions varies considerably (Figs 7.73–7.75).

Confirmation of OPA diagnosis is established at necropsy. A thorough postmortem examination must be undertaken on all ewe deaths to ascertain the significance of OPA within the flock, because many losses attributed to 'pasteurellosis' are predisposed by OPA infection. Small focal OPA lesions measuring 0.5–2 cm will not be identified unless a

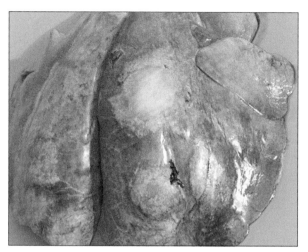

Fig. 7.74 OPA affects the right lung much more than the left lung in this case.

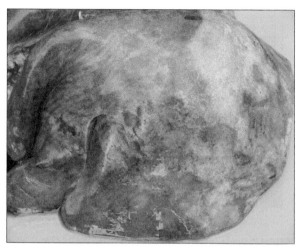

Fig. 7.75 Large OPA lesion presents in the caudo-dorsal area of the diaphragmatic lobe.

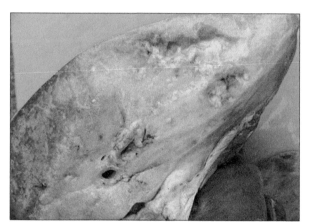

Fig. 7.76 Necropsy reveals an abscess or necrotic centre within this OPA lesion.

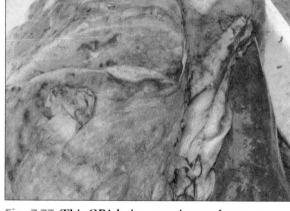

Fig. 7.77 This OPA lesion contains an abscess or necrotic centre.

methodical postmortem examination of the lungs has been undertaken. Careful palpation of the lungs should be undertaken to detect small OPA lesions before sectioning the lungs. In advanced cases the lungs are enlarged and heavy (>2 kg), with the tumours occupying the anteroventral lung fields. The tumours are solid, grey and sharply demarcated from normal lung tissue. These lesions may contain abscesses or necrotic centres (**Figs 7.76–7.79**) with associated pleurisy (**Fig. 7.80**). Compromise of the physical defence mechanism of the lungs may lead to the development of more extensive pleural abscesses (**Figs 7.81, 7.82**), but such secondary bacterial infection is uncommon. The bronchi and trachea contain copious frothy fluid. Histologically, tumour cells replace normal alveolar cells.

Treatment

There is no treatment and affected sheep must be culled as soon as clinical suspicions are confirmed by ultrasonographic examination of the chest. Antibiotic therapy, typically oxytetracycline, may temporarily improve the clinical appearance of those sheep with significant secondary bacterial infection.

Management/prevention/control measures

Currently there is no treatment for OPA and flock management practices can only reduce but not

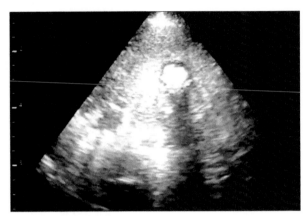

Fig. 7.78 Ultrasonography reveals an abscess or necrotic centre as a hyperechoic circular area measuring 1.5 cm in diameter, with distal shadowing within the hypoechoic OPA mass.

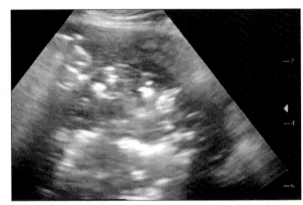

Fig. 7.79 An abscess or necrotic centre appears as a hyperechoic area measuring 1 cm in diameter, with distal shadowing within the hypoechoic OPA lesion.

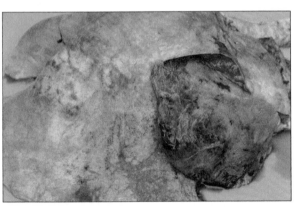

Fig. 7.80 Necropsy reveals that the fibrous pleurisy is present only over the OPA lesion; normal lung is unaffected.

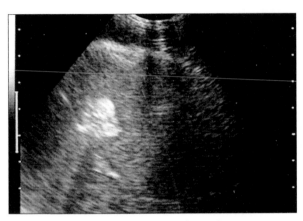

Fig. 7.81 Multiple abscesses, 1–2 cm diameter anechoic areas containing multiple hyperchoic dots, are present within the OPA lesion (see Fig. 7.82).

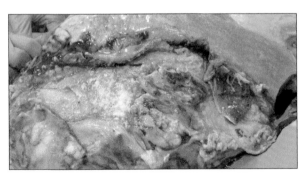

Fig. 7.82 Compromise to the physical defence mechanism of the lungs by OPA lesions may have contributed to the development of pleural abscesses.

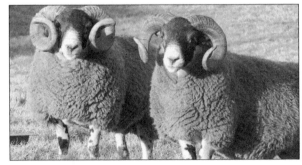

Fig. 7.83 Ultrasound screening of purchased rams should detect OPA lesions months before they cause clinical signs.

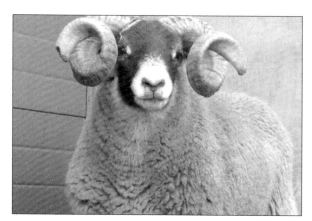

Fig. 7.84 Ram purchased 3 months earlier now presented for veterinary examination for suspected OPA. Note the bloom dip applied for the sale.

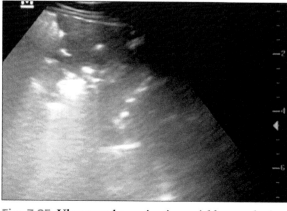

Fig. 7.85 Ultrasound examination quickly reveals significant OPA lesions affecting both lung fields (sharply demarcated hypoechoic area extending 6 cm into the lung parenchyma). This ram is a serious biosecurity risk.

eliminate losses to the disease. Therefore, good biosecurity is essential to minimize the risks of transferring OPA to unaffected farms via purchased sheep, especially rams. Ultrasound screening of introduced rams at the time of purchase should detect OPA lesions and remove potentially infectious animals; repeat examinations would be necessary at 6–12 month intervals to identify animals with undetectable lesions at the previous examination(s). With experience, it should be possible to detect lesions 2–5 cm in diameter reliably; larger lesions can be detected with accuracy approaching 100% (**Figs 7.83–7.85**).

Prevention of spread from neighbouring premises can be effected by maintaining a closed disease-free flock with double ring fencing around the perimeter of the farm. The main route of infection is by respiratory aerosol with close confinement during housing or trough feeding increasing the rate of spread of infection; therefore, housing must only be undertaken if essential for flock management purposes.

Regular flock inspection with prompt isolation and culling of lean and/or dyspnoeic sheep may identify early clinical cases and slow the spread of infection. Maintaining sheep in single age groups has been shown to be the most important management factor in reducing clinical disease. Feeding supplementary concentrates as large cubes on a clean area of pasture each day ('snacker feeding') is preferable to trough feeding. The offspring of affected sheep frequently develop OPA and must not be kept as replacement breeding stock.

A common experience is that the disease incidence in a flock appears to decline several years after the initial appearance of clinical OPA and the virus infection may appear to be 'silent'.

There appears to be a synergistic effect involving VMV and OPA and control measures should involve excluding entry of both virus conditions from the flock. De-stocking is the only practical solution when both infections exist in a flock.

Motherless rearing of lambs from an affected flock has been shown to be very useful in deriving OPA-free offspring. Recent developments in artificial rearing of lambs using automatic milk replacer feeding systems make this control measure a possibility for pedigree sheep farmers. Embryo transfer has also been mooted as a way to derive a clean flock, but is expensive and the transfer method raises welfare concerns. In the case of clinically affected ewes, their lambs should not be kept in any case as it has been shown that lambs may be infected *in utero*.

Vaccines for OPA are unlikely to be available in the foreseeable future. The failure of naturally-infected sheep to mount an immune response to JSRV has made it difficult to identify mechanisms of protective immunity that can be reproduced by vaccines.

Economics

Serious financial loss can result following the introduction of OPA into a flock, especially if the flock is housed for more than 2 months of the year. In an endemically-infected flock, OPA may contribute up to 50% of ewe deaths (up to 5% of adult sheep per annum), with considerable losses also resulting from an increased culling rate of suspected early cases and their progeny.

Welfare implications

Affected sheep must be culled for welfare reasons as soon as clinical disease is suspected.

ATYPICAL PNEUMONIA

Definition/overview

Atypical pneumonia is a non-progressive chronic pneumonia of housed sheep under 1 year old caused by *Mycoplasma ovipneumoniae* and, possibly, other organisms. The true prevalence of this disease is unknown because the clinical signs are generally mild.

Clinical presentation

The clinical presentation is reduced growth rate despite an appropriate ration, with an extended period to slaughter weights. Some lambs may show a reduced appetite but this may be difficult to discern because fattening lambs are usually fed cereals *ad libitum*. A chronic soft cough and mucopurulent nasal discharge spreads slowly through the group, most noticeable when the sheep are suddenly disturbed. Tachypnoea may be noted but this feature must be interpreted with caution as lambs fed high-concentrate rations frequently display tachypnoea. Painful infectious foot conditions in housed fattening sheep may also cause an increased respiratory rate.

Pathology

Lung changes are usually detected at the abattoir and consist of red-brown or grey collapsed areas in the apical and cardiac lobes (**Fig. 7.86**). Histology shows a lymphocytic cuffing pneumonia with pseudoepithelialization of the alveoli and hyperplasia of the bronchial epithelium. Abscessation of the lungs and pleurisy are uncommon.

Differential diagnoses
- Lungworm infestation.
- Pneumonia caused by other pathogens, such as *Pasteurella* spp.

Diagnosis

Diagnosis is based upon clinical signs and confirmed at the slaughter plant.

Treatment

Antibiotic treatment/metaphylaxis is generally not necessary because clinical signs are mild, but could be considered where growth rates are much reduced. Oxytetracycline (single long-acting intramuscular injection at 20 mg/kg) should be given to inappetent sick lambs. Mycoplasmas are sensitive to macrolide and fluoroquinolone antibiotics but such treatment is rarely needed.

Management/prevention/control measures

Control of enzootic pneumonia can be attempted by improvements in the ventilation, and reducing the stocking density. The airspace should not be shared with older sheep. Purchased lambs should be housed separately from homebred stock.

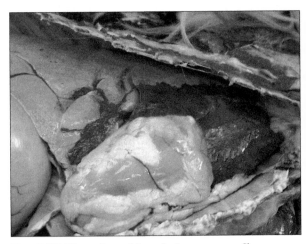

Fig. 7.86 Mycoplasmal lung lesions are usually detected at the abattoir and consist of red-brown or grey collapsed areas in the ventral apical and cardiac lobes.

Economics

Atypical pneumonia does not usually have a significant adverse effect on growth rate and profitability.

PARASITIC BRONCHITIS

Definition/overview

Unlike cattle, parasitic bronchitis is not a significant problem in sheep. Small lesions are commonly encountered at slaughter in healthy stock, and found coincidentally at necropsy.

Aetiology

The common nematodes that infest sheep lungs are *Dictyocaulus filaria*, *Protostrongylus rufescens* and *Muellerius capillaris* (**Fig. 7.87**).

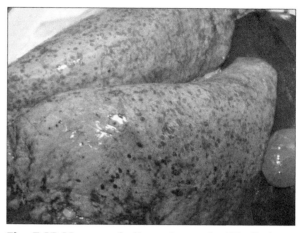

Fig. 7.87 Necropsy findings of extensive *Muellerius* spp. lesions in the lungs of a sheep.

Clinical presentation

D. filaria, and less so *P. rufescens*, may cause coughing but weight loss is very uncommon. Young stock are more likely to show clinical signs than adults, especially during late summer/early autumn. Heavy *D. filaria* infestations are commonly seen in adult sheep with clinical paratuberculosis and these may be the only sheep in the group with patent infestation. *M. capillaris* lesions are common in sheep lungs at necropsy but are of no clinical significance.

Differential diagnoses

Differential diagnoses would include atypical pneumonia in housed lambs.

Diagnosis

First stage larvae of *D. filaria* can be demonstrated by the Baermann technique in faeces of sheep with patent infestations. Adult *D. filaria* can be demonstrated in the bronchi and larger airways at necropsy (**Figs 7.88, 7.89**).

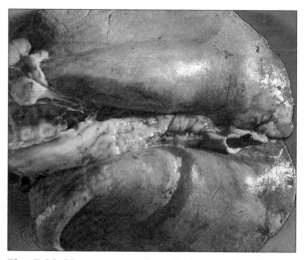

Fig. 7.88 Necropsy reveals typical consolidated lesions of *D. filaria* at the margin of the diaphragmatic lung lobes.

Management/prevention/control measures

Treatment for lungworm is not necessary and control is achieved by regular anthelmintics used in the management of parasitic gastroenteritis.

Economics

Lungworm infestation is of no economic significance.

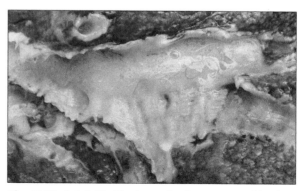

Fig. 7.89 Adult *D. filaria* can be demonstrated in the opened bronchi and larger airways at necropsy.

VISNA-MAEDI VIRUS

Definition/overview
Visna-maedi virus (VMV) infection is recognized in many countries worldwide. It was first reported in the UK in 1979, when seropositive animals were detected in sheep intended for export. The main economic effect of VMV in many countries is reported not to be overt clinical disease, but reduced production as a result of indurative mastitis and poor body condition, low reproductive efficiency, high perinatal mortality and poor lamb growth rates. In the USA the respiratory tract form of VMV infection is known as ovine progressive pneumonia.

Aetiology
A lentivirus infection causes respiratory disease (maedi), nervous disease (visna), mastitis and arthritis. The most important route of transmission of the virus is from mother to offspring in colostrum and milk. Other routes of infection may exist, but are unimportant in the overall epidemiology of the disease. The virus establishes infection in the lungs, udder, central nervous system and haematopoeitic organs, despite the immune response. The mechanisms whereby the virus escapes the immune response are complex and not fully understood. A large proportion of the flock (>60%) are likely to be seropositive when the first clinical case is diagnosed.

Clinical presentation
Clinical cases occur in sheep over 3 years old, and in some situations sheep have outlived their productive life span before overt clinical signs of maedi pneumonia develop. The earliest sign of maedi is exercise intolerance, noted during gathering. Affected sheep stand with the neck extended, flared nostrils and an increased respiratory rate, with an abdominal component to the breathing effort. As the disease progresses, wasting occurs and dyspnoea becomes obvious even at rest. Any exercise results in tachypnoea and mouth breathing, and if severely stressed, cyanosis and collapse may ensue. Auscultation of the chest is largely unrewarding. Sheep remain bright and continue to eat, despite dyspnoea and weight loss.

Although not a major presenting sign, a large number of affected sheep in the flock also have an indurative mastitis, identified as a flabby udder with diffuse hardening. Milk production is significantly decreased, although the milk produced appears normal. Associated lymph nodes are enlarged and show diffuse lymphoid infiltration and fibrosis.

VMV-associated arthritis is important in the USA, but to date has not been identified in the UK. A stiff, straight-legged gait, with swelling most commonly of the carpal joints, has been reported. There is lymphocytic proliferation over the synovial membrane.

Pathology
On gross postmortem examination, the lungs are firm, rubbery and heavy, weighing up to 2 kg (normal = 0.4–0.6 kg). On opening the chest the lungs do not collapse and impressions of the ribs may remain on their pleural surface. The lungs may exhibit mottled or grey areas. Histologically, there is smooth muscle hyperplasia with diffuse interstitial pneumonia, lymphoid infiltration and proliferation of the alveolar septae. Lesions are distributed evenly throughout the lung tissue. The caudal mediastinal lymph nodes are usually greatly enlarged with marked cortical hyperplasia.

Differential diagnoses
Differential diagnoses include:

- OPA.
- Chronic suppurative pneumonia.
- Pleuropneumonia/pleural abscess.
- Mediastinal abscess caused by CLA.

Diagnosis
Diagnosis on the basis of clinical signs alone is unsatisfactory due to the range of clinical signs of visna-maedi, and most cases occur in older sheep with concurrent infections. Death often results from secondary bacterial infection such as pasteurellosis.

Typical lung lesions may be masked at postmortem examination by pneumonic pasteurellosis or OPA. Histological diagnosis may be no more reliable as the lesions are not pathognomic, e.g. smooth muscle hypertrophy may occur with lungworm infestation and lymphoid infiltration with mycoplasma and chlamydial infections. Control can be attempted in an infected closed flock by regular 3–6 monthly serological testing, with culling of seropositive sheep and their offspring. However, this is a costly and a protracted protocol over several/many years. The sensitivity of available tests is low and sheep may seroconvert up to 2 years after acquiring infection.

Treatment
There is no effective treatment for visna-maedi.

Management/prevention/control measures
There are no vaccines, and vaccination is unlikely to be a control option within the near future due to the virus's ability to mutate around the immune response. Prevention of infection through adequate biosecurity measures and the purchase of VMV-free stock is the best option at present in the UK.

A strict culling policy and increased replacement rate can aid control in endemically infected flocks. Alternatively, control can be attempted by the removal of lambs from their dams immediately after birth before they ingest infected colostrum, thus breaking the lactogenic route of transmission. Artificial rearing systems using automated machines have greatly improved the rearing of young lambs such that this method is now a realistic option.

Economics
The true economic impact of VMV on commercial sheep farms has not been determined in the UK. Loss of VMV-accredited status would have potentially disastrous consequences in a pedigree flock selling breeding rams.

Welfare implications
Sheep showing respiratory distress should be culled for welfare reasons.

LUNG/PLEURAL ABSCESSES/CHRONIC SUPPURATIVE PNEUMONIA

Definition/overview
Lung/pleural abscesses and chronic suppurative pneumonia are common in adult sheep but are difficult to diagnose by clinical examination alone. Differentiation at necropsy is also difficult because there is often extensive fibrous and fibrinous pleurisy associated with the abscesses, such that it proves difficult to remove the lungs intact (**Figs 7.90–7.93**). The treatment for chronic bacterial infection of the lungs/pleurae is the same. Therefore, differentiation is of no clinical significance, not least as the cause of pleural abscesses remains unproven and therefore there are no specific control measures.

In young lambs pleural abscesses arise from inhalation of infection from the oropharynx, typically associated with *Fusobacterium necrophorum* infection.

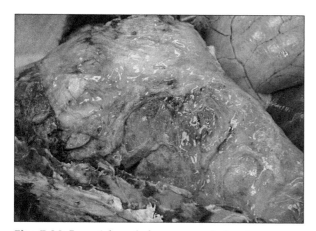

Fig. 7.90 Lung/pleural abscesses and pleurisy are common in adult sheep but are difficult to diagnose by clinical examination alone.

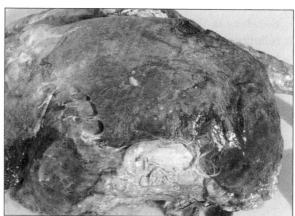

Fig. 7.91 Fibrous and fibrinous pleurisy associated with the abscesses shown at necropsy.

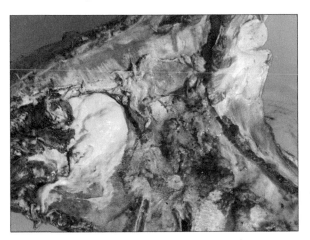

Fig. 7.92 Puncture of a superficial abscess has occurred when attempting removal of the lungs from the thoracic cavity at necropsy.

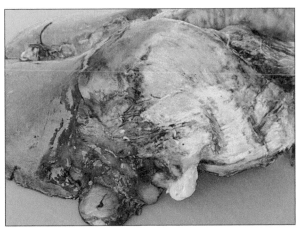

Fig. 7.93 Thick-walled abscesses and overlying fibrinous and fibrous pleurisy revealed at necropsy.

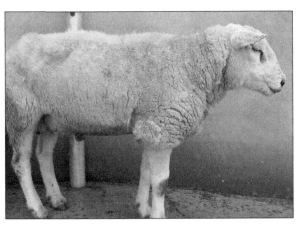

Fig. 7.94 Sheep with lung/pleural abscesses can present with a normal appetite and a normal rectal temperature.

In older sheep pleural abscesses are considered to arise from haematogenous spread from a septic focus elsewhere in the body, such as the udder, uterus or cellulitis lesion, but this assumption is unproven. In lambs, tick pyaemia is a common cause of lung abscessation.

Aetiology

Trueperella pyogenes is the most common isolate from lung/pleural abscesses and from cases of chronic suppurative pneumonia.

Clinical presentation

There is a wide spectrum of clinical presentation depending upon the number and extent of lesions (**Fig. 7.94**). Sheep with significant lesions present with a history of weight loss over several weeks to months but may only be presented for veterinary attention when they are dull and depressed (**Fig. 7.95**). Appetite may appear normal. The rectal temperature is often within the normal range or slightly elevated (up to 40.0°C). At rest affected sheep are tachypnoeic compared with normal sheep in the group, and cough occasionally with an occasional scant mucopurulent nasal discharge. Depending on the site and extent of the lesion(s), auscultation may reveal absence of normal lung sounds and muffled heart sounds. No pleuritic rubs can be heard despite extensive lesions in some cases (**Fig. 7.96**); no such sounds were generated with 10 cm of fibrinous exudate.

In sheep with unilateral pyothorax (**Fig. 7.97**), auscultation of the lung field on the affected side reveals an absence of lung sounds. Gut sounds, particularly rumen contraction sounds, are transmitted, when the

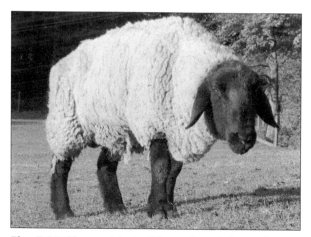

Fig. 7.95 Sheep with significant chronic lung/pleural abscesses typically present with a history of weight loss over several weeks to months.

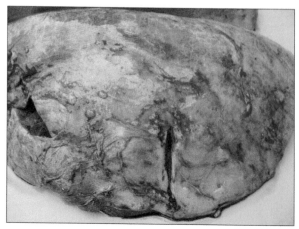

Fig. 7.96 No pleuritic rubs were auscultated in this sheep despite the extensive lesions revealed later at necropsy.

Fig. 7.97 Auscultation of the chest wall overlying this pyothorax revealed no adventitious lung sounds, only transmitted gut sounds.

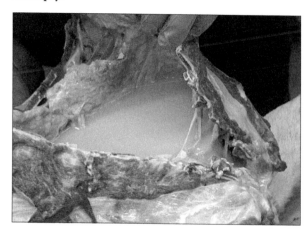

pyothorax occupies the left thorax. Auscultation of the contralateral chest reveals increased audibility of normal lung sounds. Heart sounds are increased due to displacement of the heart towards the unaffected side.

Differential diagnoses

In many cases it can prove difficult to identify the lung as the major site of bacterial infection. Therefore, the differential diagnoses should include the common causes of weight loss in individual sheep:

- OPA.
- Endocarditis.
- Mediastinal abscess caused by CLA.
- Paratuberculosis.
- Suppurative mastitis.
- Chronic parasitism including fasciolosis.

Diagnosis

Increases in acute phase proteins, including haptoglobin and fibrinogen, and serum protein concentrations may indicate inflammation caused by bacterial infection. However, these changes are not specific for respiratory disease.

Radiography: Bacteraemic spread to the lung field causing abscesses 2–3 cm in diameter could be identified by radiography (**Fig. 7.98**).

Ultrasonography: The hyperechoic linear echo representing the normal visceral pleura is lost with the

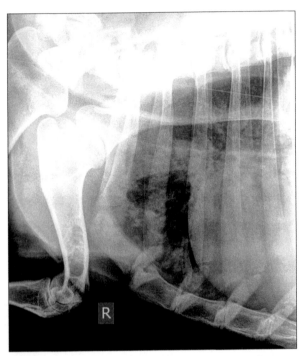

Fig. 7.98 Lateral radiograph of the chest reveals a large, well-encapsulated abscess immediately cranial to the heart.

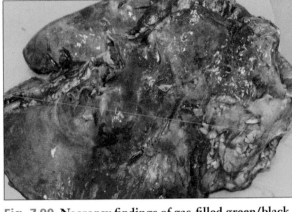

Fig. 7.99 Necropsy findings of gas-filled green/black abscesses might suggest the possible role of anaerobic bacteria in this case.

pleural abscess appearing as a uniform anechoic area containing many hyperechoic dots (see **Fig. 7.29**). These represent gas echoes and are bordered by a broad white line representing the abscess capsule. There may be focal areas of fibrous pleurisy associated with superficial lung abscessation but this is not commonly visualized.

Treatment

Penicillin is the antibiotic of choice for chronic respiratory disease in cattle and sheep because of the frequent isolation of *T. pyogenes*. Daily penicillin injection for 4–6 weeks, necessary because of the severity of chronicity of infection and time-dependent action of this antibiotic, has produced encouraging results in sheep with pleural and superficial lung abscesses identified during ultrasonographic examination. Treatment was successful in all six sheep identified with pleural/superficial lung abscesses measuring 2–8 cm in diameter, but only one of four sheep with more extensive lesions,

and one of three unilateral pyothorax cases. There have been no investigations into the possible role of anaerobic bacteria in some cases of pleural/lung abscesses (**Fig. 7.99**).

Management/prevention/control measures

Prevention is aimed at prompt treatment of bacterial infection such as mastitis, metritis and cellulitis lesions. *F. necrophorum* infection is not uncommon in orphan lambs reared in unhygienic conditions. Prolonged housing and respiratory viral infections are potential risk factors under UK management conditions.

Economics

The cost of daily administration of 44,000 IU/kg procaine penicillin for 4 or more weeks is £15–20.

Welfare implications

Sheep with significant lung pathology should be euthanased for welfare reasons.

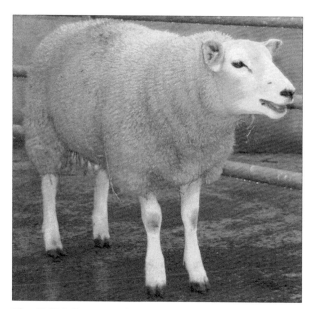

Fig. 7.100 Laryngeal chondritis is an obstructive upper respiratory tract disease characterized by severe dyspnoea, most commonly encountered in 18–24-month-old meat breed rams.

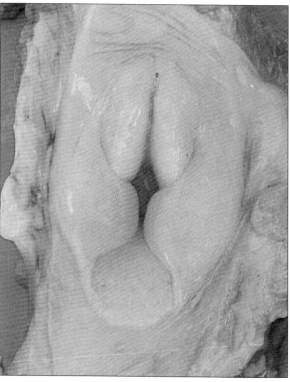

Fig. 7.101 Oedema of the arytenoid cartilages of the larynx resulting in narrowing of the lumen revealed at necropsy.

LARYNGEAL CHONDRITIS

Definition/overview
Laryngeal chondritis is an obstructive upper respiratory tract disease characterized by severe dyspnoea, most commonly encountered in 18–24-month-old meat breed rams (**Fig. 7.100**) during the late summer and autumn months. It is often associated with high levels of concentrate feeding in preparation for sale; the condition is rare in ewes.

Aetiology
T. pyogenes is a common isolate from cases of laryngeal chondritis.

Clinical presentation
There is acute onset severe respiratory distress with marked inspiratory effort and stertor caused by oedema of the arytenoid cartilages of the larynx, resulting in narrowing of the lumen (**Fig. 7.101**). Affected sheep stand with the neck extended, head held lowered with flared nostrils, mouth open and are reluctant to move due to dyspneoa. Delayed identification and/or inadequate duration of antibiotic therapy may result in abscess formation within the arytenoid cartilages (**Figs 7.102, 7.103**).

Treatment
Treatment involves intravenous/intramuscular injection of dexamethasone once only at presentation to reduce laryngeal oedema, and intramuscular injections of a broad-spectrum antibiotic for at least 7–10 consecutive days. Lincomycin is reported to be the drug of choice but may not be licensed for use in sheep in many countries.

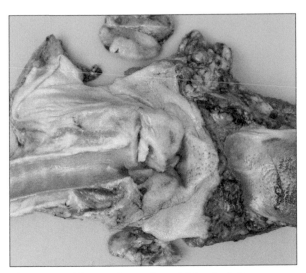

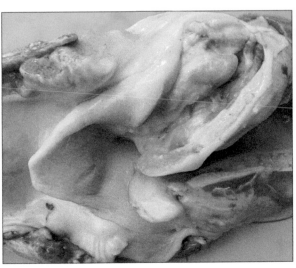

Fig. 7.102 Abscess formation within the left arytenoid cartilage and associated enlargement of the retropharyngeal lymph node revealed at necropsy.

Fig. 7.103 Swelling and abscessation of the right arytenoid cartilage revealed at necropsy.

Management/prevention/control measures

The sporadic occurrence of laryngeal chondritis means that little constructive advice can be given to breeders regarding prevention. Reducing the level of supplementary feeding may reduce the prevalence of this problem, but farmers are most reluctant not to have rams in top condition for the sales. Reducing dust in the environment is considered an important preventive measure but may be difficult, if not impossible, to achieve in practice. Some breeders recognize a higher incidence of laryngeal chondritis in certain genetic lines.

CHAPTER 8

NEUROLOGICAL DISEASES

INTRODUCTION

The central nervous system (CNS) consists of the brain (encephalo) and spinal cord (myelo). Nerve cell bodies form the grey matter (polio) and collections of nerve cell processes make up the white matter (leuco).

Rapid diagnosis permits appropriate therapy early in the clinical course of disease (**Fig. 8.1**) before irreversible changes occur (**Fig. 8.2**), as a number of factors unique to the CNS considerably hinder treatment. These factors include:

- Lack of effective drainage: the CNS is enclosed within the bony skull and vertebral column rendering the delicate nervous tissue susceptible to internal pressure changes.
- Low white cell counts in cerebrospinal fluid (CSF) restrict defences against bacterial infection.
- Lack of complement within the CSF.

- Poor penetration of the blood–brain barrier by antibiotics. Few antibiotics are capable of achieving minimum bactericidal concentrations (MBCs) within the CSF at recommended dose rates.

Increased intracranial pressure may result from pathological haemorrhage following trauma, which can be associated with dystocia in neonates or fighting injuries, especially in rams during the autumn. Cerebral oedema is classically seen in polioencephalomalacia (PEM). Increased CSF pressure associated with impaired drainage is most commonly seen associated with meningitis.

CLINICAL EXAMINATION

It is important to perform a complete clinical examination in order that important clinical signs are not overlooked. Rectal temperature is not a useful guide to infectious conditions of the CNS as most diseases

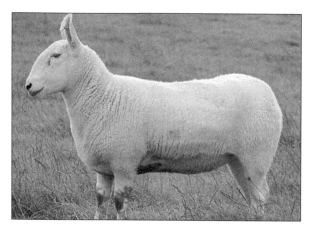

Fig. 8.1 Rapid diagnosis during the early stages of polioencephalomalacia (PEM) greatly improves prognosis (see Fig. 8.2).

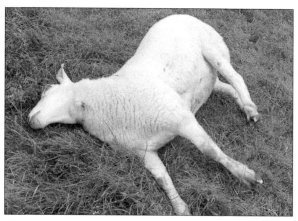

Fig. 8.2 Treatment of PEM must begin before irreversible changes take place (see Fig. 8.1).

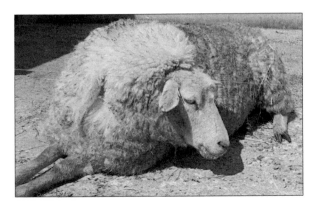

Fig. 8.3 Sheep that are comatose at veterinary examination may present with a subnormal rectal temperature.

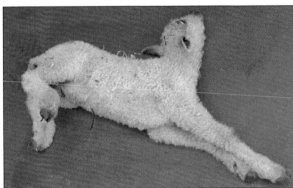

Fig. 8.4 Muscle activity and seizures, as observed in neonatal bacterial meningoencephalitis, may raise the rectal temperature.

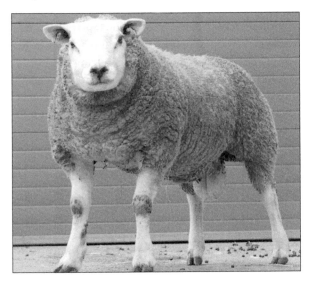

Fig. 8.5 Many neurological diseases have a breed, sex, age and management system predisposition, such as compressive cervical myelopathy in yearling Texel rams.

are afebrile. Cases of listeriosis that are comatose at veterinary examination may present with a subnormal rectal temperature (**Fig. 8.3**). Conversely, muscle activity and seizure activity, as observed in advanced PEM and neonatal bacterial meningoencephalitis (**Fig. 8.4**), may raise the rectal temperature. Many neurological diseases have a breed, sex, age and management system predisposition (**Fig. 8.5**). It is essential to inspect the group as subtle changes in others may not have been noticed by the farmer.

It is important to ascertain recent management changes, particularly changes in the animals' environment and nutrition, the duration of clinical signs and rate of deterioration in the sheep's clinical condition.

NEUROLOGICAL SYNDROMES

The brain is conveniently divided into six 'areas', each with a recognized neurological 'syndrome', although some overlap in clinical signs may result because of the complex pathways within the brain. Only four neurological syndromes – cerebral, cerebellar, pontomedullary (brainstem) and vestibular – concern the veterinary practitioner; the midbrain and hypothalamic syndromes are uncommon in ruminant species.

Cerebral syndrome

Cerebral dysfunction is the most common neurological syndrome encountered in sheep. The cerebrum is concerned with mental state, behaviour and, in conjunction with the eye and optic nerve (II), vision. Clinical signs that suggest cerebral dysfunction include:

- Blindness (**Fig. 8.6**) but with normal pupillary light reflex.
- Circling, constant chewing movements.
- Severe depression, dementia, yawning, walking forward (**Fig. 8.7**).
- Hyperaesthesia to auditory and tactile stimuli, seizures and opisthotonus (**Fig. 8.8**).
- Contralateral proprioceptive defects.

The common conditions that present with diffuse cerebral dysfunction include PEM, bacterial meningitis and ovine pregnancy toxaemia. Clinical signs attributable to a cerebral lesion localized to one cerebral hemisphere are seen in space-occupying lesions, such as a brain abscess or coenurosis, and include compulsive circling, deviation of the head (not a head tilt), and contralateral blindness and proprioceptive deficits.

Approximately 90% of efferent nerve fibres cross at the optic chiasma; therefore, animals with a left-sided space-occupying lesion would be blind in the right eye. The pupillary light reflex would be normal.

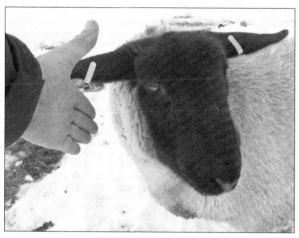

Fig. 8.6 Blindness (lack of menace response demonstrated) and altered mental state suggest cerebral dysfunction.

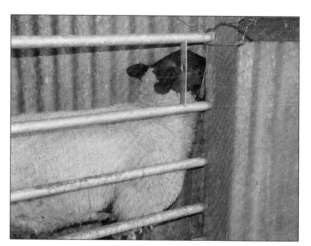

Fig. 8.7 Severe depression and walking forward are commonly associated with cerebral dysfunction.

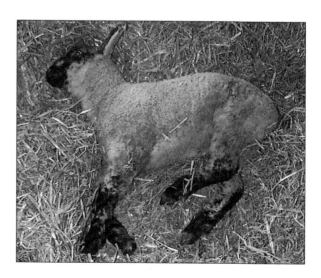

Fig. 8.8 Clinical signs of cerebral dysfunction can progress to hyperaesthesia, seizures and opisthotonus.

The menace response is not always reliable in cases of unilateral space-occupying lesions and this test can be supplemented with unilateral blindfolding.

Cerebellar syndrome

The cerebellum is primarily concerned with fine co-ordination of voluntary movement. In cerebellar disease all limb movements are spastic (rigid), clumsy and jerky. Initiation of movement is delayed and may be accompanied by tremors.

Cerebellar disease is characterized by a wide-based stance and ataxia (incoordination), particularly of the hindlimbs but with preservation of normal muscle strength. In addition to ataxia, dysmetria (problems associated with stride) may be observed. Hypermetria, or overstepping, a Hackney-type gait, is the more common form of dysmetria observed in cerebellar disease. Hypermetria may also be observed in spinal cord disease or affecting the contralateral limb in vestibular disease. With hypometria the animal will frequently drag the dorsal aspect of the hoof along the ground.

Cerebellar disease may result in jerky movements of the head, especially when the animal is aroused, or at feeding times when affected animals will often overshoot the feed bowl. This condition is often referred to as 'intention tremors'. This clinical feature is most commonly seen in general practice in cases of congenital Border disease, a virus infection affecting neonatal lambs.

Vestibular syndrome

The major clinical sign associated with a vestibular lesion is ipsilateral head tilt (**Fig. 8.9**). Circling may also be observed in vestibular disease. Rapid vertical and horizontal movements of the head in normal sheep can induce positional nystagmus, with the fast phase in the direction of head movement. Positional nystagmus may be depressed or absent in animals with a vestibular lesion when the head is moved towards the side of the lesion (head tilt). Resting nystagmus is present and permits differentiation between the two forms of vestibular disease:

- Peripheral vestibular disease – fast phase away from side of lesion.
- Central vestibular disease – fast phase in any direction including dorsal or ventral.

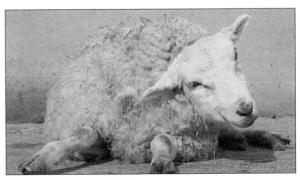

Fig. 8.9 An ipsilateral head tilt is the major clinical sign associated with a vestibular lesion.

In addition, Horner's syndrome and facial nerve paralysis is common in peripheral vestibular disease (see section on cranial nerves for further information on facial nerve paralysis), since both facial and sympathetic nerves fibres pass close to the middle ear.

Determination of a head tilt is best made when the animal is viewed from a distance of 5–10 metres. The head is normally held in the vertical plane but in vestibular disease a 5–10° tilt is present. The poll is tilted down to the affected side and may be exaggerated by blindfolding the animal. A head tilt must be differentiated from an altered head position or aversion.

Pontomedullary syndrome

As most of the cranial nerve nuclei are present within the brainstem, dysfunction referred to as the pontomedullary syndrome is characterized by multiple cranial nerve deficits (**Fig. 8.10**). In brainstem disease, depression is attributed to a specific lesion in the ascending reticular activating system of the brainstem (**Figs 8.11, 8.12**). In addition, ipsilateral hemiparesis (**Fig. 8.13**) and proprioceptive defects are common. Withdrawal and tendon jerk reflexes are present in all limbs.

In diseases affecting the brainstem, propulsive circling may result from involvement of the vestibulo-cochlear nucleus. Involvement of the facial nucleus results in ipsilateral facial nerve paralysis, evident as drooped ear, drooped upper eyelid (ptosis) and flaccid lip. Involvement of trigeminal nerve or the trigeminal motor nucleus results in paralysis of the cheek muscles and decreased facial sensation (**Fig. 8.14**).

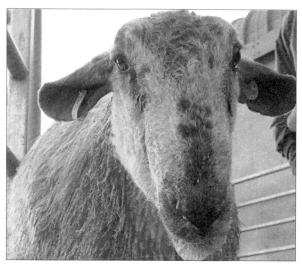

Fig. 8.10 The pontomedullary syndrome is characterized by multiple cranial nerve deficits.

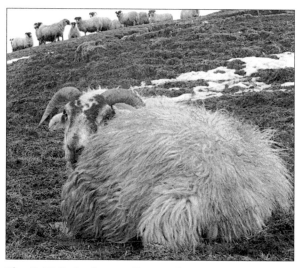

Fig. 8.11 In brainstem disease, depression is attributed to a specific lesion in the ascending reticular activating system.

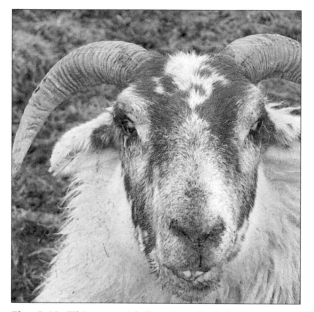

Fig. 8.12 This ewe with listeriosis is dull (involvement of the ascending reticular activating system) and shows multiple (left-sided) cranial nerve deficits (V and VII).

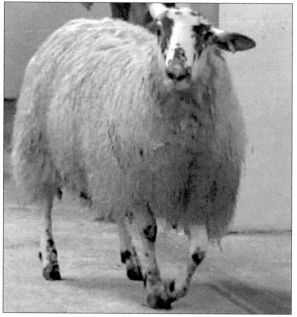

Fig. 8.13 Ipsilateral (left) hemiparesis and proprioceptive defects are commonly observed in unilateral brainstem disease.

Abnormal respiratory patterns may result from damage to the respiratory centre in the medulla.

Cranial nerves

Cranial nerves leave the forebrain and brainstem and have a variety of specialized functions (*Table 8.1*).

Olfactory nerve (I): Assessment of the olfactory nerve has little clinical application in ruminant species.

Optic nerve (II): The visual pathway can be tested by observing the sheep encountering obstacles and by evaluating the menace response – the eyelids close quickly in

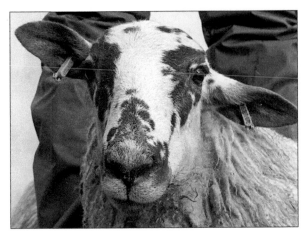

Fig. 8.14 Involvement of the trigeminal motor nucleus results in paralysis of the cheek muscles and decreased facial sensation.

response to a rapidly approaching object. The menace response can be difficult to evaluate in depressed animals and should be interpreted with caution.

Up to 90% of optic nerve fibres decussate at the optic chiasma; therefore, vision in the left eye is perceived in the contralateral (right) cerebral hemisphere.

The signal generated by the menace response in the left eye travels along the left optic nerve to the optic chiasma, then crosses to the right optic tract and right occipital cortex. The motor (efferent) pathway is from the right visual cortex to the left facial nucleus, resulting in closure of the left eye.

Lesions of the eye and optic nerve result in ipsilateral blindness. Lesions of the optic tract or nucleus cause contralateral blindness. Therefore, an abscess in the right cerebral hemisphere affecting the nucleus will result in blindness of the left eye.

Oculomotor nerve (III): Pupillary diameter is controlled by constrictor muscles innervated by the parasympathetic fibres in the oculomotor nerve, and by dilator muscles innervated by the sympathetic fibres from the cranial cervical ganglion.

The normal response to light directed in one eye is constriction of both pupillary apertures, with a direct response in the stimulated eye and a consensual response in the contralateral eye.

A dilated pupil in an eye with normal vision (menace response) would suggest a lesion in the

Table 8.1 **Assessment of function associated with cranial nerves and brain centres**	
ASSESSMENT OF NORMAL FUNCTION	**CRANIAL NERVES AND ASSOCIATED CENTRES**
Vision	Eye, II, cerebrum (contralateral)
Pupillary light response (pen torch)	II, III
Pupil size and symmetry (pen torch)	II, III, brainstem, sympathetic nervous system
Menace response (rapidly approaching object)	II, VII, cerebrum, brainstem, cerebellum
Eyeball position	III lateral strabismus IV dorsal and medial VI medial strabismus
Normal head/cheek muscle tone	V
Touch cornea, eyeball retracts	V, VI
Touch medial canthus, eye closes	V, VII
Ears held in normal position	V, VII
Nostrils – normal sensation	V
Eyelids in normal position	III, VII, sympathetic nervous system
Hearing	VIII
Normal head position	VIII, cerebrum
Deglutition, tongue movement	IX, X, XII

oculomotor nerve (III). The contralateral eye with normal oculomotor nerve (III) function will respond to both direct and consensual stimulation. If a lesion involves primarily one cerebral hemisphere, increased pressure to one oculomotor nerve presents as different pupillary aperture diameters (anisocoria), with the affected side displaying pupillary dilation.

Horner's syndrome: Horner's syndrome refers to the clinical appearance of damage to the sympathetic nerve supply to the eyeball causing slight ptosis (drooping of upper eyelid), constriction of the pupil (miosis) and slight protrusion of the nictitating membrane. The menace response (vision) and pupillary light response are normal.

Oculomotor (III), trochlear (IV) and abducens (VI) nerves: These cranial nerves are responsible for normal position and movement of the eyeball within the bony socket. Abnormal position of the eyeball is rarely seen as an acquired syndrome in sheep. An abnormal eyeball position is referred to as strabismus:

- Paralysis of the oculomotor nerve – lateral strabismus.
- Paralysis of the trochlear nerve – dorsomedial strabismus.
- Paralysis of the abducens nerve – medial strabismus.

Many cerebral lesions can result in strabismus. If there is a unilateral cerebral lesion, the strabismus is directed to the ipsilateral side. Dorsomedial strabismus is classically seen in PEM and acute bacterial meningitis of neonates (**Fig. 8.15**) as a reflection of cerebral oedema involving upper motor neuron pathways.

Trigeminal (V) nerve: The trigeminal nerve has three branches: mandibular, maxillary and ophthalmic. They supply the motor fibres to the muscles of mastication and sensory fibres to the face.

Loss of motor function of the mandibular branch of the trigeminal nerve results in rapid atrophy of the temporal and masseter muscles that are responsible for mastication. Unilateral lesions result in deviation

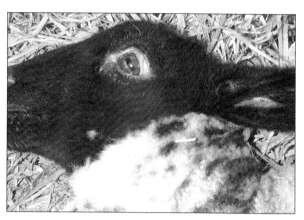

Fig. 8.15 Many cerebral lesions can result in strabismus; in this case, caused by bacterial meningoencephalitis.

of the lower jaw and muzzle away from the affected side. Responses to stimulation of the skin around the face are mediated through sensory fibres in the trigeminal nerve and motor fibres in the facial nerve. These reflexes require intact cranial nerves V and VII, trigeminal and facial nuclei and brainstem.

Abducens (VI) nerve: Lesions of the abducens nerve result in constant medial strabismus and loss of the ability to retract the eyeball into the bony socket (corneal reflex).

Facial (VII) nerve: The facial nerve is concerned primarily with motor supply to the facial muscles. The facial nerve contains the lower motor neurons for movement of the ears, eyelids, nares and muzzle and the motor pathways of the menace and palpebral reflexes.

When the periocular skin is touched, the normal reflex is that the animal will close the palpebral fissure. The lack of the palpebral reflex may indicate a lesion in:

- The trigeminal nerve or nucleus (sensory pathway).
- The facial nerve or facial nucleus (motor pathway).
- Both nerves or nuclei involved.

If the facial (VII) nerve only is involved, skin sensation of the face is normal due to normal trigeminal nerve function.

Facial nerve paralysis is characteristically seen as drooping of the upper eyelid and ear. With a unilateral lesion there is deviation of the muzzle towards the unaffected side due to loss of facial muscle tone in the affected side.

Differentiation between central or peripheral facial nerve involvement can be attempted by identifying involvement of other central structures such as the trigeminal and vestibulo-cochlear nuclei.

Vestibulocochlear (VIII) nerve: Deafness in sheep may be difficult to determine. The vestibular system controls orientation of the head, body and eyes. Nystagmus refers to movement of the eyeball within the bony socket. Normal vestibular nystagmus refers to horizontal movement of the eyeball as the head is turned laterally, with the fast movement phase toward the side to which the head is turned. Pathological change causing nystagmus originates in the vestibular system.

Spontaneous nystagmus refers to nystagmus when the head is held in the normal position. Positional nystagmus results when the head is held in various abnormal positions.

Glossopharyngeal (IX) and vagal (X) nerves: Damage to these nerve nuclei results in dysphagia and associated salivation. Affected animals cannot swallow or drink.

Accessory (XI) nerve: In ruminants, the accessory nerve appears to have little specific function.

Hypoglossal (XII) nerve: The hypoglossal nerve provides motor supply to the muscles of the tongue. With a unilateral lesion there is atrophy of musculature but the sheep is still able to retract the tongue within the buccal cavity. In the case of a bilateral lesion the sheep is unable to prehend and masticate food and the tongue remains protruded.

Midbrain syndrome

The midbrain syndrome is relatively uncommon in ruminants and is characterized by depression/coma, possible limb rigidity and opisthotonus. Most affected animals have normal vision, ventrolateral strabismus and a mydriatic pupil that is unresponsive to light. The most common causes of midbrain syndrome in ruminants are cranial trauma or a hepatic encephalopathy.

Hypothalamic syndrome

This is a relatively uncommon syndrome in sheep. There are multiple cranial nerve deficits (II–VII) depending on which nerve roots are affected by the lesion. The defect(s) is typically due to an abscess or tumour of the pituitary gland.

MENINGITIS

The CNS is covered by three membranous layers: dura, arachnoid mater and pia mater. Inflammation of the meninges is divided into pachymeningitis involving the dura mater, and leptomeningitis, involving the arachnoid mater, subarachnoid space containing CSF and pia mater.

Most cases of meningitis involve the leptomeninges with extension to involve the underlying cerebral cortex. Such infections are more correctly referred to as meningoencephalitis. For clinical purposes, the meningitis lesion is of primary importance due to the development of hypertensive hydrocephalus.

COLLECTION AND ANALYSIS OF CEREBROSPINAL FLUID

CSF collection and gross inspection provides rapid in some situations instant, information to the veterinary clinician investigating a disease problem in the living animal. CSF analysis is particularly useful for confirming the presence of an inflammatory lesion and differentiation of spinal cord lesions.

To collect CSF it is necessary to puncture the subarachnoid space in the cerebellomedullary cistern (cisternal sample) or at the lumbosacral site (lumbar sample). In the absence of a focal spinal cord compressive lesion there is usually no substantial difference between the composition of cisternal and lumbar CSF samples. While theoretically it may be desirable to collect CSF from the site nearer the suspected lesion, this is not always possible in farm animal practice.

When correctly performed under local anaesthesia, lumbar CSF collection is a safe procedure and there are no observed harmful sequelae; there are few indications for cisternal collection. Adequate restraint and identification of bony landmarks are essential during the sampling procedure. In order to appreciate the relevant anatomical structures it is recommended that the technique is first attempted on cadavers.

Collection of lumbar CSF is facilitated when the animal is positioned in sternal recumbency with the hips flexed and the hindlimbs extended alongside the abdomen. A version of the head against the flank may assist in maintaining sternal recumbency during the CSF collection procedure. Sedation of the animal is not usually necessary but can be achieved using 10 μg/kg detomidine injected intravenously (note extra label use). Intramuscular xylazine (0.04–0.07 mg/kg bodyweight) produces very variable sedation and is not recommended.

The site for lumbar CSF collection is the midpoint of the lumbosacral space (**Fig. 8.16**), which can be identified as the midline depression between the last palpable dorsal lumbar spine (L6) and the first palpable sacral dorsal spine (S2). (See also p. 390 [Chapter 17, Anaesthesia] for identification of lumbosacral space.) The site must be clipped, surgically prepared and 1–2 ml of local anaesthetic injected subcutaneously. An internal stylet is not required.

The needle is slowly advanced at a right angle to the plane of the vertebral column or with the hub directed 5° caudally. It is essential to appreciate the changes in tissue resistance as the needle point passes sequentially through the subcutaneous tissue and interarcuate ligament, and then the sudden 'pop' due to the loss of resistance as the needle point finally penetrates the ligamentum flavum into the extradural space. Once the needle point has penetrated the dorsal subarachnoid space, CSF will well up in the needle hub within 2–3 seconds. Failure to appreciate the change in resistance to needle travel may result in puncture of the conus medullaris. This may elicit an immediate pain response and cause unnecessary discomfort to the animal and must be avoided.

A sample of 1–2 ml of CSF is sufficient for laboratory analysis; while the sample can be collected by free flow, it is more convenient to employ gentle syringe aspiration over 10–30 seconds. Care must be taken not to dislodge the needle point from the dorsal subarachnoid space when the syringe is attached to the needle hub. Stabilizing the position of the needle can be assisted by firmly resting the wrist on the sheep's vertebral column. The seal on the syringe should be broken before it is connected to the needle hub, which must be anchored firmly between the thumb and index finger (**Fig. 8.17**). Selection of the correct needle length (*Table 8.2*)

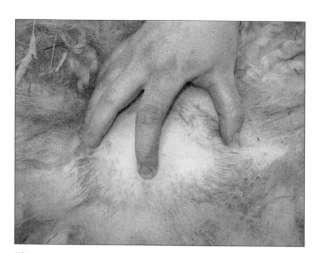

Fig. 8.16 **The site for lumbar CSF collection is the midpoint of the lumbosacral space.**

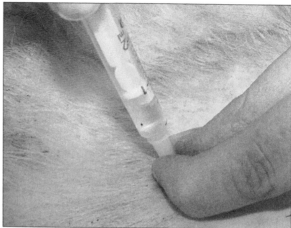

Fig. 8.17 **The needle hub must be anchored firmly between the thumb and index finger when collecting cerebrospinal fluid (CSF).**

Table 8.2 **Guide to needle length and gauge for lumbar CSF sampling**			
Neonatal lambs		1 cm	21–23 gauge
Lambs	<30 kg	2.5 cm	21 gauge
Ewes	40–80 kg	4 cm	19 gauge
Rams	>80 kg	5 cm	19 gauge

ensures that the needle hub is close to the skin, thereby assisting stabilization.

Failure to obtain fluid is most commonly caused by incorrect direction of the needle. The reference bony landmarks must then be rechecked and the needle correctly aligned. A new needle must be used on each occasion but no more than two attempts should be made to collect CSF.

Analysis of CSF
Specific gravity
Specific gravity results are not sufficiently precise to be useful in the investigation of ovine neurological disease.

Protein concentration
Many CSF samples have first to be concentrated due to low protein content. CSF protein concentration can be quoted in mg/dl or g/l units (multiply concentration in g/l by 100 for concentration in mg/dl). The normal range for CSF protein concentration is <0.4 g/l.

A rapid approximation of CSF globulin concentration can be made using the Pandy test whereby one drop of CSF is added to 1 ml of saturated phenol solution. A blue/white turbidity indicates a significant increase in the CSF globulin concentration. A urinary protein dipstick test is not sufficiently sensitive to determine low CSF protein concentration, and should only be relied upon to estimate CSF protein concentrations >2.0 g/l.

White cell concentration
White cell concentration in CSF can be determined using a haemocytometer. Cytological examination of CSF is performed within 2 hours of collection and is greatly facilitated if the sample is first concentrated by cytospin. The sample is then air-dried and stained with Leishman stain. The differential white cell count should be based on a minimum of 20 cells. Alternatively, a sedimentation chamber can be used to examine CSF cellular morphology.

Presence of bacteria in cerebrospinal fluid
Samples of CSF can be examined microscopically for the presence of bacteria following preparation with Gram's stain.

Positive bacteriological culture of CSF has only been reported in cases of neonatal bacterial meningitis. CSF bacteriology is unlikely to assist the clinician in the immediate diagnosis and choice of treatments, due to the time taken for results and antibiotic sensitivity testing. A provisional result of bacterial meningitis could be provided by a direct Gram's stain.

Other cerebrospinal fluid constituents
Concentrations of glucose, creatine kinase, lactate dehydrogenase and other CSF constituents are not routinely performed as they provide little additional information in the diagnosis of the common CNS diseases.

Interpretation of results
Red blood cells (RBCs) may be present in the CSF following pathological haemorrhage into the subarachnoid space, but this is very uncommon in the author's experience. More commonly, the presence of RBCs in the CSF sample results from needle puncture of blood vessels on the dura, and particularly the leptomeninges, during the sampling procedure. Accidental trauma resulting in intrathecal haemorrhage is more common following repeated attempts to obtain CSF. Haemorrhage caused by the sampling technique will appear as streaking of blood in clear fluid and gradually clears as more CSF is allowed to flow freely from the needle hub. Turbidity caused by recent haemorrhage into the CSF will clear after centrifugation to leave a clear supernatant. Alternatively, if the sample is left to stand for approximately 2 hours the RBCs gravitate and form a small plug at the bottom of the

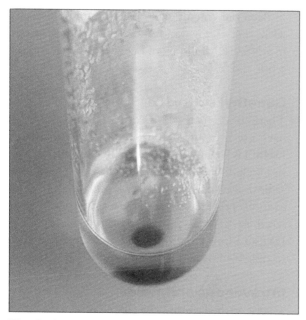

Fig. 8.18 Iatrogenic haemorrhage – red blood cells in the CSF have gravitated to form a small plug at the bottom of the collection tube.

collection tube (**Fig. 8.18**). Pathological haemorrhage within the CSF is most confidently diagnosed by the presence of phagocytosed RBCs within macrophages.

A yellow discoloration of the CSF, referred to as xanthochromia, appears within a few hours after subarachnoid haemorrhage and may persist for 2–4 weeks. Xanthochromia is caused by release of pigment following lysis of RBCs, resulting from membrane fragility of RBCs as a consequence of the low CSF protein concentration.

Normal CSF contains $<0.012 \times 10^9/l$ white cells, which are predominantly lymphocytes with occasional neutrophils. As a general rule, a predominantly polymorphonuclear intrathecal inflammatory response is found in acute CNS bacterial infections, whereas a mononuclear response is seen in viral CNS infections. Macrophages are seen following destruction of cerebral tissue or following haemorrhage and are variably seen in PEM. There are few reports in the veterinary literature of a consistent association between an increased CSF eosinophil concentration and parasitic infection of the CNS.

TREATMENT OF CENTRAL NERVOUS SYSTEM INFECTIONS

More than any other organ system, effective treatment of bacterial infections of the CNS necessitates early detection of abnormal signs by the farmer, rapid diagnosis by the veterinarian and aggressive antibiotic treatment and supportive therapy. Unfortunately there are few studies in the veterinary literature which report the outcome of such treatments.

The important factors to consider in the treatment of CNS infections include the bacterial pathogen, duration and extent of the disease process. The antibiotic must be selected on its ability to penetrate the blood–brain barrier and achieve concentrations 10–30 times the minimum bactericidal concentration (MBC) in order to sterilize the CSF.

Supportive treatments include corticosteroids, diuretics and non-steroidal anti-inflammatory drugs (NSAIDs). In addition, certain situations necessitate appropriate intravenous and oral fluid replacement therapy to correct fluid disturbances.

For an antibiotic to be effective in bacterial meningitis, it must penetrate into the CSF in sufficient concentration to be bactericidal to the invading organism. Few broad-spectrum bactericidal antibiotics are capable of penetrating the intact blood–brain barrier; it is generally assumed that the disruption of the blood–brain barrier occurs in bacterial CNS diseases, allowing increased antibiotic penetration. Such increased permeability may be sufficient to allow MBCs to be achieved within the CSF, but few studies have been undertaken in animals with naturally-occurring CNS infections to validate such assumptions.

Antibiotic penetration of the blood–brain barrier depends on:

- Lipid solubility– the greater the degree of ionization of an antibiotic in plasma, hence reduced lipid solubility, the lower the penetration through the blood–brain barrier.
- Degree of protein binding – large molecular weight antibiotics, such as aminoglycosides, achieve very poor CSF concentrations even in the presence of meningeal inflammation.

In addition to the choice of antimicrobial agent, there is considerable debate regarding the duration of treatment for CNS diseases. In farm animal practice the cost of antibiotic is the most important limiting factor in the animal's treatment and high-dose/short-duration therapy is the best compromise in many situations.

Penicillins

In man, penicillin and ampicillin are usually considered the antibiotics of choice for meningitis caused by *Listeria monocytogenes*. High-dose penicillin treatment of 'confirmed' cases of ovine listeriosis (typical clinical signs and CSF changes) and oxytetracycline treatment of mild cases of ovine listeriosis have been reported.

Chloramphenicol/florfenicol

In veterinary medicine chloramphenicol was stated to be the antibiotic of choice for the treatment of bacterial meningoencephalitis as it is capable of crossing the intact blood–brain barrier. Chloramphenicol is no longer licensed for food producing animals in many countries and, as yet, there are no published data that report the efficacy of florfenicol in the treatment of bacterial meningitis in lambs.

Ceftiofur

Third and fourth generation cephalosporins are widely used for the treatment of bacterial meningo-encephalitis in human medicine but there are no data relating to their field use in sheep. While good results have been achieved with ceftiofur in the treatment of streptococcal meningitis in pigs, equally good results have been achieved with procaine penicillin.

Anti-inflammatory agents

In certain neurological diseases, particularly PEM and bacterial meningitis, the control of cerebral oedema affects prognosis. The recommended treatment for cerebral oedema is either 1–2 mg/kg dexamethasone given intravenously, 1–2 g/kg of dimethyl sulphoxide (DMSO) as a 40% solution given intravenously (where licensed) or furosemide 1–2 mg/kg given intravenously. Unfortunately, there are no comparative field investigations of corticosteroid treatment in ovine CNS disease.

Bacterial meningitis is commonly associated with septicaemia and intravenous administration of a NSAID would be of benefit in the treatment of septic shock.

Dimethyl sulfoxide

There is no licensed DMSO product for veterinary use in many countries, but analytical quality DMSO is frequently used. DMSO has many properties including reduction of cerebral oedema and free radical scavenging; however, special handling precautions preclude its use in most situations encountered in general practice. In veterinary practice DMSO administration would probably be restricted to valuable hospitalized animals.

Intravenous/oral fluids

Severe dehydration can be corrected by the intravenous infusion of isotonic saline. Metabolic acidosis, which may be encountered in listeriosis cases caused by saliva loss, can be corrected by daily administration of solutions containing sodium bicarbonate by orogastric tube.

SWAYBACK

Definition/overview

Swayback is a congenital condition affecting newborn lambs; delayed swayback (enzootic ataxia) most commonly affects lambs aged 2–4 months. The incidence depends upon geographical area, soil type, land and pasture improvements through drainage and lime application, breed and weather conditions during the period corresponding to mid-trimester.

Aetiology

Swayback is associated with low copper status of the dam and/or growing lamb. The condition occurs within well-defined geographic areas, usually upland and hill pastures, where it is often related to pasture improvement including liming, fertilizer application and re-seeding. Swayback occurs more commonly after mild winters because less supplementary feeding is provided to sheep during mid- and late gestation, resulting in ingestion of copper antagonists

Neurological Diseases

199

in soil. It has been proposed that copper deficiency reduces the activity of copper-dependent enzymes such that the cell is unable to maintain the metabolic requirements of structure, growth and function.

Clinical presentation

Congenital form: Severely affected lambs are small and weak and may be unable to raise themselves or maintain sternal recumbency. Depressed corneal and pupillary reflexes and blindness have been reported. Some affected lambs show fine head tremor, which is increased during periods of activity such as feeding. Less severely affected lambs have normal birthweight and are bright and alert. These lambs have poor co-ordination and have difficulty finding the teat, leading to starvation. Failure of adequate passive antibody transfer predisposes these lambs to watery mouth disease and localized infections of liver, joints and meninges after bacteraemia.

Delayed form: In the delayed form of swayback (enzootic ataxia) the lambs are normal at birth but show progressive weakness of the hindlimbs from 2–4 months (**Figs 8.19, 8.20**). Weakness is often first noted during gathering when affected lambs lag behind the remainder of the flock.

The hindlimbs are weak, with reduced muscle tone and reflexes, and show muscle atrophy.

Diagnosis

Clinical diagnosis of swayback is based upon clinical findings, and flock details such as geographical area, copper supplementation and supplementary feeding during mid-gestation.

Diagnosis of swayback is confirmed by histopathological examination of the brain and spinal cord, and supported by liver copper determination where concentrations below 80 mg/kg indicate low copper status. Care must be exercised that cases of enzootic ataxia have received no copper supplementation prior to liver copper determinations.

Differential diagnoses

Congenital form: Differential diagnoses of the congenital form of swayback include:

- Septicaemia.
- Hypoglycaemia/hypothermia.
- Border disease.

Septicaemic lambs present with depression, reluctance to suck, injected scleral vessels; they deteriorate

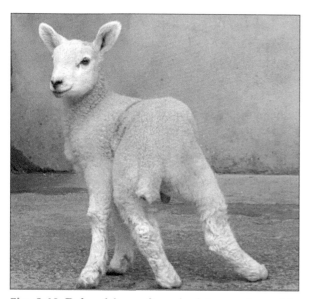

Fig. 8.19 Delayed form of swayback (enzootic ataxia); affected lambs show progressive weakness of the hindlimbs from 2–4 months old.

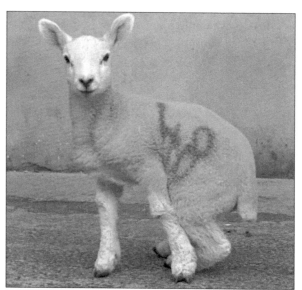

Fig. 8.20 The hindlimbs are weak, with reduced muscle tone and reflexes, and show muscle atrophy.

rapidly to stupor and death with 24–36 hours. Hypothermic/hypoglycaemic lambs appear gaunt and hunched with no palpable abomasal content but respond well to appropriate supplementary feeding and warming. Border disease presents with clinical signs indicative of cerebellar dysfunction including intention tremors, a wide-based stance, lowered head carriage and hypermetria with preservation of limb strength. Severely affected lambs may present with opisthotonus resulting from damage to the rostral cerebellum.

Delayed form: Compressive lesions affecting the thoracolumbar spinal cord (T2–L3) resulting from vertebral body empyema are common in 2–4-month-old lambs following pyaemia. Vertebral body abscessation may be associated with tick-borne fever and tick pyaemia on infested upland and hill pastures where delayed swayback is also more common. The clinical course associated with thoracolumbar vertebral abscessation (T2–L3) is progressive over 4–7 days (**Fig. 8.21**) with upper motor neuron signs to the hindlimbs. This condition differs from the lower motor neuron signs typically observed in enzootic ataxia. Lesions compressing the thoracolumbar spinal cord cause an elevated protein concentration in lumbar CSF, which aids differentiation from enzootic ataxia. Hindlimb paresis has been reported in sheep with thoracolumbar spinal cord lesions associated with *Sarcocystis* spp. infestation and coenurosis.

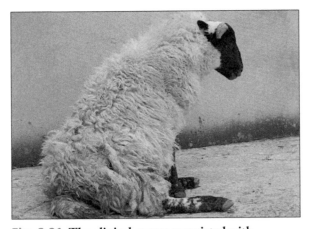

Fig. 8.21 The clinical course associated with thoracolumbar vertebral abscessation (T2–L3) is progressive over 4–7 days.

Pathology

The pathogonomic lesions of swayback are microscopic and present in the brainstem and spinal cord. Nerve cell changes, including swelling, vacuolation and chromatolysis proceeding to a 'hyaline-like' necrosis, are most evident in the large neurones of the red and vestibular nuclei, the reticular formation and the ventral horns of the spinal cord.

In the spinal cord altered nerve fibres mainly occupy the peripheral zones of the dorsal and ventral parts of the lateral funiculi and the sulco-marginal funiculi. There is pallor of myelin in the affected areas and a positive Marchi reaction. There is evidence of Wallerian-type degeneration, myelin degradation and reduced myelin synthesis.

Treatment

Treatment of lambs with congenital swayback is hopeless and affected lambs must be humanely destroyed for welfare reasons. There is limited evidence that copper supplementation of lambs with enzootic ataxia slows the progress of the condition. Lambs with enzootic ataxia should be confined in small paddocks to allow appropriate supervision and fed a high-concentrate ration in an attempt to achieve marketable weights.

Management/prevention/control measures

There is a great breed variation in susceptibility to copper toxicity; Texel and certain rare breeds such as the Soay and North Ronaldsay are highly susceptible. Indeed, reports have detailed copper toxicosis in Texel sheep that had received neither supplementary feeding nor parenteral copper administration. Prevention of swayback by copper supplementation must therefore be carefully considered. Factors that should be considered before supplementation include the prevalence of confirmed or suspected swayback cases in the flock, breed of sheep, supplementary feeding during gestation and geographical area including soil analysis.

Determination of serum copper and copper-dependent enzyme concentrations, such as superoxide dismutase, in pregnant ewes provides some indication of copper status but liver copper concentration is the most useful measurement. The subcutaneous or intramuscular injection of chelated copper presents the most convenient method for supplementation of extensively-managed ewes during mid-gestation but, as stated above, is not without risk.

Economics

Swayback is controlled by administration of copper either by injection or administration of copper oxide needles to ewes during mid-gestation. If the prevalence of swayback is low in a particular flock the decision to supplement is based upon disease forecasts, which take into account prevailing weather conditions and supplementary feeding of the flock.

Welfare implications

Newborn lambs with swayback fail to thrive and should be euthanased for welfare reasons, and a healthy lamb fostered onto the ewe. Lambs with delayed swayback should be confined to low-ground pastures and not returned onto hill ground. Supplementary feeding will aid finishing, and these lambs should be slaughtered at the nearest slaughter plant to limit transport distances.

POLIOENCEPHALOMALACIA

(syn. cerebrocortical necrosis [CCN])

Definition/overview

PEM is an acute neurological disease of weaned lambs but is seen sporadically in adult sheep.

The disease is characterized by blindness, initial depression and aimless wandering, dorsiflexion of the neck, progressing rapidly to hyperexcitability, seizures and opisthotonus.

Clinical presentation

PEM is most commonly seen in weaned lambs aged 4–8 months but disease does occur in adult sheep. Sucking lambs are rarely affected. Individual lambs are usually affected approximately 2 weeks after movement to another pasture or other dietary change; either event may be associated with routine anthelmintic treatment. During the early stages of PEM affected sheep become isolated from the group, are blind (**Fig. 8.22**) and may wander aimlessly (**Fig. 8.23**). There may be marked dorsiflexion of the neck ('star-gazing') when sheep are stationary (**Fig. 8.24**). If untreated, the condition progresses over 12–24 hours to seizure activity (**Fig. 8.25**) and opisthotonus. Affected sheep are hyperaesthetic to auditory and tactile stimuli, which may precipitate seizure activity during handling. Dorsomedial strabismus and spontaneous horizontal nystagmus are frequently observed. Trauma to the peripheral facial nerve on the dependent side may result in ptosis and drooped ear. Death follows within 3–5 days in untreated sheep.

Pathology

The cerebral hemispheres are swollen, pale and soft with yellow discoloration of some gyri, especially in

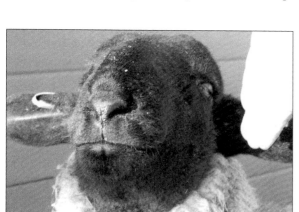

Fig. 8.22 **During the early stages of polioencephalomalacia (PEM) affected sheep become isolated from the group and are blind, shown here as a lack of menace response.**

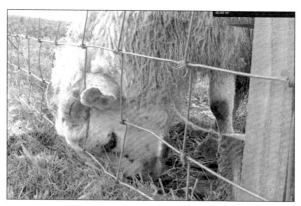

Fig. 8.23 **PEM affected sheep wander aimlessly and may become trapped in fences and hedgerows.**

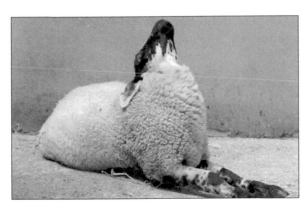

Fig. 8.24 Marked dorsiflexion of the neck ('star-gazing') is often observed during the early stages of PEM.

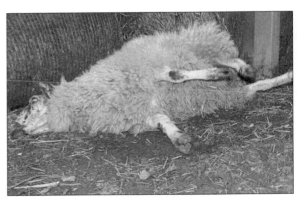

Fig. 8.25 If untreated, the clinical signs of PEM progress within 12–24 hours to seizure activity and opisthotonus.

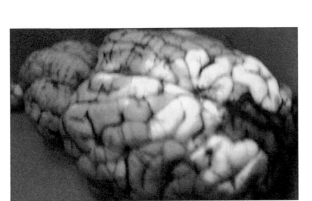

Fig. 8.26 At necropsy, areas of the cortex affected by PEM exhibit a bright white autofluorescence when viewed under ultraviolet light (Wood's lamp; 365 nm).

the frontal, dorsolateral and dorsomedial areas of the cortex. The posterior vermis may appear cone-shaped due to herniation through the foramen magnum. PEM-affected areas of the cortex may exhibit a bright white autofluorescence (**Fig. 8.26**) when cut sections of the cerebrum are viewed under ultraviolet light (Wood's lamp; 365 nm). This property has been attributed to the accumulation of lipofuchsin in macrophages but not all PEM cases fluoresce. Definitive diagnosis relies upon the histological findings in the cortical lesions of vacuolation and cavitation of the ground substance, with astrocytic swelling, neuronal shrinkage and necrosis.

Differential diagnoses

A common differential diagnosis is focal symmetrical encephalomalacia (FSE) in unvaccinated weaned lambs. Very occasionally, the occurrence of numerous lambs in lateral recumbency caused by drenching gun injury progressing to involve the cervical spinal cord may briefly be confused with PEM, as the latter condition often follows anthelmintic treatment and change of pasture. Pregnancy toxaemia, acute coenurosis and listeriosis represent the more common differential diagnoses in adult sheep.

Diagnosis

Diagnosis is based upon clinical findings and response to parenteral administration of thiamine (10 mg/kg bid). Diagnostic biochemical parameters for PEM including thiaminase activities in blood, rumen fluid or faeces are rarely used in farm animal practice.

Treatment

The treatment response during the early clinical stages of PEM to high doses of thiamine (10 mg/kg bid administered intravenously for the first occasion) is generally good (**Figs 8.27, 8.28**). Successfully treated sheep are able to stand and commence eating within 24 hours although normal vision may not return for 5–7 days. Treatment should be continued for 3 consecutive days. The intravenous injection of

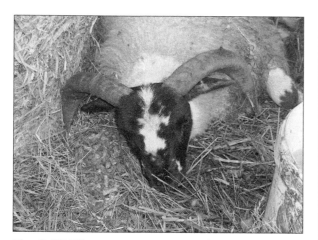

Fig. 8.27 The treatment response during the early clinical stages of PEM is generally good (see Fig. 8.28).

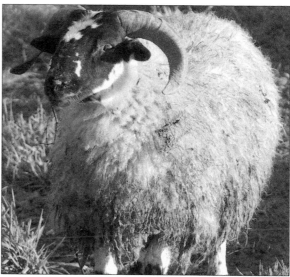

Fig. 8.28 Successful treatment of PEM (Fig. 8.27); the sheep was able to stand and commenced eating within 24 hours of thiamine injection.

a high dose of soluble corticosteroid such as dexamethasone (1 mg/kg) at the first treatment to reduce cerebral oedema remains controversial.

Management/prevention/control measures
The sporadic occurrence and good treatment response of PEM cases mean that prevention measures are rarely attempted under most grazing systems in the UK.

Economics
The low financial value of commercial sheep results in few suspected PEM cases presented to veterinary surgeons. Cost considerations result in suboptimal therapy, including intramuscular injection rather than intravenous thiamine administration on the first occasion, and once-daily treatment, both situations contribute to a reduced recovery rate.

Welfare implications
Affected sheep should be housed in a quiet, dark, well-bedded pen and propped in sternal recumbency between straw bales or similar (**Fig. 8.27**). If unable to maintain sternal recumbency, the sheep must be turned regularly to prevent urine scalding. Sheep unable to stand unaided after 2 days' treatment are unlikely to recover fully and should be euthanased for welfare reasons.

SULPHUR TOXICITY

Definition/overview
Several outbreaks of a disease not dissimilar to PEM but affecting large numbers of weaned lambs or yearlings fed high levels of concentrates have been recorded in the literature.

Aetiology
An outbreak of sulphur toxicity has been reported affecting 21 of 71 weaned lambs aged 4–6 months 15–32 days after they were introduced to an *ad libitum* concentrate ration containing 0.43% sulphur. No further cases were identified after all the remaining lambs were given a single intramuscular injection of vitamin B1. Similarly, an outbreak of sulphur toxicity was reported in a group of fattening lambs fed a ration containing ammonium sulphate as a urinary acidifier.

Clinical presentation
The clinical signs reported were acute in onset and included depression and bilateral lack of

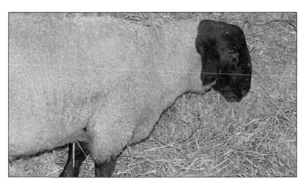

Fig. 8.29 **The clinical signs of sulphur toxicity include dullness and bilateral lack of menace response.**

menace response (**Fig. 8.29**). Affected sheep would walk forward until contacting a solid object and appeared unable to reverse themselves out of corners. However, hyperaesthesia, nystagmus, dorsiflexion of the neck and opisthotonus, typical of spontaneous cases of PEM, were not observed.

Differential diagnoses
- PEM.
- Hepatic encephalopathy associated with cobalt deficiency.
- Acidosis/grain overload.
- Urolithiasis.

Diagnosis
The treatment response to the standard regimen for PEM is poor. The diagnosis is confirmed on histopathological examination of brain tissue.

Pathology
The pathology of sulphur toxicity cases includes widespread areas of malacia in the brain with a clearly defined periphery. Areas of the thalamus and mid-brain are also involved but no lesions are observed in the cerebellum or hippocampus.

Treatment
There is a poor response to intravenous treatment with vitamin B1 and dexamethasone. Affected lambs may regain a normal appetite but remain dull with impaired vision.

Management/prevention/control measures
Care should be taken when formulating intensive rations for fattening lambs and rams being prepared for sale. While no further cases have been identified in some outbreaks after all the remaining lambs were given a single intramuscular injection of vitamin B1, some reports have questioned such a metaphylactic approach.

Economics
Whilst not commonly reported, production losses to sulphur toxicity can be considerable and care must be taken when formulating intensive rations for fattening lambs.

Welfare implications
Those sheep not responding to treatment should be slaughtered for welfare reasons.

BACTERIAL MENINGOENCEPHALITIS

Definition/overview
Bacterial meningoencephalitis occurs sporadically in young lambs, rarely exceeding 0.5% of lambs at risk. The true incidence of disease, however, has not been accurately determined because affected lambs may simply be found dead.

Aetiology
Bacterial meningoencephalitis most commonly affects young lambs aged 2–4 weeks after localization of bacteraemia arising from the upper respiratory tract or tonsils. Failure of passive antibody transfer predisposes neonates to bacteraemia with subsequent localization of pathogenic bacteria. The umbilicus as a route of infection remains uncertain as few affected lambs with bacterial meningoencephalitis have concurrent omphalophlebitis, and few lambs with omphalophlebitis/liver abscessation develop meningoencephalitis. Furthermore, the 2–4 week interval between umbilical infection acquired within the first few hours of life and clinical signs of meningoencephalitis suggests another route of bacterial invasion. There is little experimental evidence to support the hypothesis that the umbilicus is the major portal of entry for pathogenic bacteria. Studies in neonatal lambs have revealed bacteraemia in 34% of neonates with severe watery mouth disease.

Escherichia coli, *Pasteurella* spp., *Staphylococcus pyogenes* and *Trueperella pyogenes* have all been isolated from clinical cases of meningoencephalitis.

Clinical presentation

Initial clinical signs include depression (**Fig. 8.30**), lethargy, a gaunt appearance and separation from the dam. Affected lambs are often found isolated, sheltering behind hedgerows and walls. Affected lambs are rarely pyrexic. The head is often held lowered in rigid extension and gentle forced movement of the neck causes pain and vocalization. As the disease progresses, affected lambs are hyperaesthetic to tactile and auditory stimuli and seizure activity may be precipitated (**Fig. 8.31**) during intravenous antibiotic injection. Episcleral injection, congested mucous membranes and dorsomedial strabismus are consistent findings (**Fig. 8.32**). The menace response may be reduced or absent but can be difficult to interpret in depressed or stuporous lambs. Advanced stages of the disease process are characterized by lateral recumbency with seizure activity, opisthotonus and odontoprisis. There may be evidence of concurrent focal bacterial infection of other organ systems, particularly the limb joints, with associated swelling of drainage lymph nodes.

Differential diagnoses

Differential diagnoses of bacterial meningoencephalitis in young lambs include cerebellar hypoplasia (caused by Border disease virus), infection of the atlanto-occipital joint causing recumbency, hepatic necrobacillosis, starvation, septicaemia and nephrosis.

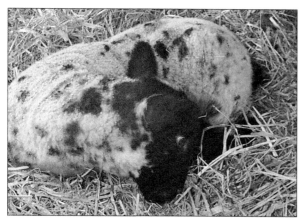

Fig. 8.30 Initial clinical signs of bacterial meningoencephalitis include depression and aversion of the head against the flank.

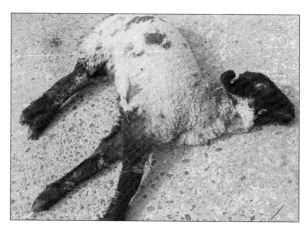

Fig. 8.31 As bacterial meningoencephalitis progresses, affected lambs become hyperaesthetic and show seizure activity.

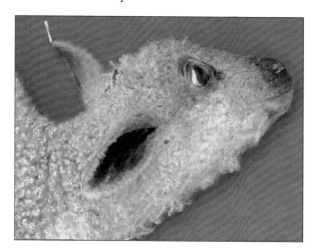

Fig. 8.32 Episcleral injection, congested mucous membranes and dorsomedial strabismus are consistent findings of bacterial meningoencephalitis.

Diagnosis

Diagnosis is based upon a thorough clinical examination. Lumbar CSF can be readily collected in field situations under local anaesthesia using hypodermic needles. Gross CSF inspection reveals a turbid sample caused by the huge influx of white cells, and a frothy appearance visible after gentle sample agitation due to the increased protein concentration. If necessary, laboratory analysis reveals an average 100-fold increase in white cell concentration comprised mainly of neutrophils (neutrophilic pleocytosis) and five-fold or greater increase in protein concentration. Culture of lumbar CSF is largely unrewarding.

Treatment

The treatment response is hopeless and affected lambs should be humanely destroyed once the diagnosis has been confirmed by CSF inspection. Antibiotics that could be used include trimethoprim/sulphonamide combination, ceftiofur and florfenicol (note off-label use). The role of high doses of soluble corticosteroid, such as 1.1 mg/kg dexamethasone, remains controversial in the treatment of bacterial meningoencephalitis in lambs.

Management/prevention/control measures

The isolation of gram-negative enteric bacteria from bacteraemic neonates supports the hypothesis that the environment is an important source of infection. Control should be directed at general preventive measures for all bacterial infections in the perinatal period including high standards of hygiene in the lambing environment and timely passive antibody transfer.

BRAIN ABSCESSATION

Definition/overview

Brain abscesses are very occasionally diagnosed in lambs aged 2–4 months.

Aetiology

Brain abscesses presumably arise following bacteraemic spread from a septic focus, but it is unusual to find evidence of another pyogenic disease except for the almost ubiquitous superficial docking and/or castration wounds caused by elastrator rings. Superficial lesions affording bacterial entry may simply not be detected at necropsy or have healed by the time the space-occupying nature of the brain lesion is noted.

Clinical presentation

Clinical signs are slowly progressive and result from the space-occupying nature of the lesion rather than any associated inflammatory response. Depression is commonly observed with the head turned towards the lamb's chest. There may be compulsive circling but affected sheep often stand motionless or appear trapped with the head pushed into a corner. The gait may appear ataxic. The lesion commonly affects one cerebral hemisphere; as a consequence the animal often presents with contralateral blindness and proprioceptive deficits but normal pupillary light reflexes. Proprioceptive deficits, with hyperflexion of the fetlock joint (knuckling) of the contralateral limbs, are commonly observed.

Pituitary abscesses (basilar empyema) occur rarely in adult sheep. Clinical findings include depression and multiple cranial nerve deficits.

Differential diagnoses

The common differential diagnoses causing depression/stupor of some days' duration in growing lambs include nephrosis, possibly sulphur toxicity and coenurosis, although coenurosis is uncommon in lambs less than 6 months old. PEM has a more acute clinical course than brain abscessation.

Diagnosis

Diagnosis is based upon a careful neurological examination. Evidence of other localized bacterial infection is uncommon and, unless present, there are no changes in routine haematology values, fibrinogen or serum globulin concentrations. Lumbar CSF analysis may reveal a small increase in protein concentration and increased white cell concentration.

Treatment

Treatment of brain abscesses is hopeless and affected lambs should be euthanased for welfare reasons.

Management/prevention/control measures

Good husbandry practices in the neonatal period ensure adequate passive antibody transfer and low environmental bacterial challenge.

COENUROSIS

Definition/overview
Coenurosis is an uncommon disease of the CNS in sheep in the UK. It is a considerable problem in many southern European countries. Education programmes detailing correct treatment of farm dogs with appropriate anthelmintics, and correct disposal of sheep carcases, have all combined to break the sheep–dog cycle in the UK, although not all farmers strictly adhere to the latter practice, especially in hill areas.

Aetiology
Coenurus cerebralis is the larval stage of *Taenia multiceps*, a tapeworm that infests the small intestine of carnivores. Contamination of pastures grazed by sheep with dog faeces can result in larval migration to the CNS and clinical disease. The life cycle is completed when the carnivorous definitive host ingests infested sheep's brain.

Clinical presentation
Both acute and chronic forms of coenurosis have been described, although chronic disease is more readily identified and more frequently reported.

Acute coenurosis has been reported in a flock of sheep introduced on to a pasture heavily contaminated by dog faeces. Clinical signs appeared within 10 days and ranged from mild to severe, with death occurring within 3–5 days of onset of neurological dysfunction. Acute coenurosis has also been reported in 6–8-week-old lambs where clinical signs ranged from pyrexia, listlessness and head aversion to convulsions and death within 4–5 days.

Chronic coenurosis is more commonly reported in growing sheep aged 6–18 months, where it presents as a slowly progressive focal lesion of the brain, typically involving one cerebral hemisphere. Chronic coenurosis has rarely been reported in sheep over 3 years of age. The time taken from larval hatching and migration to the brain to evidence of neurological dysfunction ranges from 2–6 months. The cyst is located in one cerebral hemisphere in 80% of cases, the cerebellum in approximately 10% and affects multiple locations in 8%. Individual cases of coenurosis cyst within the spinal cord have been reported

but such cases could be more prevalent as the clinical presentation is similar to vertebral empyema.

Localization of the coenurus cyst: Compulsive circling behaviour is commonly observed in sheep with coenurosis. Narrow diameter circles (1–2 m) suggest involvement of the basal nuclei at a deep location within the forebrain, whereas wide circles are suggestive of a more superficial location for the cerebral cyst. There is the tendency for sheep to circle towards the side of superficial cysts and away from the side of more deep-sited cysts. Depression and head-pressing behaviour occur with cysts involving the frontal lobe of the cerebrum.

The presence of a cyst in one cerebral hemisphere causes loss of the menace response in the contralateral eye; therefore, blindness in the right eye indicates that the lesion is in the left hemisphere. Blindness can also be investigated by unilateral blindfolding. Unilateral proprioceptive deficits suggest a contralateral cerebral cyst, whereas bilateral deficits more probably indicate a cerebellar cyst.

A head tilt towards the affected side may result if the cyst involves either the vestibular or cerebello-vestibular pathways. Cerebellar lesions are characterized by dysmetria, ataxia, but with preservation of strength, and a wide-based stance. Bilateral postural deficits and lack of menace response are usually also present with a cerebellar cyst. Deterioration of the clinical condition occurs more rapidly with a cerebellar cyst.

Differential diagnoses
Listeriosis, louping-ill and PEM should be considered when formulating a diagnosis of acute coenurosis. Brain abscessation should be included in the differential diagnosis list but the clinical signs tend to remain relatively static and do not deteriorate as occurs in chronic coenurosis.

Diagnosis
The presumptive diagnosis is confirmed at surgery after the lesion has been localized to either the right or left cerebral hemisphere or the cerebellum, following a thorough neurological examination. Softening of the frontal bone, as a consequence of a generalized increase in intracranial pressure, may be palpable but is not a reliable guide to the precise location of the cyst.

The bone softening may be either ipsilateral or contralateral to the cyst position, and in some cases there is softening on both sides in the presence of only a unilateral cyst. Real-time B-mode ultrasonography has been described as an aid to *C. cerebralis* cyst localization. Ancillary tests, such as the intradermal injection of coenurus cyst fluid, do not give consistent results and false-positive results are common.

Treatment

Many farmers may elect to slaughter those sheep fit for marketing for economic reasons. An 85% surgical success rate for removal of the coenurus cyst can be achieved after accurate localization of the lesion.

There are no general anaesthetic agents licensed for use in sheep in the UK, but this author has used pentobarbitone sodium for a variety of surgical procedures in sheep with good success. The dose of pentobarbitone sodium administered by intravenous injection is 20 mg/kg with two-thirds of the computed dose given over 20–30 seconds, and the remaining volume given to effect after an interval of 60 seconds. The duration of surgical anaesthesia is approximately 1–2 hours. It has been recommended that the dose rate of pentobarbitone sodium for sheep with coenurus cysts should be approximately two-thirds of the normal calculated dose.

Whenever possible, the sheep should be starved for 24 hours before surgery. The sheep is placed in sternal recumbency with the head held lowered to allow drainage of saliva from the mouth throughout the operation. Preoperative intravenous dexamethasone injection is recommended in an attempt to reduce brain oedema, which may result from the surgical procedure and complicate the animal's recovery. Procaine penicillin should be administered at 44,000 IU/kg 2 hours before surgery; alternatively crystalline penicillin can be given intravenously 20–30 minutes before surgery. Preoperative analgesia should include a NSAID, and be continued for 3 consecutive days thereafter.

The surgical approach is based upon the neurological findings. For a cerebral cyst the trephine site is 1–2 cm lateral to the mid-line and immediately rostral to the coronal (parietofrontal) suture line. The trephine site for a cerebellar cyst is mid-line between the nuchal line and the suture line between the occipital and parietal bones. The dura mater is incised once the 1 cm diameter bone core has been removed. At this point the increased intracranial pressure caused by the cyst forces brain tissue into the trephine hole. An 18 gauge intravenous catheter connected to a 20 ml syringe is used to drain the cyst and withdraw a portion of the cyst wall to the trephine hole, where it can be grasped with forceps and the entire cyst wall and protoscolices carefully removed. Recovery after successful surgical cyst removal is rapid and there is a return to full neurological function within 1 week.

Pathology

During the acute phase of coenurosis pale yellow tracts are visible on the surface of the brain, and in cut sections of brainstem and cerebellum. On microscopic examination, the tracts are comprised of necrotic tissue surrounded by haemorrhage and leucocyte infiltration. Eosinophils and giant cells predominate in the inflammatory reaction surrounding these tracts.

In chronic coenurosis the increased intracranial pressure from the cyst compresses surrounding brain tissue and may result in softening of an area of the skull. Such changes may not occur in bone immediately overlying the cyst. Hydrocephalus may result from a coenurus cyst in a ventricle or the cerebral aqueduct. Increased intracranial pressure may cause herniation of the vermis of the cerebellum through the foramen magnum or the cerebrum may become herniated beneath the tentorium.

Management/prevention/control measures

Control of coenurosis can be effected by regular dosing of farm dogs at 6–8 week intervals with an effective taenicide. Correct disposal of all sheep carcases will prevent scavenging by dogs belonging to the general public that may not receive regular anthelmintic treatment. Foxes are not considered to be an important definitive host of *T. multiceps*.

Economics

While the recovery rate following removal of a cerebral cyst is good, the poor clinical condition of the sheep at presentation to the veterinary surgeon and low financial value relative to the cost of general anaesthesia cause most farmers to slaughter those sheep fit for marketing for economic reasons, and euthanase those in poor condition.

Welfare implications

Timely treatment, slaughter and/or humane destruction resolve any welfare concerns.

SARCOCYSTOSIS

Definition/overview

The prevalence of neurological disease caused by *Sarcocystis* spp. in the UK is probably under-diagnosed, because the clinical signs are easily mistaken for vertebral empyema. All ages of sheep may be affected but neurological signs of spinal cord disease are more commonly observed in 6–12-month-old lambs.

Aetiology

Sarcocystis spp. are obligate two-host parasites. The two potentially pathogenic microcyst species in sheep (*S. arieticanis* and *S. tenella*) have either a sheep–dog (**Fig. 8.33**) or sheep–fox cycle. Other sporozoan parasites such as *Neospora caninum*, which has a probable cattle–dog life cycle, may also infect sheep.

Clinical presentation

All ages of sheep may be affected but neurological signs are more commonly observed in 6–12-month-old lambs. Anecdotal reports have described outbreaks following movement from hillgrazing onto pastures regularly used by walkers for exercising their dogs, with subsequent contamination with dog faeces. Some reports describe disease in young sheep housed in close proximity to a litter of puppies, with direct contamination of feed supplies (**Fig. 8.34**).

Affected sheep remain bright and alert with a normal appetite. Hindlimb ataxia and paresis have been described (**Fig. 8.35**) with affected sheep adopting a dog-sitting posture. Some sheep recover with supportive care. Peracute disease with seizure activity and death within 24 hours has also been reported (**Fig. 8.36**).

Differential diagnoses

* Compressive lesions affecting the thoracolumbar spinal cord (T2–L3).
* Sarcocystosis.

Diagnosis

Diagnosis in farm animal practice is difficult because compressive spinal cord lesions, including

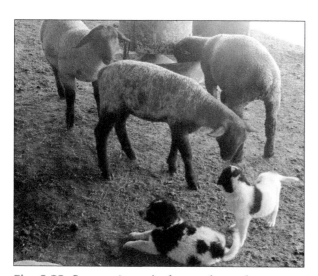

Fig. 8.33 *Sarcocystis* species have a sheep–dog life cycle.

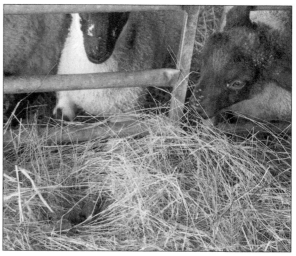

Fig. 8.34 Reports describe sarcocystis in young sheep housed in close proximity to a litter of puppies, where infection follows faecal contamination of sheep feedstuffs.

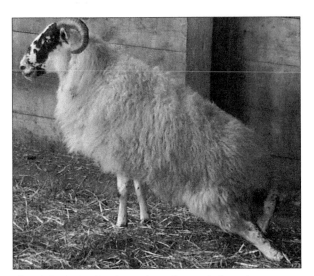

Fig. 8.35 Hindlimb ataxia and paresis have been described in sheep with sarcocytosis.

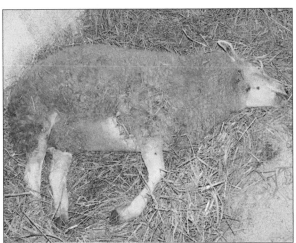

Fig. 8.36 Peracute disease with seizure activity and death within 24 hours has also been reported in sheep with sarcocytosis.

vertebral body empyema, present with similar neurological findings. Serology is not helpful as the majority of sheep have titres to *Sarcocystis* spp, and the provisional diagnosis can only be confirmed by demonstration of characteristic histological lesions in the CNS. An increased lumbar CSF eosinophil count/percentage is suggestive of parasitic infestation of the CNS but there are few supporting data. The use of CSF *Sarcocystis* spp. antibody titres has not been determined.

Pathology
There are few gross pathological changes. There is a non-suppurative encephalomyelitis characterized by multifocal perivascular cuffing and gliosis in the brain. Histopathological examination of the spinal cord has revealed axonal swelling and oedema but no significant demyelination. Despite intensive searches, few cells containing protozoa may be found and further investigations using immunocytochemistry may be necessary.

Treatment
Treatment of naturally-occurring cases is unlikely to be effective, although there are anecdotal claims of cure following drenching sheep with diclazuril daily for 6 weeks at the dose rate quoted for coccidiosis treatment. Such a regimen is expensive.

Management/prevention/control measures
Macroscopic *Sarcocystis* spp. lesions are commonly observed in slaughter plants but neurological disease occurs sporadically. Control is based upon preventing completion of the sheep–dog life cycle, including prevention of faecal contamination of pasture and bedding material by dogs, especially litters of puppies, correct disposal of sheep carcases (a legal requirement in some countries) and not feeding uncooked sheep meat or offal to dogs.

Economics
The disease occurs sporadically but may have a significant financial impact if neurological disease occurs in pedigree breeding stock.

Welfare implications
Sheep with hindlimb paralysis should be confined to deep-bedded straw pens and given supportive care including being turned regularly. If there is no improvement within 10 days the affected sheep should be euthanased for welfare reasons.

VESTIBULAR DISEASE

Definition/overview
Peripheral vestibular disease occurs sporadically in sheep of all ages but particularly growing and

weaned lambs. It is commonly misdiagnosed as listeriosis by farmers.

Aetiology

Unilateral peripheral vestibular lesions are commonly associated with otitis media and ascending infection of the eustachian tube is not uncommon in growing lambs. *Pasteurella* spp, *Streptococcus* spp. and *T. pyogenes* have been isolated from infected lesions.

Clinical presentation

The vestibular system helps the animal maintain orientation in its environment, and maintain the position of the eyes, trunk and limbs with respect to movements and positioning of the head.

Sheep with unilateral vestibular disease present with loss of balance, which may cause recumbency, a head tilt towards the affected side (**Fig. 8.37**) and horizontal nystagmus with the fast phase directed away from the side of the vestibular lesion. Eye droop on the affected side is usually present. Ipsilateral peripheral facial nerve paralysis frequently results from otitis media, causing ptosis and drooping of the ear. There may be evidence of otitis externa and a purulent aural discharge in some cases but rupture of the tympanic membrane is not a common portal of infection.

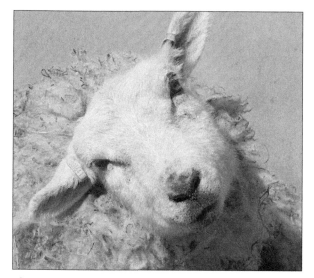

Fig. 8.37 **Sheep with unilateral vestibular disease present with loss of balance and a head tilt towards the affected side.**

Differential diagnoses

Unilateral peripheral vestibular lesions with associated peripheral facial nerve paralysis should be differentiated from listeriosis because of the different treatment regimen and control measures.

Diagnosis

Diagnosis is based upon the clinical examination.

Treatment

When the disease is recognized during the early stages, a good treatment response is achieved with 5 consecutive days' treatment with procaine penicillin. Alternatively, trimethoprim-sulphonamide combination can be used to similar effect.

Management/prevention/control measures

The disease occurs sporadically and there are no specific control measures.

LISTERIOSIS

Definition/overview

Listeriosis is primarily a winter-spring disease most commonly, but not exclusively, associated with silage feeding; the less acidic pH of spoiled silage (pH >5.0) enhances multiplication of *Listeria monocytogenes*. The number of sheep clinically involved in an outbreak is usually less than 2% but in exceptional circumstances may reach 10% in a flock. Outbreaks may occur within 10 days of feeding poor-quality silage (**Figs 8.38–8.40**). Removal or change of silage in the ration often halts the appearance of listeriosis but cases can still occur for a further 2 weeks.

Aetiology

L. monocytogenes is a ubiquitous saprophyte that lives in a plant-soil environment. The natural reservoirs of *L. monocytogenes* appear to be soil and mammalian gastrointestinal tract, both of which contaminate vegetation. It has been postulated that listeria-contaminated silage results in numerous latent infections in the intestinal wall, often approaching 100% of the exposed flock, but clinical listeriosis in only a few animals. *Listeria* spp. that are ingested or inhaled tend to cause septicaemia, abortion and latent infection. Those that gain entry to tissues

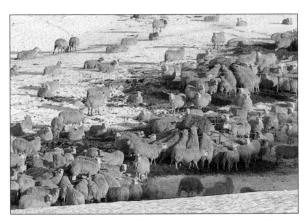

Fig. 8.38 Outbreaks of listeriosis may occur within 10 days of feeding poor-quality silage.

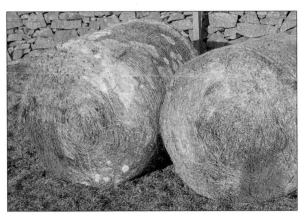

Fig. 8.39 Silage with obvious mould growth suggests poor storage conditions.

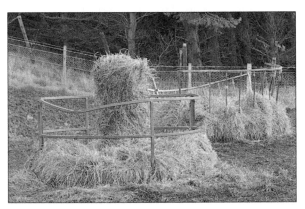

Fig. 8.40 Big bales of grass silage in ring feeders may not be eaten for up to 10–14 days, allowing rapid bacterial multiplication.

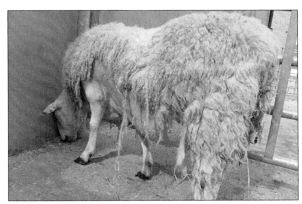

Fig. 8.41 Sheep with listeriosis are depressed, disorientated and may walk forward into corners and not reverse away.

have a predilection to localize in the intestinal wall, medulla oblongata and placenta. Infection can cause encephalitis via minute wounds in buccal mucosa with ascending infection of the trigeminal nerve.

Clinical presentation

Listeriosis is found classically in sheep fed poorly-conserved silage and it affects all ages and both sexes, sometimes as an epidemic, in feedlot sheep. In the UK, sheep aged 18–24 months are most commonly affected. This is associated with cheek teeth eruption facilitating infection of buccal lesions and silage feeding during the winter months. Listeriosis can be encountered in young lambs that have access to silage.

Listeric encephalitis is essentially a localized infection of the brainstem that occurs when *L. monocytogenes* ascends the trigeminal nerve. Clinical signs are generally unilateral in sheep more than 4 months old, and vary according to degree of dysfunction of the damaged cranial nerve nuclei. Signs also include depression, due to involvement of the ascending reticular activating system, and circling (vestibulo-cochlear nucleus).

Initially, affected animals are anorexic, depressed, disorientated and walk forward into corners or under gates (**Figs 8.41–8.43**). This behaviour is not 'head pressing' but occurs because the brainstem in ruminants is programmed to have slow forward walking as the default. They may lean against objects due to hemiparesis (weakness affecting the same side of the body), with knuckling at the fore fetlock joint occasionally present. Affected animals may move in a circle towards the affected side but this is by no means pathognomic of listeriosis; it may simply reflect the confines of the pen with the sheep walking around the boundary.

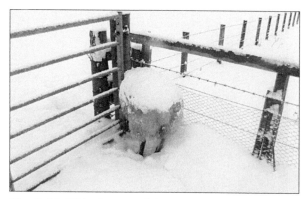

Fig. 8.42 This sheep with listeriosis has pushed itself into the corner of a fence.

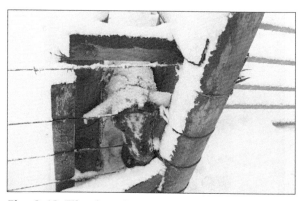

Fig. 8.43 The sheep is not caught it simply fails to reverse out of the corner.

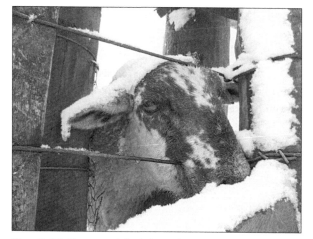

Fig. 8.44 Stupor with right-sided facial and trigeminal nerve paralysis caused by listeriosis.

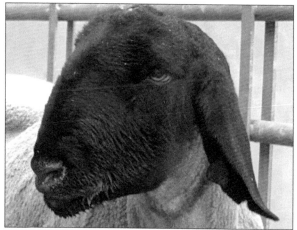

Fig. 8.45 Facial paralysis results in drooping ear, deviated muzzle, flaccid lip and lowered eyelid on the affected (left) side.

There is profuse, almost continuous, salivation, with food material impacted in the cheek of the affected side due to trigeminal nerve paralysis which also results in loss of skin sensation of the face. Facial paralysis results in drooping ear, deviated muzzle, flaccid lip and lowered eyelid on the affected side (Figs 8.44–8.47). There is unilateral lack of blink response and exposure keratitis may arise after 2–3 days. During the terminal stages affected animals are unable to rise or maintain sternal recumbency, and lie on the same side. Involuntary running movements are common leading rapidly to the development of superficial trauma.

Some sheep can present with clinical signs of initial stupor and recumbency (Fig. 8.48), with rapid progression to seizure activity more consistent with meningitis than encephalitis. Where treatment is successful there is a rapid response with few residual signs of cranial nerve deficits (Fig. 8.49).

Differential diagnoses

Trauma to the peripheral facial nerve frequently results after short periods spent in lateral recumbency caused by a number of conditions, and it is important that the drooped ear and ptosis that can result are not mistaken for involvement of the facial nerve nucleus present in listeriosis.

Pregnancy toxaemia commonly affects multigravid ewes during the last 4 weeks of pregnancy. Clinical examination reveals diffuse cerebral signs including central blindness, head pressing and depression, but frequently hyperaesthesia to tactile stimuli during administration of treatments. There is

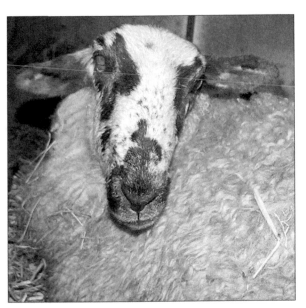

Fig. 8.46 Right-sided facial paralysis results in drooping ear, deviated muzzle, flaccid lip and lowered eyelid on the affected side.

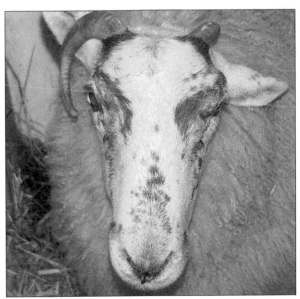

Fig. 8.47 Left-sided facial paralysis results in drooping ear, deviated muzzle, flaccid lip and lowered eyelid on the affected side.

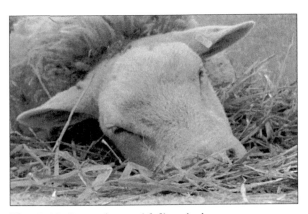

Fig. 8.48 Some sheep with listeriosis can present with initial stupor and recumbency more consistent with meningitis than encephalitis (see Fig. 8.49).

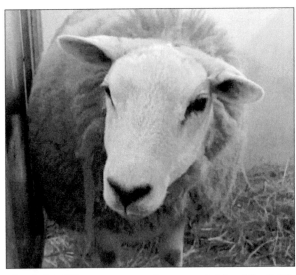

Fig. 8.49 Where treatment is successful (see Fig. 8.48), there is a rapid response with few residual signs of cranial nerve deficits.

no trigeminal or facial nerve paralysis associated with pregnancy toxaemia. 3-OH butyrate concentrations exceed 3.0 mmol/l, often >5.0 mmol/l. There are no CSF changes associated with pregnancy toxaemia.

Peripheral vestibular lesions can present with head tilt, loss of balance, spontaneous horizontal nystagmus and, commonly, damage to the facial nerve due to lateral recumbency causing ptosis and drooped ear. However, the sheep's appetite remains good, and there is neither depression nor signs indicative of trigeminal nerve involvement. The response to conventional-dose antibiotic therapy is very good.

Brain abscesses and coenurosis generally involve only one cerebral hemisphere. Affected sheep commonly present with circling, contralateral blindness and proprioceptive deficits, but no trigeminal and facial nerve deficits.

Radial nerve paralysis should not be mistaken for hemiparesis observed in some sheep with listeriosis.

Diagnosis

Diagnosis of listeriosis is based upon a thorough clinical examination, supported by CSF collection and analysis and, in fatal cases, by histopathological examination of the brainstem and bacteriology. Samples of lumbosacral CSF can readily be collected under local anaesthesia using a 19 gauge 4 cm hypodermic needle (75–85 kg ewe; see *Table 8.2*). Gross examination of CSF reveals no abnormality and laboratory examination must be undertaken. Cases of listeriosis present with an elevated CSF protein concentration, 0.8–4.0 g/l (normal = <0.3 g/l), and a mild increase in white cell concentration (pleocytosis) comprised of large mononuclear cells. To reduce laboratory costs urinary protein dipsticks can detect protein concentrations >2.0 g/l; but a large percentage of false-negative results will occur.

Listeriosis can be confirmed only by isolation and identification of *L. monocytogenes*. Specimens of choice are brain from animals with CNS involvement and aborted placenta and foetus. If primary isolation attempts fail, ground brain tissue should be held at 4°C for several weeks and recultured weekly. Serology is not used routinely for diagnosis because many healthy sheep have high listeria titres.

Treatment

Recovery of sheep from listerial encephalitis (**Fig. 8.50**) depends on early detection of illness by the shepherd, and accurate diagnosis with prompt aggressive antibiotic treatment by the veterinary practitioner. *L. monocytogenes* is susceptible to various antibiotics including penicillin, ceftiofur, erythromycin and trimethoprim/sulphonamide; this author's choice is penicillin. Oxytetracycline is not considered to be an appropriate antibiotic for the treatment of listeriosis; while occasional studies report good results after its use in sheep, there are questions regarding the accuracy of the provisional diagnosis.

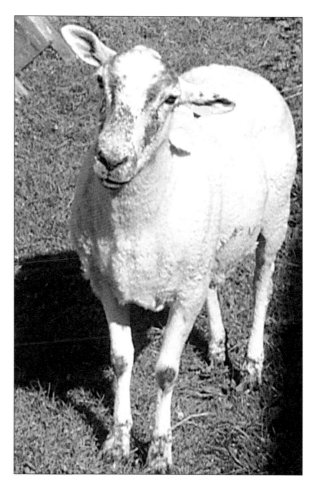

Fig. 8.50 Recovery of sheep from listerial encephalitis depends on early detection of illness and prompt aggressive antibiotic treatment.

High doses of antibiotic are required to achieve MBCs within brain tissue. It is likely that cost will become a consideration in most commercial farm situations before optimum penicillin dosages are achieved. The initial dose requirement may be as high as 300,000 IU/kg. As the best compromise to treat commercial sheep, emphasis should be placed on administering the maximum dose of penicillin that costs will permit at the first visit, rather than the duration of subsequent daily penicillin injections. The overall recovery rate in sheep can be up to 30% when sheep are presented early in the clinical course. However, if signs of meningitis are present (lateral recumbency, seizure activity) death usually occurs despite treatment.

This author's treatment for a 75 kg ewe affected by listeriosis comprises one 5 mega vial of crystalline penicillin (intravenously) plus 5 ml procaine penicillin (300,000 IU/ml injected intramuscularly sid) for the next 5 days. A single intravenous injection of soluble corticosteroid, such as dexamethasone at a dose rate of 1.1 mg/kg, may reduce the associated severe inflammatory reaction and improve prognosis. However, this treatment is based upon clinical observations and there are no supportive clinical studies reported in the literature. High-dose corticosteroid treatment is expensive, but could be considered for valuable individual sheep. (NB: injection of more than 16 mg of dexamethasone after day 136 of pregnancy will cause abortion/premature birth). Propylene glycol, or a concentrated oral rehydration solution containing dextrose, should be administered as per the manufacturer's data sheet to prevent development of a severe energy deficit and the possibility of pregnancy toxaemia in multigravid ewes. Fresh palatable foods and clean water must always be available. A topical antibiotic eye ointment should be applied qid.

The response to successful antibiotic treatment is slow, and initially appears only to arrest deterioration of clinical signs. After a few days the sheep attempts to eat but may experience difficulty masticating food and swallowing. Soft foods such as soaked sugar beet pulp plus some rolled barley in a shallow bowl placed at shoulder height is helpful. Rumen impaction is common after prolonged periods of inappetance and large volumes of warm water and 'rumen stimulants' by orogastric tube assist restoration of rumen function. If available, the transfer of rumen contents from a healthy animal aids recovery. Facial paralysis slowly improves over some weeks.

Management/prevention/control measures

Outbreaks may occur more than 10 days after feeding poor-quality silage. In an outbreak affected animals should be segregated. If silage is being fed, use of that particular silage should be discontinued whenever possible. Spoiled silage should be discarded routinely (or fed to growing cattle at the farmer's risk).

The use of additives for grass silage is likely to produce a more acidic pH, which discourages multiplication of *L. monocytogenes*. Silage clamps must be rolled continuously during filling then sheeted to prevent entry of air. A block cutter operating along a short silage face limits air entry and secondary fermentation once the clamp has been opened. Every effort must be taken not to puncture wrapped silage bales during handling and storage (**Figs 8.51, 8.52**), and all punctures sealed immediately. Stores of wrapped silage bales must be fenced against farm stock and vermin.

The usefulness of a single intramuscular injection of procaine penicillin or other antibiotic to all at-risk sheep during an outbreak of listeriosis (antibiotic metaphylaxis) has not been reported.

Results with vaccines in sheep are limited and the sporadic nature of the disease questions the benefit:cost of vaccination. Some researchers have reasoned that available vaccines are contraindicated for listeriosis.

Economics

Listeriosis generally causes only sporadic losses, rarely greater than 2%, typically in silage-fed flocks. The cost of conserving grass as good quality silage is cheaper than the risks associated with hay making. Farmers acknowledge the risk posed by listeriosis when feeding silage but these can be limited by attention to detail when ensiling grass, and by prompt recognition and appropriate treatment of clinical cases. Consideration should be given to feeding hay to at-risk sheep (those aged around 2 years) should listeriosis cases persist, even after following the adoption of good silage-making practice.

Welfare implications

Sheep presenting with seizure activity and unable to maintain sternal recumbency, and those animals that deteriorate despite 2–3 days' antibiotic therapy, should be humanely destroyed.

VISNA-MAEDI VIRUS

Definition/overview

Visna is a very uncommon manifestation of visna-maedi virus (VMV) infection in the UK, although there are few reliable surveillance data. Clinical disease is rarely reported until the flock seroprevalence rate exceeds 70%.

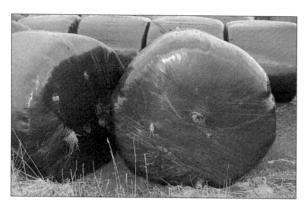

Fig. 8.51 All silage bale wrap punctures must be sealed immediately.

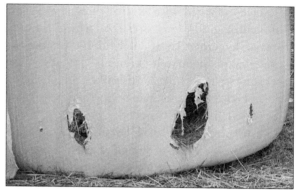

Fig. 8.52 Stores of wrapped silage bales must be fenced against farm stock and vermin.

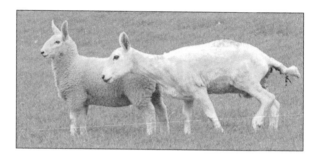

Fig. 8.53 Unilateral hindlimb conscious proprioceptive deficit progressing to paralysis in the spinal cord form of visna.

Aetiology

VMV is a lentivirus related to caprine arthritis encephalitis virus, with cross infection possible between species.

Clinical presentation

The incubation period is protracted and clinical disease is more common in sheep 4–5 years old. Visna has been a very uncommon manifestation of VMV infection in the UK, often appearing some years after the diagnosis of maedi in the flock.

Two forms of visna are reported but poorly defined: an uncommon brain form and a spinal form. In each form of visna the neurological signs are insidious in onset with gradual deterioration over several months.

Brain form: The neurological signs are insidious in onset and present as head tilt approximately 5–10° from the vertical plane and circling towards the affected side. These clinical signs result from lesions within the lateral ventricles. Some affected animals may display hypermetria and hindlimb ataxia.

There is a slow deterioration of neurological signs and affected sheep are usually destroyed for humane reasons within 2 months of initial recognition.

Spinal cord form: The initial neurological signs are hypometria, with reduced flexion of the distal limb joints, conscious proprioceptive deficits and reduced weight-bearing affecting one hindlimb (**Fig. 8.53**). On casual visual examination, these signs could easily be mistaken for lameness originating from the hip or stifle joint. As the condition progresses, the dorsal surface of the hoof remains in contact with the ground when the limb is weight-bearing, with characteristic knuckling of the fetlock joint.

Differential diagnoses

Brain form: A peripheral vestibular lesion causing head tilt, often with ipsilateral facial nerve paralysis, is an important differential diagnosis of the brain form of visna but is more commonly seen in sheep less than 1 year old. Affected animals remain bright and alert with a normal appetite and there is a good response to antibiotic therapy.

Sheep affected with scrapie show a wide range of neurological signs, some of which (hindlimb ataxia; hypermetria; wide-based stance, but with preservation of muscle strength) are observed in certain visna cases. Head tilt and circling behaviour are not observed in scrapie. Scrapie sheep also have a depressed, detached attitude.

Space-occupying brain lesions, such as abscess formation or *Coeneurus cerebralis* cyst, have a chronic course and generally affect one cerebral hemisphere causing contralateral blindness and proprioceptive deficits. Circling toward the affected side is commonly observed in coenurosis.

Spinal cord form: The initial unilateral hindlimb involvement excludes many focal spinal cord lesions, such as epidural or vertebral body compressive lesions, that would affect both hindlimbs. Joint lesions of the hindlimb can be excluded by careful palpation with absence of joint distension, normal joint capsule and joint excursion. Peroneal nerve paralysis is uncommon in adult sheep, and is characterized by overextension of the hock joint, knuckling of the fetlock joint and the absence of skin sensation over the craniolateral aspect of the limb distal to the stifle joint.

Diagnosis

Diagnosis is based upon the clinical examination findings supported by positive VMV serology (usually agar gel immunodiffusion [AGID] test).

Treatment

There is no treatment. All clinical cases, seropositive stock and their progeny should be culled, although this recommendation must be tempered by the VMV status in particular countries, especially those where VMV infection is considered endemic.

Management/prevention/control measures

The impact of VMV on sheep production is disputed between countries. This, in addition to national seroprevalence rate, largely determines the adoption of prevention and control measures. In countries such as the UK, VMV flock control measures are limited to a relatively small number of pedigree flocks.

Economics

Loss of VMV accreditation status prevents the sale of pedigree rams to other pedigree breeders and this incurs a severe financial penalty. There are no recent reliable UK data on potential losses from VMV infection in commercial flocks. Such losses in VMV infected flocks could accrue from culling of clinical cases, poor lamb growth rate resulting from the dam's chronic indurative mastitis and possibly lameness.

Welfare implications

There are no specific welfare problems related to VMV infection other than timely culling during the early stages of clinical disease.

GENETIC DISORDERS

Dandy-Walker malformation
Definition/overview

Dandy-Walker malformation (agenesis of the caudal cerebellar vermis) has been reported in Suffolk sheep in the UK. The prevalence of Dandy-Walker malformation can be high, with reports of 16 affected lambs from 22 ewes, and 17 lambs from 60 ewes. Cases have included twins in which either both lambs were affected or only one lamb, the unaffected twin lamb growing normally. The associated hypertensive hydrocephalus and doming of the skull (**Figs 8.54, 8.55**) frequently causes dystocia. Many affected lambs are either stillborn or die during the neonatal period.

Aetiology

The occurrence of Dandy-Walker malformation (agenesis of the caudal cerebellar vermis) in Suffolk flocks following the introduction of a particular ram indicates a strong genetic component.

Pathology

There is marked distension of the ventricular systems including the lateral, third and fourth ventricles. The cerebellum is abnormal with no visible vermis.

Clinical presentation

The associated hypertensive hydrocephalus and doming of the skull frequently causes dystocia even when the lamb is presented normally. Many affected lambs are either stillborn or die during the neonatal period

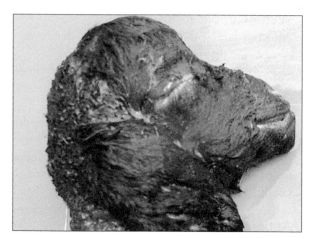

Fig. 8.54 Hypertensive hydrocephalus and doming of the skull are seen in lambs with Dandy-Walker malformation.

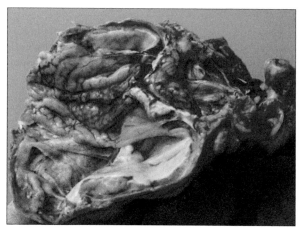

Fig. 8.55 Necropsy reveals the Dandy-Walker malformation with agenesis of the caudal cerebellar vermis and hypertensive hydrocephalus.

caused by failure to ingest colostrum, with death resulting from starvation/hypothermia and/or septicaemia.

Differential diagnoses
Causes of hypertensive hydrocephalus.

Diagnosis
The occurrence of numerous progeny of one ram with doming of the skull is strongly suggestive of Dandy-Walker malformation.

Treatment
The marked doming of the skull frequently causes dystocia even when the lamb is presented normally because the skull is too large to enter the maternal birth canal. The veterinary surgeon is presented with two options: either deliver the lamb by caesarean operation or crush the thinned cranium and deliver the lamb *per vaginam*. While this author has always selected the former course of action, it is reported that crushing the thinned bones comprising the cranium requires little force because of the pressure exerted by the hypertensive hydrocephalus during foetal development. Affected lambs delivered alive must be humanely destroyed.

Management/prevention/control measures
In an investigation of Dandy-Walker malformation in three flocks, the condition only occurred in Suffolk sheep and was associated with particular rams, although exposure to an unidentified teratogen could not be excluded. Careful examination of breeding records in pedigree flocks may identify the affected lambs as the progeny of a ram introduced into the flock for that breeding season. It is important that this ram and his progeny are not used for further breeding.

Economics
Sale of related stock, especially stud rams, may result in the occurrence of Dandy-Walker malformation in the purchaser's flock. The occurrence of Dandy-Walker malformation has serious financial implications for a pedigree flock offering stud rams for sale.

Daft lamb disease
Definition/overview
Daft lamb disease is a poorly-defined disease of neonatal lambs with an uncertain mode of inheritance. Estimation of disease prevalence is limited by the poor disease definition, prevalence of other neonatal lamb neurological diseases with predominantly cerebellar signs and other causes of neurological dysfunction in neonatal lambs, including hypoglycaemia, Border disease and congenital swayback.

Aetiology
Daft lamb disease is considered an inherited disorder by some authors, although the mode of inheritance has not been determined.

Clinical presentation

The clinical signs are observed within the first 2–3 days of life and are typical of cerebellar disease, including wide-based stance with lowered head carriage, ataxia but with preservation of strength and dysmetria. Severely affected lambs have difficulty in searching for the teat but suck vigorously when bottle-fed.

Pathology

Degenerative changes, swelling, pallor or hypochromasia, vacuolation and necrosis have been observed in Purkinje cells and Type II Golgi cells of the cerebellar cortex, the nerve cells of the dentate nucleus and the central cerebellar nuclei.

Differential diagnoses

Differential diagnoses include those more common neonatal lamb neurological diseases with predominantly cerebellar signs, including Border disease, congenital swayback and other causes of neurological dysfunction, such as hypoglycaemia and septicaemia in neonatal lambs. Bacterial meningitis rarely affects lambs less than 1 week old. *In utero* Akabane and Schmallenberg virus infection can cause congenital defects of arthrogryposis, cerebellar hypoplasia and hydranencephaly.

Diagnosis

A tentative diagnosis of cerebellar disease can be based upon the clinical findings. Histological examinations are required to differentiate this disease from Border disease, idiopathic hydrocephalus and congenital swayback.

Management/prevention/control measures

Since the disease has a genetic basis, an increased disease prevalence will occur after the introduction of replacement breeding stock, usually a ram. The suspected heterozygote and all progeny should be sold for slaughter and not kept as breeding replacements.

Economics

It is important that any ram with affected progeny is not used for further breeding and that his progeny are not presented for sale. This could result in considerable loss for a pedigree breeder.

Welfare implications

Affected lambs should be humanely destroyed as soon as the diagnosis has been established.

Cerebellar abiotrophy

Definition/overview

Cerebellar abiotrophy is a familial syndrome which has been described occasionally in Charollais sheep in the UK. Problems with establishing an accurate diagnosis probably lead to under-reporting of this condition.

Aetiology

At necropsy the major histological findings include widespread degeneration of Purkinje cells, with associated hypocellularity of the granular layer and degeneration of myelin in cerebellar foliae and peduncles. There is widespread loss of Purkinje cells, with individual remaining cells being angular and showing condensed, eosinophilic cytoplasm and loss of nuclear detail.

Clinical presentation

Clinical signs of cerebellar abiotrophy may be present from birth or occur in adults. More recent reports in the UK have described lambs with a normal gait for the first 4–8 weeks of life; thereafter, there is progressive deterioration in clinical signs. The clinical signs are typical of cerebellar dysfunction and include lowered head carriage, intention tremors, a wide-based stance, ataxia but with preservation of strength and dysmetria. The hindlimb ataxia may result in the animal falling over, especially when turning quickly. Fine muscle fasciculations, present in the head and neck, may become more pronounced following arousal and resemble coarse muscle tremors causing frequent vigorous jerky movements of the head.

Differential diagnoses

In utero infections, such as Border disease and Akabane and Schmallenberg viruses, cause neurological signs at birth. Compressive cervical spinal lesions, caused by either infection of the atlanto-occipital joint or vertebral body empyema, result in tetraparesis after several days and deteriorate more rapidly than abiotrophy cases. Delayed swayback should also be considered in the differential diagnosis list.

Diagnosis

Clinical diagnosis is based upon the history of progressive deterioration in neurological function with signs indicative of a cerebellar lesion. There is no antemortem test. Confirmation of the diagnosis of cerebellar abiotrophy requires histological demonstration of widespread Purkinje cell degeneration in the cerebellum. Collection of normal CSF helps to eliminate focal bacterial meningoencephalitis from the differential diagnoses list.

Treatment

There is no treatment.

Management/prevention/control measures

The possible inherited nature of this metabolic defect stresses the importance of an accurate diagnosis, especially in a stud ram, which may contribute significantly to the genetic profile of the flock. The parents and siblings of the affected lamb should be sold for slaughter and not kept as breeding replacements.

PITUITARY ABSCESS

(syn. basilar empyema)

Definition/overview

Haematogenous spread of bacteria gives rise to a localized infection of the rete mirabile (a complex of blood capillaries surrounding the pituitary gland), extending into the cranial cavity and along the floor to affect cranial nerves II–VII (**Fig. 8.56**). The prevalence of this disease is not known because it is commonly mistaken for listeriosis.

Aetiology

Localized infection of the frontal sinuses (**Fig. 8.57**) is considered to be one source of haematogenous spread to the rete mirabile that gives rise to basilar empyema (**Figs 8.58, 8.59**). Fighting injuries causing infected head wounds may explain the more common occurrence in rams.

Clinical presentation

Clinical findings include multiple cranial nerve deficits, particularly bilateral cranial nerve deficits involving II–VII, ataxia and bradycardia.

Differential diagnoses

Listeriosis is the primary differential diagnosis because of involvement of multiple cranial nerves, but it is unusual to find bilateral cranial nerve deficits in adult sheep and lack of menace response.

Diagnosis

Diagnosis is based on (bilateral) involvement of cranial nerves II–VII.

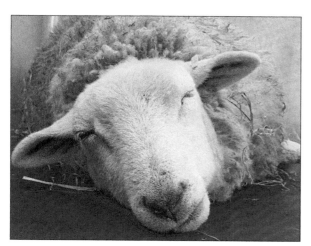

Fig. 8.56 **Basilar empyema causes bilateral deficits in cranial nerves II–VII.**

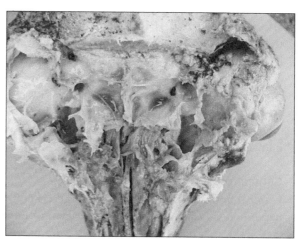

Fig. 8.57 **Localized infection of the frontal sinuses is considered to be one source of haematogenous spread to the rete mirabile.**

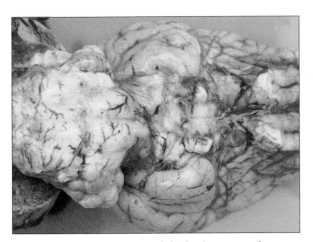

Fig. 8.58 Ventral surface of the brain removed at necropsy showing pus around the roots of cranial nerves II–VII.

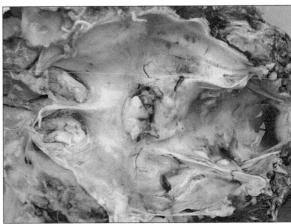

Fig. 8.59 Cranial cavity showing infection tracking caudally from the pituitary fossa to involve the cranial nerve roots.

Treatment

The treatment protocol is the same as for listeriosis but the advanced pathology at presentation, and lack of drainage from within the cranium, results in a guarded prognosis.

Management/prevention/control measures

There are no specific control measures.

PITUITARY TUMOUR

Definition/overview

There is slow growth of the tumour (**Fig. 8.60**) to affect cranial nerves II and III. The prevalence of this disease is not known because the condition is likely to be commonly mistaken for either PEM or a cerebral abscess.

Aetiology

The cause of the tumour affecting older sheep is not known.

Clinical presentation

Clinical findings include bilateral II and III cranial nerve deficits causing blindness and lack of pupillary light reflexes (**Figs 8.61, 8.62**). Compression of the cerebral hemispheres may cause altered mentation.

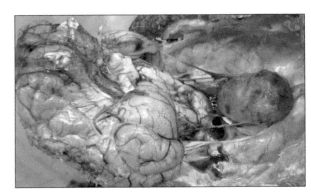

Fig. 8.60 The pituitary tumour causes compression of cranial nerves II and III and the cerebral hemispheres.

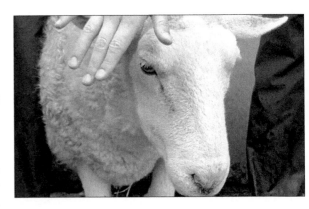

Fig. 8.61 An aged ewe with a pituitary tumour shows a lack of menace response.

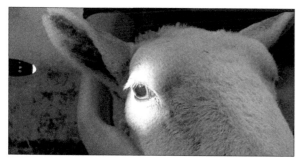

Fig. 8.62 There is no papillary light reflex in this aged ewe with a pituitary tumour.

Differential diagnoses

PEM, basilar empyema and cerebral abscess should be considered in the differential diagnoses and closantel toxicity if treated within the past 10 days.

Diagnosis

Diagnosis is based upon bilateral involvement of cranial nerves II and III.

Treatment

There is no treatment and affected sheep should be euthanased for welfare reasons.

Management/prevention/control measures

There are no control measures.

CLOSANTEL TOXICITY

Definition/overview

Closantel is toxic to small ruminants even in moderate overdose (1.5–2 times) and incidents of closantel toxicity in sheep have been reported worldwide. The speed of onset and severity of clinical signs appear to be dose dependent; a much higher prevalence has been reported (22%) and shorter 1–3 days' interval to onset, after a three- to six-fold overdose. The increasing prevalence of triclabendazole resistance in *Fasciola hepatica* has resulted in an increased use of closantel in the UK.

Aetiology

The proposed mechanism of toxicity involves disruption of cells with tightly packed cell membranes, leading to retinopathy, myelinic oedema and white matter vacuolation.

Clinical presentation

There is sudden onset blindness approximately 1–8 days after drenching with closantel. Clinical findings also include lack of pupillary light reflexes and hyperaesthesia but normal appetite. Higher dose rates are reported to cause a wider range of clinical signs, including ataxia, colic, opisthotonus and collapse. There is no improvement over time.

Differential diagnoses

Differential diagnoses include PEM, sulphur toxicity and pregnancy toxaemia; pituitary tumour would be unlikely to affect several sheep simultaneously.

Diagnosis

Diagnosis is based upon (bilateral) involvement of cranial nerves II and III. At necropsy, histopathology reveals extensive loss of nerve structure and replacement with fibrosis in the intracanalicular section of the optic nerve. Wallerian degeneration of axons is visible within the optic chiasm.

Treatment

There is no treatment; the changes are irreversible.

Management/prevention/control measures

Accurate dosing is essential; sheep should be weighed and divided into narrow weight categories before drenching.

SPINAL CORD LESIONS

Definition/overview

Traumatic and infective lesions of the vertebral column causing spinal cord compression and dysfunction are common in sheep. Infective lesions are more common in growing lambs 1–4 months old but can occur in all age groups. Infection of the atlanto-occipital joint is common in neonatal lambs following *Streptococcus dysgalactiae* infection. Fracture of the cervical vertebrae is not uncommon in rams following fighting during the breeding season. Compressive cervical myelopathy is common in Texel and Beltex sheep in the UK.

Aetiology

Vertebral body empyema arises from an infectious focus; however, macroscopic evidence of the initiating infection is not commonly found at necropsy. A high flock prevalence of vertebral body empyema may be associated with tick-bite pyaemia in areas with tick-borne fever. *T. pyogenes* and *Staphylococcus* spp. have been isolated from typical lesions. Lesions caused by dosing gun injuries, and those associated with intramuscular injection of a potentially-irritating substance into the neck muscles, may give rise to infective lesions tracking to involve the cervical spinal canal.

Traumatic lesions involving the cervical region occur in rams caused by fighting injuries prior to the seasonal breeding period. Tumour conditions affecting the spinal cord, such as meningioma, have occasionally been reported.

Compressive cervical myelopathy is common in certain bloodlines of Texel and Beltex sheep suggestive of a hereditary susceptibility (**Fig. 8.63**).

Differential diagnoses

Recumbency can be caused by a variety of conditions including limb fractures and painful joint lesions from bacterial polyarthritis, osteoarthritis and associated with endocarditis.

Metabolic conditions causing recumbency and altered mentation, including ovine pregnancy toxaemia and hypocalcaemia, should be carefully considered in recumbent ewes during late gestation.

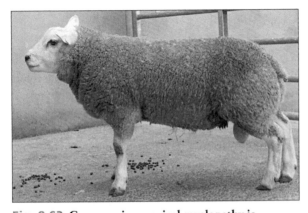

Fig. 8.63 Compressive cervical myelopathy is common in certain bloodlines of UK Texel and Beltex sheep.

Clinical presentation

Localization of a spinal cord lesion involves evaluation of withdrawal and tendon jerk reflexes of the hind- and forelimbs, and assessment of the panniculus reflex. The simple spinal reflex arc is the basis to the spinal cord examination. Under field situations it may prove difficult to undertake a satisfactory examination in large rams and heavily pregnant ewes that are recumbent.

Upper/lower motor neuron disease terms refer to the responses obtained to stimulation of local reflex arcs. The presence of a lesion at the level of a reflex arc results in lack of muscle contraction in response to stimulation. Denervation of the effector muscle results in flaccid paralysis with atony. This type of lesion is referred to as lower motor neuron disease.

The presence of a lesion cranial to the reflex arc removes the normal inhibitory controlling inputs from the descending upper motor neuron pathways and results in spastic paralysis (stiffness). There is similar loss of voluntary motor function but stimulation of the reflex arc results in an exaggerated response referred to as upper motor neuron disease. Determination of fore- and hindlimb responses aids in the localization of a spinal lesion. Flexion of the stimulated limb but extension of the contralateral limb is referred to as 'crossed extensor reflex' and indicates the presence of a CNS lesion above the reflex arc.

The clinical signs depend upon the degree and location of spinal cord compression. Localization of a spinal cord lesion is achieved by evaluating the reflex pathways.

Cervical spinal lesions (C1–C6): Cervical spinal lesions may result from *S. dysgalactiae* infection of the atlanto-occipital joint in neonatal lambs, vertebral body fractures associated with fighting injuries in rams, dosing gun injuries involving abscessation of the intervertebral body of the atlanto-occipital joint or C1/C2 articulation and vertebral body empyema associated with a pyaemia/septicaemia (**Fig. 8.64**).

In mild cervical lesions (C1–C6) there is ataxia and weakness involving all four limbs but the hindlimbs are more severely affected. There are

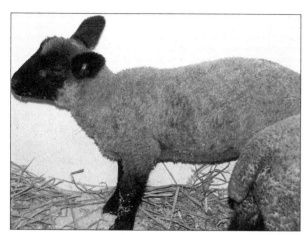

Fig. 8.64 Cervical lesions (C1–C6) present with ataxia, weakness involving all four limbs and possibly signs of pain with the head held rigidly.

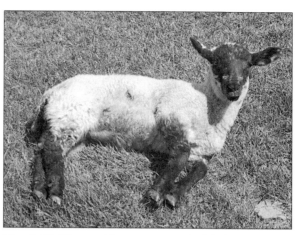

Fig. 8.65 Sheep with a severe cervical lesion (C1–C6) may not be able to maintain sternal recumbency.

hopping, placing and conscious proprioceptive deficits. The fore- and hindlimb reflexes are increased (upper motor neuron signs). Severely affected sheep may not be able to maintain sternal recumbency and must be supported (**Fig. 8.65**).

Compressive cervical myelopathy: Clinical findings typical of cervical spinal cord compression have been reported in 12–18-month-old Texel and Beltex sheep, more commonly in males than females. Sheep with mild signs make minor errors in placing the hindlimbs and stand with a wide-based stance at rest. The sheep often sway on the hindlimbs when turning. Frequent stumbling is noted in the forelimbs when the sheep is forced to trot. Withdrawal reflexes in the hindlimbs are exaggerated. Sheep with moderate signs have more obvious hindlimb ataxia and weakness, and often show dysmetria of the forelimbs. Hopping deficits are present in one or more forelimbs and usually in all four limbs. Withdrawal reflexes are exaggerated in hind- and forelimbs. Sheep with severe signs tend to collapse when handled. When placed in lateral recumbency, more severely affected sheep often have prominent extensor tone of the hindlimbs. Hyper-reflexia with clonus and crossed-extensor reflexes are present in the hindlimbs.

CSF specific gravity, total protein content and cell count are within normal ranges. Radiographic examination of the cervico-thoracic vertebral column fails to demonstrate any gross bony abnormalities; however, radiographic myelograms have revealed extradural lesions at the level of C6–C7 where the dorsal contrast column ends abruptly at C6–C7.

No bony abnormalities are identified as described in cases of canine and equine wobbler syndrome. Postmortem examinations reveal discrete, smooth, nodular to polypoid projections of adipose tissue prolapsing through the dorso-lateral intervertebral space at C6–C7, causing localized spinal cord compression. Histopathology of the nodules confirms that they are composed of well-differentiated adipocytes typical of fatty tissue. There is marked Wallerian degeneration at the site of compression, with milder changes present cranial and caudal to the lesion.

Atlanto-occipital joint: Infection of the atlanto-occipital joint caused by *S. dysgalactiae* infection has become increasingly reported in flocks lambing indoors in the UK over the past 10 years. Lambs appear normal for the first 4–7 days then show lowered head carriage, neck pain and progressive weakness of all four limbs over 1–3 days, progressing to recumbency (**Fig. 8.66**). This condition is often misdiagnosed as muscular dystrophy. Early cases (**Fig. 8.67**) respond within 6 hours to intravenous dexamethasone and parenteral procaine

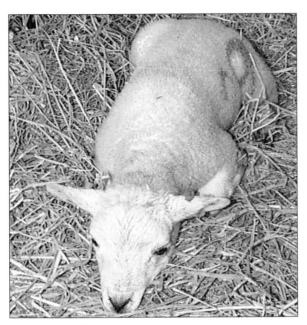

Fig. 8.66 Infection of the atlanto-occipital joint caused by *Streptococcus dysgalactiae* infection causes lowered head carriage, neck pain and progressive weakness of all four limbs.

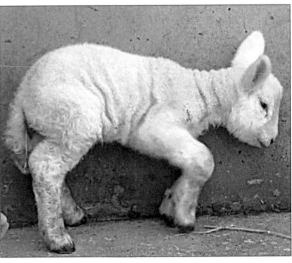

Fig. 8.67 Infection of the atlanto-occipital joint is often misdiagnosed as muscular dystrophy.

penicillin (**Fig. 8.68**); 5–10 days consecutive days' penicillin injections are necessary to prevent relapse. There may be no evidence of polyarthritis in affected lambs but other lambs in the group may show infection of the carpal, fetlock and hock joints.

Brachial intumescence (C6–T2): The term intumescence refers to the concentration of neurons in the grey matter of the spinal cord at the level of the fore- and hindlimbs (**Fig. 8.69**). Lesions affecting this length of spinal cord cause reduced forelimb reflexes (lower motor neuron signs) and increased hindlimb reflexes (upper motor neuron signs). Forelimb weakness is judged by the resistance to lateral movement of the animal by pushing the animal's shoulder away.

T2–L3: Animals with a spinal lesion caudal to T2 have normal forelimb function. These animals frequently adopt a dog-sitting posture with the hips flexed and the hindlimbs extended alongside the abdomen, rather than the normal flexed position underneath the body (**Fig. 8.70**). The clinician's attention is immediately drawn to this abnormal posture because sheep always raise themselves with the hindlimbs first.

The presence of a spinal cord lesion in the thoraco-lumbar region T2–L3 results in upper motor neuron signs of increased tendon jerk and withdrawal reflexes in the hindlimbs. There are conscious proprioceptive deficits and weakness of the hindlimbs.

Scoliosis (deviation of the spine) may occur in cases of asymmetric myelopathies, with the concave side opposite the lesion due to the maintenance of muscular tone on the unaffected (contralateral) side.

The panniculus reflex is a useful means of localizing a focal thoraco-lumbar spinal lesion. The sensory stimulus travels to the spinal cord at the level of stimulation. The absence of reflex muscle contraction would indicate the caudal aspect of the spinal lesion.

L4–S2: Lesions in the region L4–S2 result in flaccid paralysis of the hindlimbs, with reduced or absent reflexes.

S1–S3: Lesions affecting S1–S3 cause hypotonia of the bladder and rectum, resulting in distension with urine and faeces, respectively.

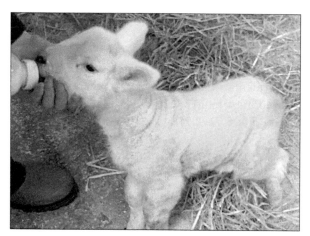

Fig. 8.68 Early cases (see Fig. 8.67) respond within 6 hours to intravenous dexamethasone and parenteral procaine penicillin.

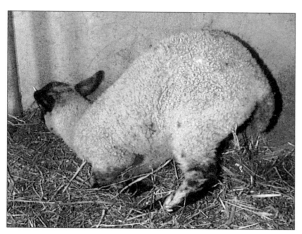

Fig. 8.69 Forelimb weakness caused by a lesion at C6–T2.

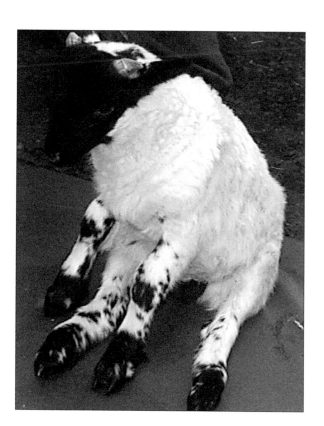

Fig. 8.70 Sheep with a lesion at T2–L3 frequently adopt a dog-sitting posture.

Diagnosis

A careful neurological examination should identify the section of the spinal cord involved in the disease process. Rapidity of onset, duration and change in clinical presentation, in addition to age and recent management practices of the animal, such as mixing mature rams, may provide some useful information.

Inflammatory lesions extending into the vertebral canal causing spinal cord compression result in an elevated protein concentration in lumbar CSF. Cranial CSF flow is blocked by the compressive lesion and prevents equilibration within the lateral ventricles. This phenomenon caused by blockage of cranial CSF flow is not dissimilar to Froin's syndrome in man, which has been reported as a result of localized spinal meningitis.

Once the suspected lesion has been localized to a region of the spinal cord, radiography may allow identification of vertebral osteomyelitis. Myelography can be undertaken under general anaesthesia (**Fig. 8.71**), but these more specific diagnostic procedures are too expensive except for particularly valuable breeding stock. Radiography may be helpful to identify suspected fracture(s) of a cervical vertebra in valuable rams.

In general practice a diagnosis of an infective lesion causing significant spinal cord compression is based on the clinical signs described above of greater than 5 days' duration without improvement despite antibiotic therapy, plus a lumbar CSF sample with an elevated protein concentration.

Treatment

The extent of the vertebral body empyema that precedes spinal cord compression and the appearance of neurological dysfunction is so severe that antibiotic treatment will never effect a cure; therefore, affected sheep must be humanely destroyed for welfare reasons (**Figs 8.72–8.74**).

Management/prevention/control measures

The disease occurs sporadically, thus there are no specific prevention or control measures.

Economics

Significant losses may occur when infective lesions arise from tick-bite pyaemia. Valuable breeding rams may occasionally be lost to cervical vertebral body fracture.

Welfare implications

Lambs with vertebral body empyema should be humanely destroyed once the condition has been determined. Predation may occur in extensive systems.

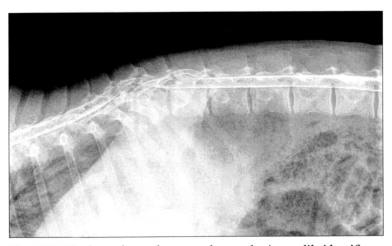

Fig. 8.71 Myelography, under general anaesthesia, readily identifies spinal cord compression.

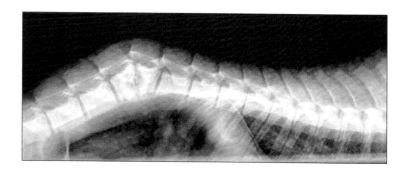

Fig. 8.72 Radiography reveals the extent of bone lysis in this case of vertebral body empyema.

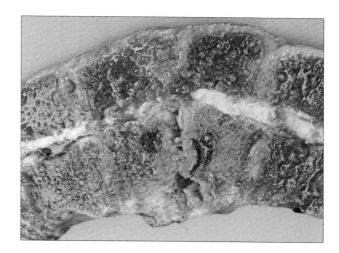

Fig. 8.73 Necropsy reveals the extent of this vertebral body empyema lesion; antibiotic treatment will not effect a cure.

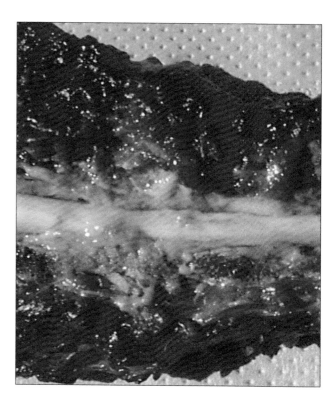

Fig. 8.74 Necropsy reveals the extent of this vertebral body empyema lesion; affected sheep must be humanely destroyed for welfare reasons.

INTRODUCTION

The musculoskeletal system comprises the skeleton, joints, ligaments, tendons and muscles. Together with the nervous system, it is responsible for the animal's stance and gait. Infections of the musculoskeletal system are common in sheep; polyarthritis is common in neonates, interdigital dermatitis in growing lambs and footrot in adults; all cause serious welfare concerns. Osteoarthritis, commonly predisposed by trauma, is largely confined to the elbow and stifle joints. Clinical involvement of the musculoskeletal system is manifest as lameness, and much less commonly as weakness.

ASSESSMENT OF THE PROBLEM(S)

The extent of the lameness problem within the group must be defined by the veterinarian before the sheep are penned, otherwise lameness shown by many sheep will be masked by their close confinement. It is best to walk quietly through the sheep while they are still

at pasture to quantify accurately the prevalence and severity of the lameness problem (**Figs 9.1, 9.2**).

It may be possible to select lame sheep from the group by slowly walking the sheep through a gate into another field; lame sheep will trail behind their sound peers and may even lie down if the lameness is severe, so the majority of the lame sheep can be separated from the group. This method is not always successful as the flocking instinct and fear of separation may temporarily overcome the pain of the lameness in some sheep. Diseases of other organ systems, such as respiratory disease, may also cause exercise intolerance.

ASSESSMENT OF THE HANDLING FACILITIES

It is advisable to check the sheep handling facilities used for footbathing on the farm (**Fig. 9.3**), their suitability for the number of sheep and maintenance. Treatment records should be consulted but are not always kept up to date.

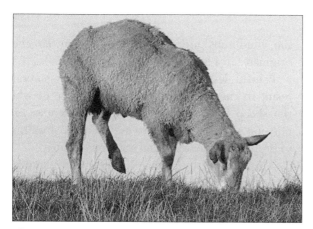

Fig. 9.1 The severity of the lameness problem is best assessed before sheep are confined in a pen.

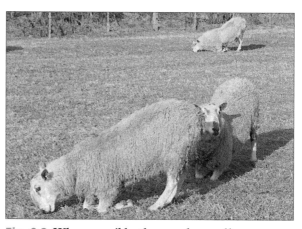

Fig. 9.2 Where possible, the prevalence of lameness should be assessed before the sheep are gathered. Note all three rams are lame and grazing on their knees.

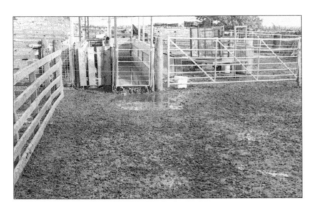

Fig. 9.3 The farmer may need advice regarding the sheep handling and footbathing facilities.

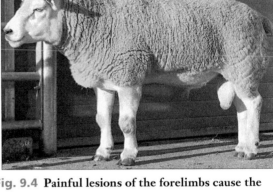

Fig. 9.4 Painful lesions of the forelimbs cause the sheep to graze on its knees, leading to abrasions and thickening of the skin overlying the knees.

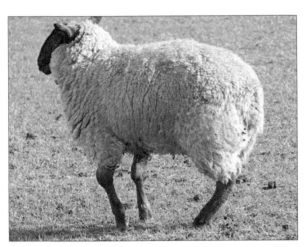

Fig. 9.5 Painful forelimb lesions result in the hind feet being drawn forward and extended under the body to bear more weight.

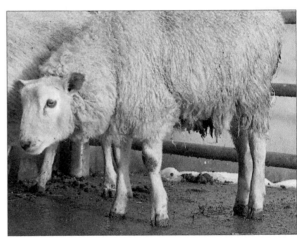

Fig. 9.6 The hindlimbs are held straight when lameness originates in a hindlimb.

OBSERVATION

Sheep with moderate to severe lameness and weakness spend increased time in sternal, or even lateral, recumbency. Painful lesions affecting the foot and distal joints, but also elbow arthritis, cause the sheep to graze on its knees leading to abrasions and thickening of the skin overlying the knees (**Fig. 9.4**). Repeated skin trauma over the cranial aspect of the carpal joints may result in discoloration of the hairs at the periphery of these callused areas; typically black hairs regrow grey or white (**Fig. 9.4**). Painful forelimb lesions result in the hind feet being drawn forward and extended under the body to bear more weight (**Fig. 9.5**) whereas

the hindlimbs are held straight when lameness originates in a hindlimb (**Fig. 9.6**).

Painful lesions affecting a hindlimb generally result in the affected limb being uppermost when the sheep is resting in sternal recumbency. This position allows the sheep to use the lower hindlimb to propel itself forward and up during rising.

The extent of the lameness is subjectively scored on a 10 point scale, 1 being slight lameness to 10 which is non-weight-bearing even at rest (**Fig. 9.7**), with the sheep unwilling to take even one or two steps forward. Typically, long bone fractures and septic joints result in severe (10/10) lameness but so too can white line abscesses, especially those that track up to the coronary band. Therefore, the degree of lameness does not necessarily determine prognosis.

CLINICAL EXAMINATION

The clinician must always remember that lameness originates from a painful lesion and that manipulations should be kept to a minimum and undertaken with care and empathy. In particular, joint lesions are especially painful; manipulations to elicit crepitus are unnecessary. The clinical examination must not exacerbate the degree of lameness; this merely reflects poor examination technique. Gentle digital palpation will reveal much more information regarding joint effusion and thickness of the joint capsule (**Fig. 9.8**) than trying to elicit crepitus by forceful movement of the joint. The more sensitive the palpation process, the more information gleaned. Erosion of articular cartilage to such an extent as to cause 'joint crepitus' with bone surfaces grinding against one another would probably only occur after many months of severe lameness and neglect (**Fig. 9.9**).

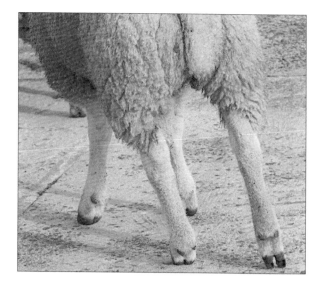

Fig. 9.7 The extent of the lameness is subjectively scored on a 10 point scale; 10 is non-weight-bearing even at rest (this case).

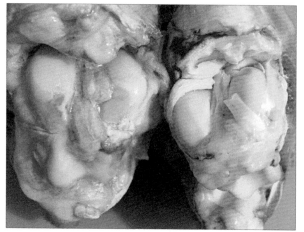

Fig. 9.8 Despite considerable joint pathology (and resultant pain) evident as proliferation of synovial membrane and thickening of the joint capsule of the stifle joint shown on the left side compared to normal, movement of this joint would not have generated crepitus.

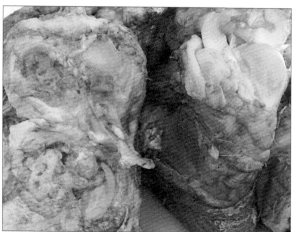

Fig. 9.9 Erosion of articular cartilage to cause 'joint crepitus' with bone surfaces grinding against one another (left side) only occurs after many months of severe lameness and neglect.

The extent of muscle wastage depends upon both the severity and duration of lameness. Muscle wastage can be reliably detected after 5–7 days' moderate to severe lameness (**Figs 9.10, 9.11**) by careful palpation over bony prominences such as the spine of the scapula and head of the femur for forelimbs and hindlimbs, respectively. Visual detection of muscle wastage is usually prevented by the presence of the full fleece. Comparison of changes with the contralateral limb, if sound, is recommended. In the case of elbow arthritis where there is considerable enthesophyte formation, the breadth of the affected joint should be measured with callipers and compared with measurements from sound sheep of similar breed, sex and age.

Enlargement of the prescapular lymph node (two to five times normal size) can be readily appreciated within 3–7 days of bacterial infection of forelimb joints and cellulitis lesions. White line and sole abscesses and footrot lesions do not usually cause such obvious drainage lymph node enlargement. Infected lesions distal to the stifle joint cause enlargement of the popliteal lymph node but this node is not readily palpable unless there is considerable muscle atrophy. Infection proximal to the stifle joint results in enlargement of the deep inguinal lymph nodes within the pelvic canal.

Casting the sheep to permit detailed examination of the foot/feet is undertaken as the last component of the examination. This must not be undertaken if there is a painful joint lesion or suspected fracture. Turning crates are commonly used to facilitate turning and restraint in dorsal recumbency to examine the feet and are generally well tolerated by sheep. The interdigital space is examined and any impacted foreign material removed. Grossly overgrown horn from the abaxial wall and toe of the foot of the lame limb is carefully removed with shears or a sharp hoof knife to check for a white line abscess or toe granuloma. Over-paring of the hoof horn of the wall must be avoided because this action simply transfers weight to the sole, which is abnormal. Foot paring must not be undertaken where there is separation of the horn from the corium caused by footrot or contagious ovine digital dermatitis (CODD).

While routine foot trimming was once considered an essential part of flock management, particularly for rams, this practice may cause altered weight distribution from the wall to the sole.

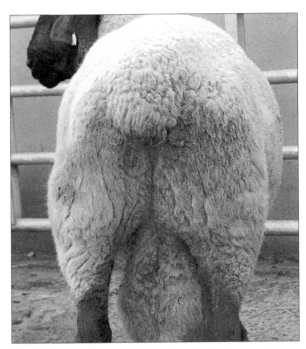

Fig. 9.10 Muscle wastage can be reliably detected (rear view) after 5–7 days' moderate to severe lameness.

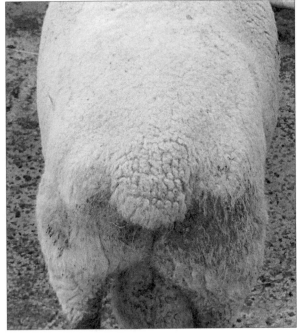

Fig. 9.11 Muscle wastage can be reliably detected (dorsal view) after 5–7 days' moderate to severe lameness.

Under-running of the horn associated with foot-rot or CODD is very painful and it is best treated with parenteral antibiotics, such as oxytetracycline or a macrolide drug, such as tilmicosin. Field studies show better results are achieved with tilmicosin but this drug is restricted for veterinary administration in many countries. Other macrolide antibiotics such as gamithromycin are increasingly used for treating footrot and CODD because no such restriction applies although there is presently no license for their use in sheep in many countries. It is essential not to damage the sensitive corium as this will delay regeneration of epithelium and extend healing time. Foot trimming 5–7 days later when the lesions appear less aggressive is not necessary and could delay healing. Exposure of the sensitive corium to irritant chemicals, such as formalin in footbaths, may result in excess granulation tissue and the formation of a toe fibroma.

ARTHROCENTESIS

Arthrocentesis is not commonly undertaken in sheep because joint infection with the common bacterial pathogens *Streptococcus dysgalactiae* and *Erysipelothrix rhusiopathiae* rarely causes marked joint effusion (**Fig. 9.12**). Attempts can be made to collect synovial fluid from distended joints under local anaesthesia but anaesthetic can only be given subcutaneously; the infected joint capsule/synovial membrane cannot be readily desensitized. Intravenous regional anaesthesia can be used to anaesthetize the hock, fetlock and distal limb joints.

The arthrocentesis site is shaved and aseptically prepared. The approach depends on the anatomy of a particular joint; in general, the joint capsule is punctured where it is most distended as this 'pouching' occurs away from structures such as ligaments and tendons.

Normal synovial fluid is pale yellow, viscous, clear and does not clot. The protein concentration is <18 g/l, with a low white cell concentration comprised mainly of lymphocytes. Septic arthritis is characterized by a turbid sample caused by increased white cell concentration that is comprised almost exclusively of neutrophils. The protein concentration is increased above 40 g/l.

Samples collected from chronically infected joints frequently fail to grow bacteria. Direct smears of the aspirate can be made onto a glass slide and stained with Gram's stain to gain some information on the potential pathogen(s) involved. In the investigation of a flock outbreak, the best means of establishing the cause is to sacrifice a typical early case which has received no antibiotic therapy and submit a sample of inflamed synovial membrane from several affected joints to the laboratory.

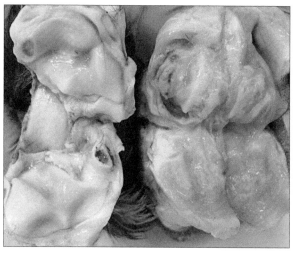

Fig. 9.12 **The common bacterial pathogens of ovine joints rarely cause marked effusion.**

RADIOGRAPHY

Radiography is most useful in the identification of greenstick fractures in young lambs (**Fig. 9.13**) and the investigation of long bone fractures (**Fig. 9.14**). Sedation, or preferably general anaesthesia, may be required to allow correct positioning of the sheep for radiography of the humerus and femur. Enthesophyte formation is common in the elbow joint of adult sheep and the best radiographic results are obtained from an oblique view (**Fig. 9.15**). Radiography may prove useful in the investigation of some early cases of septic pedal arthritis, especially where the lesion has not progressed to cause a discharging sinus at the coronary band (**Fig. 9.16**).

Radiography adds little new information to the investigation of most cases of septic arthritis other than to reveal widening of the joint space. Indeed, radiography of a septic joint revealing only slight widening of the joint space (**Figs 9.17, 9.18**) may be mistakenly interpreted to mean there is little pathology present.

ULTRASONOGRAPHY

Ultrasonography using a 7.5 or 10 MHz linear array scanner can provide useful information regarding the thickness of the joint capsule and extent and nature of any joint effusion. The skin overlying the joint is shaved to ensure good contact; a stand-off may be required for examination of smaller joints. Affected joint(s) should be compared with the contralateral joint, where normal. Ultrasonography has many advantages over radiography for joint

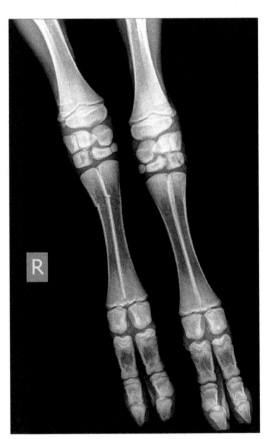

Fig. 9.13 Dorso-palmar view. Radiography is especially useful in the investigation of greenstick fractures in neonatal lambs; proximal third metacarpal bone of the right forelimb in this case.

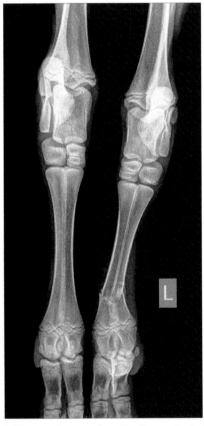

Fig. 9.14 Dorso-plantar view. Radiography is helpful in the investigation of long bone fractures to identify potential involvement of the physes; distal third metatarsal bone of the left hindlimb in this case.

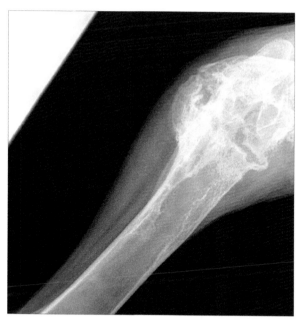

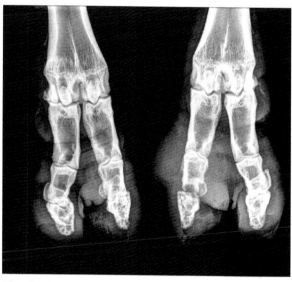

Fig. 9.16 Loss of the articular surfaces of the distal interphalangeal joint of the medial claw of the left foot. Note also the soft tissue swelling in this region.

Fig. 9.15 Enthesophyte formation is common in the elbow joint of adult sheep; best radiographic results are obtained from an oblique view.

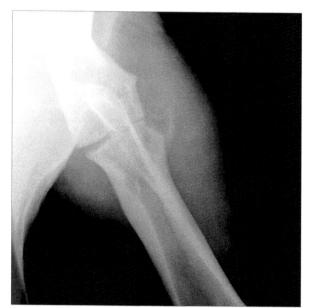

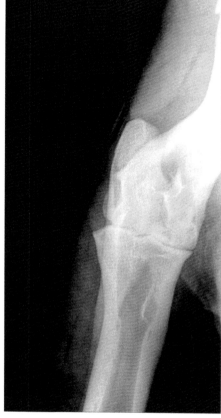

Fig. 9.17 Radiography of acute joint sepsis reveals only slight widening of the (elbow) joint space (see Fig. 9.18).

Fig. 9.18 Radiograph of the normal elbow joint space.

examination in that the procedure is cheap, reveals more detail of soft tissue, involves no health and safety concerns and is readily portable for on-farm examinations. Ultrasound examination of the joint can be undertaken prior to arthrocentesis to determine the presence of an effusion.

NERVE BLOCKS

Unlike horses, nerve blocks and intra-articular anaesthesia are rarely used in sheep.

FOOTROT

Footrot, presenting as interdigital dermatitis (**Fig. 9.19**) or progressing to hoof horn separation from the corium (**Fig. 9.20**), is caused by *Dichelobacter nodosus*; consequently both presentations of disease should be managed together.

Footrot – interdigital dermatitis
Definition/overview
Interdigital dermatitis is an acute necrotizing infection of the interdigital skin. In the UK, it is most commonly seen affecting intensively managed, densely-stocked lambs aged 4–10 weeks, causing considerable lameness (**Fig. 9.21**). The morbidity rate can rapidly exceed 50% in less than 1 week. Infection is much more common during periods of warm wet weather.

Aetiology
Ovine interdigital dermatitis is caused by *D. nodosus* and predisposed by wet conditions and trauma to the interdigital skin. *D. nodosus* is an obligate organism found only in the feet of ruminants affected by footrot and can only survive in the environment for 7–14 days. Thus disease is introduced into a flock by the purchase of infected carrier sheep. This carrier state may persist for 2–3 years.

Clinical presentation
Ovine interdigital dermatitis commonly affects large numbers of lambs aged 4–10 weeks. There is sudden onset severe lameness such that lambs may not put the affected foot to the ground; some lambs may graze on their knees (**Fig. 9.22**). Close examination

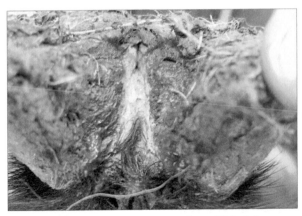

Fig. 9.19 Footrot may present as interdigital dermatitis, which is an acute necrotizing infection of the interdigital skin.

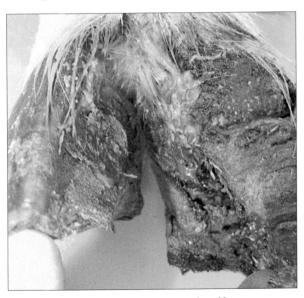

Fig. 9.20 Footrot may progress to hoof horn separation from the corium and under-running of the sole.

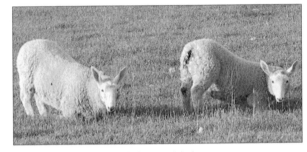

Fig. 9.21 Interdigital dermatitis is most commonly seen affecting intensively managed, densely-stocked lambs aged 4–10 weeks and causes severe lameness.

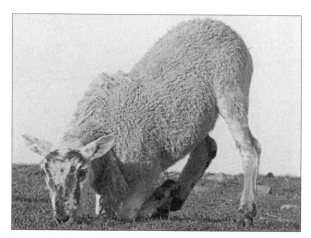

Fig. 9.22 Interdigital dermatitis causes sudden onset lameness such that lambs may graze on their knees.

reveals marked hyperaemia of interdigital skin with superficial accumulations of moist whitish necrotic material (**Fig. 9.23**).

Differential diagnoses
Sudden onset severe lameness affecting one or more growing lambs could also be caused by erysipelas; however, this can readily be differentiated on clinical examination. Following hedge cutting thorns can lead to a high prevalence of foot abscesses.

Diagnosis
The diagnosis is based on the clinical examination and rapid response to topical oxytetracycline spray, or other bactericidal agent.

Treatment
If possible the flock should be moved to dry pasture where spontaneous recovery may occur, but this is not an option in most situations. In the UK the method of choice is to turn every lamb and treat all affected feet with topical oxytetracycline aerosol, but this is very labour intensive. Affected lambs are identified and topical treatment repeated 2 days later if necessary. Surprisingly, despite the severe lameness, there is return to full soundness within 1–2 days of first treatment.

The use of 5% formalin footbaths produces acceptable results but young lambs do not go through a footbath easily. Lambs are often considerably more lame for a short period after formalin footbathing.

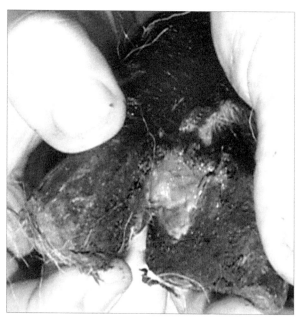

Fig. 9.23 Interdigital dermatitis causes hyperaemia of interdigital skin, with superficial accumulations of moist, whitish necrotic material.

Zinc sulphate, as a 10% solution with sodium lauryl sulphate added as a wetting agent, has largely replaced formalin footbaths.

Some farmers report that where there are fewer ewes with footrot, epidemics of interdigital dermatitis in lambs are less likely.

Management/prevention/control measures
Footbaths can be used at weekly intervals to control infection, although less frequent footbathing will usually contain the problem.

Economics
Interdigital dermatitis can cause severe lameness and an abrupt check in growth rate in growing lambs, with consequent extended interval to marketing if left untreated for 1 week or more. Footbaths are an inexpensive means of treatment, although extra labour may be necessary to handle young lambs when passing through the footbath for the first time.

Welfare implications
Interdigital dermatitis can cause severe lameness in a large number of lambs, necessitating immediate treatment.

Footrot with hoof separation
Definition/overview
Footrot is the term commonly used to describe the highly contagious foot disease caused by *D. nodosus* with extensive under-running of hoof horn. Footrot accounts for approximately 90% of foot lameness in the UK where the prevalence of lameness is around 10%. Footrot causes serious welfare concerns and leads to significant lost production due to lameness. Losses result from reduced wool production, poorer wool quality, lowered live-weight gain/poorer body condition and reduced reproductive performance. Lameness during the breeding season can cause a significant reduction in reproductive performance with rams reluctant/unable to serve ewes.

Footrot eradication schemes are in operation in a number of countries, most notably Australia where climatic and environmental conditions are more conducive to such programmes than in the UK or New Zealand. Whole flock gamithromycin injection has successfully eradicated footrot from many flocks.

Aetiology
Strains of *D. nodosus* vary in the extent to which they produce keratinolytic proteases and this property directly determines their invasive capacity. Strains of *D. nodosus* with low protease activity cause mild lesions affecting only the interdigital skin and hoof of the axial wall; strains of *D. nodosus* with high protease activity cause separation of the hoof from the corium, with considerable under-running of the hoof capsule in severe cases.

Clinical presentation
Footrot lesions start at the junction of the interdigital skin and axial wall horn (**Fig. 9.24**) and spread abaxially to under-run the sole (**Fig. 9.25**) and possibly the abaxial wall (**Fig. 9.26**). The axial hoof horn margin becomes separated from the skin, appearing as a thin irregular white strip 2–3 mm wide. There is a characteristic smell of necrotic horn/exudate. The whole hoof capsule may become completely under-run in severe cases (**Fig. 9.27**). Chronic infection leads to grossly misshapen hooves.

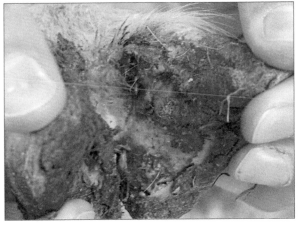
Fig. 9.24 Footrot lesions start at the junction of the interdigital skin and axial wall horn.

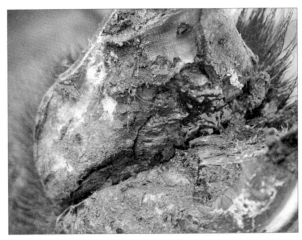
Fig. 9.25 Footrot lesions spread abaxially to under-run the sole.

Differential diagnoses
In individual sheep, the differential diagnosis of severe lameness caused by footrot includes white line abscess and septic pedal arthritis. CODD may also present as an outbreak of severe lameness affecting a large percentage of sheep in the group, but separation of the hoof horn occurs at the coronary band.

Diagnosis
Diagnosis is based upon clinical examination with under-running of hoof horn of the sole extending up the wall. A polymerase chain reaction (PCR)-based

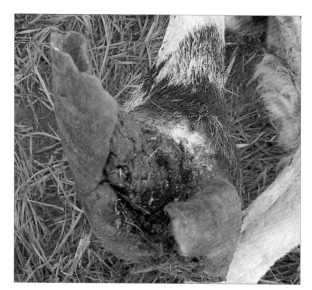

Fig. 9.26 Footrot lesions spreading to under-run the hoof wall.

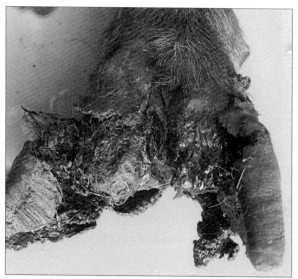

Fig. 9.27 The whole hoof capsule may become completely under-run in severe cases of footrot.

assay can be used to identify and group *D. nodosus* from footrot lesions, although strain typing is rarely undertaken in practice.

Treatment

Given a suitable hard standing, footbathing sheep before housing and after gathering can kill bacteria on the surface of the foot. Footbathing is most successful in preventing footrot and will also treat interdigital dermatitis. There is no evidence that any one type of bath treatment formulation is more effective than another. Footbathing is not an appropriate treatment for sheep already with footrot although, if used correctly, it may limit the spread of the disease. Such sheep will not recover or will recover slowly, by which time production losses will have occurred and their welfare will have been compromised.

The most commonly used treatment for individual sheep with footrot is an injection of long-acting oxytetracycline at10 mg/kg, together with removal of all debris from the interdigital space and application of an antibacterial spray. Treatment of sheep with footrot within 3 days of onset of lameness minimizes spread of the disease to other sheep. Pain relief in the form of a non-steroidal anti-inflammatory drug (NSAID) should also be administered in all cases where the sheep is markedly lame. In many countries

this regimen involves the use of a product off-licence and attention must be paid to meat withdrawal time for those animals going for slaughter. Recent large scale field studies have demonstrated that gamithromycin injection is more effective than oxytetracycline but is considerably more expensive.

Segregating those sheep with footrot from sound sheep at the earliest opportunity helps to reduce the spread of footrot; this should be done at every gathering, and especially at housing and at turnout.

Traditionally, sheep feet were trimmed routinely once or twice a year. Indeed, this practice was recommended in advisory literature. However, there is no scientific evidence that routine foot trimming is beneficial in the treatment or prevention of footrot and recent veterinary advice is that the feet of all sheep should not be trimmed routinely (**Figs 9.28, 9.29**). Trimming horn should only be undertaken in individual sheep to reshape excessively overgrown feet. Overzealous paring and exposure of the sensitive corium in combination with frequent formalin footbath treatments may result in the generation of toe fibromas.

Management/prevention/control measures

For most causes of foot lameness there are effective treatments that, if applied promptly, can reduce the

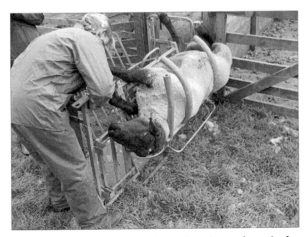

Fig. 9.28 Sheep's feet should not be trimmed routinely.

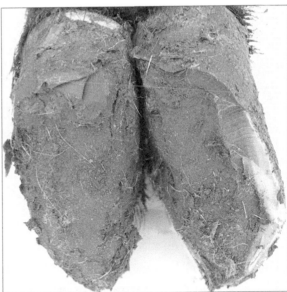

Fig. 9.29 Excessive trimming of the hoof wall merely transfers weight to the sole causing abnormal loading.

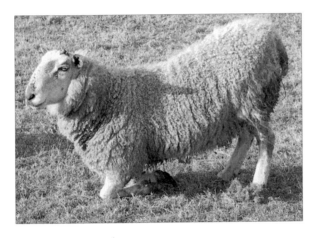

Fig. 9.30 More should be done to minimize lameness as a cause of poor welfare in sheep.

prevalence of lameness in a flock to less than 2%. The current high prevalence in the UK suggests that much more could be done by shepherds to minimize lameness as a cause of poor welfare in sheep (**Fig. 9.30**).

The UK's climate predisposes to the spread of footrot for 10–11 months of the year and, even indoors, footrot can spread via bedding. Footrot spreads under wet, warm conditions. Treatment programmes are much more likely to be successful during non-transmission stages if such environmental conditions exist at some stage in the year.

Whilst footrot can be eliminated from individual flocks, its ubiquitous nature makes any footrot-free flock very vulnerable to reinfection. The risks of reintroduction should be carefully considered before a farmer opts for attempted eradication of

footrot. Whole flock gamithromycin treatment has produced very encouraging results in Denmark and the UK, with flocks having remained free of footrot for up to 2–3 years at the time of publication of this book. The critical factor is that every single sheep must be treated and this appears to require veterinary attendance so no sheep are left untreated – typically sheep intended for sale in several weeks/months are often untreated and act as reservoirs of infection.

There is little evidence that Australian eradication programmes for footrot would be successful in the UK because of the climate, structure of sheep breeding and lack of co-ordination between farmers.

Wherever possible sheep producers should maintain a closed flock to prevent purchasing diseased sheep. If purchases are essential, ewe lambs should be bought from known sources rather than old ewes, which are often chronic carriers. All purchased stock must be quarantined for 1 month and examined for footrot before introduction into the main flock. Swabs for PCR testing of *D. nodusus* would be advisable. Footbathing should be undertaken during this quarantine period. Treatment of all introduced sheep with a macrolide antibiotic, such as gamithromycin, could be considered on veterinary advice.

Prior infection does not confer any appreciable immunity. There are few reported split-flock trials of footrot vaccines in the UK, but there is anecdotal evidence that vaccination can contribute to footrot control measures in flocks. Disadvantages associated with vaccination include cost (£1.50 per dose), short duration (booster vaccinations required every 6 months or before the anticipated challenge period) and occasional severe localized reaction at the injection site. Poor injection technique has resulted in infection tracking into the extradural space in the cervical region, causing tetraparesis in a small number of cases. Accidental self-injection is a serious concern and it is recommended that the operator report immediately to the nearest Accident and Emergency Department with the data sheet should this occur.

In the UK, the vaccine contains 10 strains of inactivated *D. nodosus* with an oil adjuvant. It is recommended that all sheep are vaccinated, thereby limiting future environmental contamination and challenge. A single dose of vaccine is given which can be boosted 4–6 weeks later if significant levels of disease still remain in the flock. Subsequent doses should be administered according to prevailing conditions or in anticipation of climatic conditions that favour disease.

All breeds are susceptible to footrot. In the UK Suffolk sheep are more susceptible than most other breeds when co-grazed. In New Zealand British breeds are more resistant than Merino sheep. Breeding sheep that are more resistant to footrot is desirable and possible. This can be achieved through selectively breeding from families of animals with greater resistance to footrot. Advances in genotyping will greatly facilitate selection of sheep with greater resistance to footrot.

While cattle are suitable hosts for *D. nodosus*, these strains are usually benign for sheep, allowing some degree of control by alternate grazing or co-grazing.

Economics

The financial impact of footrot varies between farms within a region, between regions and between countries. In many situations, particularly in Australia, footrot is regarded as the single most important disease of sheep-limiting production. The successful eradication of footrot following whole flock gamithromycin injection offers considerable potential in closed flocks with effective biosecurity.

Welfare implications

Footrot is a very painful condition indeed (**Fig. 9.31**). For reasons of its high prevalence, severity, and chronicity with extended convalescence after treatment, virulent footrot is considered to be the most important welfare issue in the UK. Welfare problems arise with footrot in the UK because:

- High-dose antibiotic therapy is expensive (£2–3) relative to the value of many commercial value sheep, particularly store lambs.

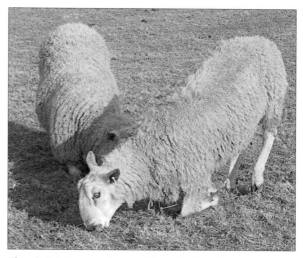

Fig. 9.31 Footrot is considered to be the most important welfare issue in the UK sheep industry because of its high prevalence, severity and chronicity, with extended convalescence after treatment.

- Labour requirements: footbathing is time-consuming because few farmers have invested in adequate facilities. In particular, few farms have sufficient dry standing areas after footbathing. When not undertaken correctly, gathering and inappropriate footbathing may simply serve to spread infection further.
- Distant grazings: sheep are often grazed considerable distances away from centralized footbathing facilities. While mobile facilities can be used, there are rarely dry standing facilities after footbathing.

CONTAGIOUS OVINE DIGITAL DERMATITIS

Definition/overview

Contagious ovine digital dermatitis (CODD) is a severe foot condition first described in sheep in the UK in 1997.

Aetiology

The isolation of spirochaetes resembling those involved in digital dermatitis in cattle from some, but not all, suspected clinical cases in sheep has led to the adoption of the current name CODD. However, the isolation of the same spirochaetes from apparently normal feet, and the occurrence of mixed infections of ovine foot lesions with the causal agent of footrot, provide ample opportunity for confusion.

Clinical presentation

Affected sheep show severe lameness (**Fig. 9.32**) affecting one or both digits of one foot in most animals, with the affected foot held well above the ground. The lesion starts at the coronary band of the abaxial wall with subsequent invasion and under-running of the hoof wall from the coronary band extending distally, causing detachment (**Figs 9.33–9.35**) then shedding of the horn capsule (**Figs 9.36, 9.37**). Typically, there is also loss of hair extending proximally 3–5 cm above the coronary band but no interdigital skin involvement (**Fig. 9.38**). The damage to the corium may be so severe that regrowth of the horn appears permanently affected (**Fig. 9.39**). Some affected digits show no evidence of new horn production, and at necropsy sagittal sections through affected digits show considerable resorption of the third phalanx (**Figs 9.40, 9.41**).

Differential diagnoses

The major differential diagnosis is severe lameness caused by footrot (**Fig. 9.42**). It may not be possible to differentiate CODD from footrot and indeed mixed infections are possible.

Diagnosis

Diagnosis is based on clinical examination, with findings of under-running of the hoof capsule starting at the coronary band and extending distally. Attempted isolation of spirochaetes is rarely undertaken in practice.

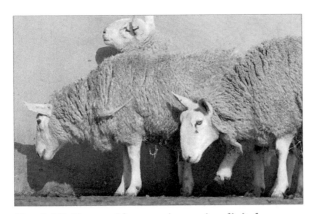

Fig. 9.32 Sheep with contagious ovine digital dermatitis (CODD) show severe lameness.

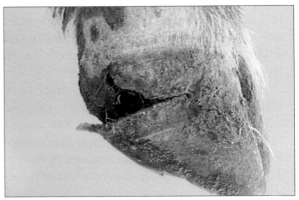

Fig. 9.33 The CODD lesion starts at the coronary band of the abaxial wall, with subsequent under-running of the hoof wall from the coronary band extending distally.

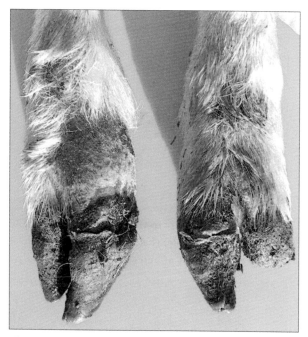

Fig. 9.34 One or both digits can be affected with CODD.

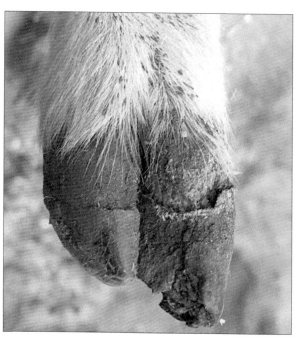

Fig. 9.35 CODD causes under-running of the hoof wall from the coronary band extending distally, causing detachment of the hoof capsule.

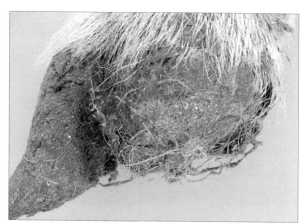

Fig. 9.36 CODD has caused shedding of the horn capsule.

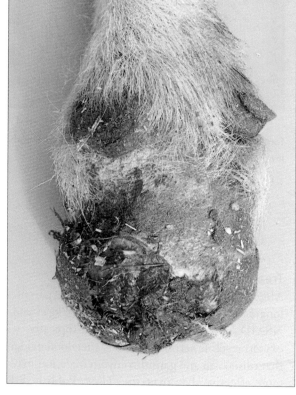

Fig. 9.37 Shedding of the horn capsule and loss of hair extending proximally 3–5 cm above the coronary band, associated with CODD.

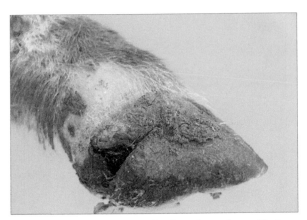

Fig. 9.38 Lateral view of the foot shows loss of hair extending proximally 3–5 cm above the coronary band.

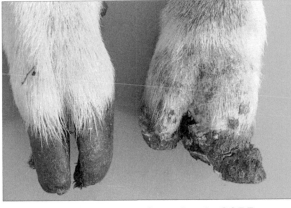

Fig. 9.39 The damage to the corium in CODD may be so severe (right side) that regrowth of the horn appears permanently affected (left side normal).

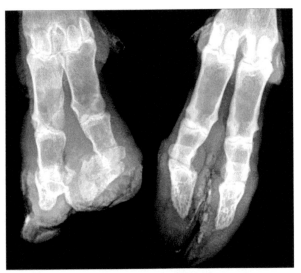

Fig. 9.40 Dorso-plantar view of a CODD-affected foot; there is considerable resorption of the third phalanges (left side, right side normal).

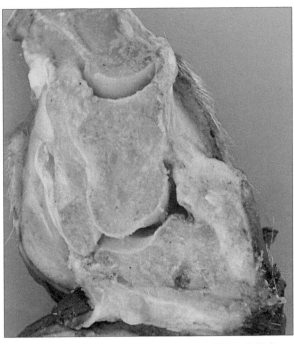

Fig. 9.41 Sagittal section through an affected digit (P1, P2 and P3 all shown) at necropsy shows considerable resorption of the third phalanx.

Treatment

Affected sheep should be treated with parenteral long-acting oxytetracycline (10 mg/kg) and a NSAID and skin lesions treated topically with oxytetracycline aerosol. There is anecdotal evidence that tilmicosin and gamithromycin injection may be more effective than oxytetracycline. Published data on comparative treatment regimens are needed. There is limited evidence that whole group metaphylactic antibiotic injection may reduce the appearance of new cases in the group.

No antibiotic is licensed for use in footbaths, although lincomycin/spectinomycin soluble powder and tylosin soluble powder (each at a concentration of

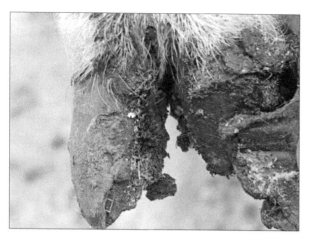

Fig. 9.42 Severe lameness and loss of the hoof capsule can also be caused by footrot.

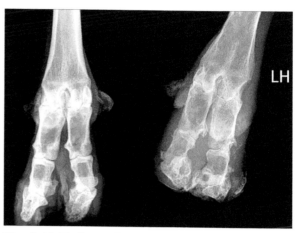

Fig. 9.43 Radiographic evidence of considerable resorption/remodelling of the third phalanx, and disarticulation of the distal interphalangeal joint (LH), raises considerable welfare concerns.

100 g per 200 litres of water) have been used in sheep following success of this treatment protocol in cattle.

Management/prevention/control measures

Strict biosecurity is essential to prevent introducing CODD onto the farm.

Economics

The high prevalence of disease after introduction into a flock, treatment costs and protracted convalescence cause serious financial losses.

Welfare implications

The radiographic evidence of resorption/remodelling of the third phalanx (**Fig. 9.43**), and disarticulation of the distal interphalangeal joint in some sheep, is of particular concern because pain and lameness would probably persist should regrowth of the hoof horn occur. Further study is necessary of these chronic bone changes in CODD.

WHITE LINE ABSCESSES

Definition/overview

Abscesses arise following impaction of dirt and bacteria in the white line. It is more common in misshapen hooves with hoof horn separation after footrot infection. White line abscesses occur sporadically in sheep in all countries worldwide.

Aetiology

Entry of bacteria with multiplication to form an abscess which may ascend the white line to rupture at the coronary band.

Clinical presentation

Affected sheep often present with sudden severe lameness of the affected limb with the foot held off the ground. Pressure on the overlying hoof wall will elicit a pain response and immediate foot withdrawal. The lesion is especially painful if it has extended to the coronary band causing swelling; rupture of this abscess some days later often relieves the pain with a dramatic reduction in lameness.

Careful foot paring reveals separation and impaction of the white line, with dirt leading to an abscess that may spurt pus upon release. There is a marked improvement in locomotion within 2 days. Care must be taken not to expose the sensitive corium, which could lead to granuloma formation and persistence of lameness. Granuloma formation is more common following exposure of the corium at the toe.

Differential diagnoses

White line abscess can be differentiated from septic pedal arthritis by lack of interdigital involvement and swelling localized to a small area of the abaxial coronary band.

Diagnosis
The abscess is confirmed upon release of pus.

Treatment
The abscess is treated by releasing the pus, through careful foot paring with removal of impacted dirt and under-run horn (**Fig. 9.44**).

Management/prevention/control measures
There are no specific control measures for white line abscesses but control measures for footrot should also limit the incidence of white line abscesses.

Economics
Painful foot lesions result in rapid weight loss with resultant delays to marketing. Ram lameness during the mating period can result in failure to mate ewes, with an extended lambing period and more barren ewes than usual.

Welfare implications
White line abscesses can cause marked lameness and necessitate immediate attention.

TOE FIBROMA/GRANULOMA

Definition/overview
Toe fibromas most commonly result from over-zealous foot paring, with exposure of the corium (**Fig. 9.45**) and excessive use of formalin footbaths. Toe fibromas can occur in association with virulent footrot where horn separation results in exposure of the corium. Toe fibromas are in themselves not painful being comprised of granulation tissue without nerve endings, but exposure and infection of the adjacent corium leads to lameness.

Aetiology
Repeated insult to the exposed corium leads to granulation tissue proliferation.

Clinical presentation
There is a large fibrous growth protruding from the toe, which may be overlain by overgrown hoof horn (**Fig. 9.46**). Careful paring of the hoof wall often reveals a narrow stalk attaching the fibroma to the corium.

Differential diagnoses
Foot lameness may result from abscess formation in the white line, footrot, penetrating foreign body, septic pedal arthritis and CODD.

Diagnosis
The diagnosis is confirmed by careful foot paring.

Treatment
This condition can be resolved by careful foot paring, excision of the growth then applying a pressure

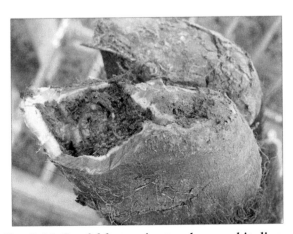

Fig. 9.44 Careful foot paring to release a white line abscess followed by removal of under-run horn of the abaxial wall. There is neither bleeding nor damage to the corium.

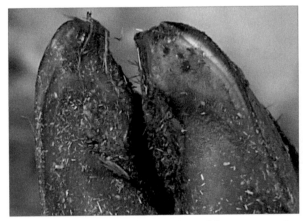

Fig. 9.45 **Overzealous foot paring with exposure of the corium may lead to formation of a toe fibroma.**

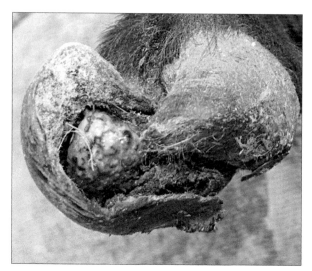

Fig. 9.46 A large toe fibroma is covered by hoof horn (see Fig. 9.47).

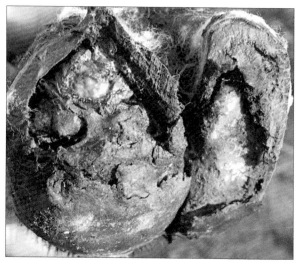

Fig. 9.47 One week after excision of the fibroma and application of a pressure bandage to inhibit further granulation tissue. The overgrown horn has been removed to facilitate the pressure bandage.

bandage to the affected area. The toe fibroma is comprised of exuberant granulation tissue without a nerve supply; therefore, the fibroma can be excised without the need for any analgesia. The fibroma is cut off level with the sole using a scalpel blade (a hoof knife is not sharp enough for this procedure). A pressure bandage is carefully applied over the exposed corium and removed after 3–5 days. While some authors have recommended cautery to prevent regrowth of the fibroma, such action may be counter-productive as it destroys the surrounding healthy corium and thereby delays healing. A pressure bandage inhibits granulation tissue formation and achieves more rapid healing (**Fig. 9.47**).

Management/prevention/control measures

Careful foot paring to drain a foot abscess must not damage the sensitive corium. Sheep with exposed corium must not be put through formalin footbaths. These sheep should be treated with topical oxytetracycline and rechecked 3–5 days later and retreated if necessary. Any toe with granulation tissue present should be bandaged to prevent fibroma formation.

Economics

Toe fibromas can be treated by the shepherd and are not a serious economic concern.

Welfare implications

Toe fibromas indicate either neglect of footrot (**Fig. 9.48**) and/or unskilled and over-enthusiastic foot paring.

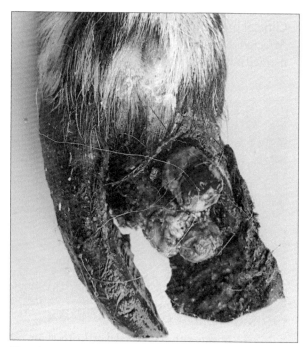

Fig. 9.48 Toe fibromas are often associated with chronic cases of footrot.

SEPTIC PEDAL ARTHRITIS

Definition/overview

Septic pedal arthritis occurs sporadically in adult sheep in many flocks but such lame sheep are often ignored. Ankylosis between P2 and P3 may eventually result after months of suffering and lameness. While this condition generally has a very low prevalence, it raises important animal welfare concerns. There are reports of severe outbreaks of septic pedal arthritis in flocks in Australia and New Zealand caused by prolonged periods of heavy rain leading to interdigital infection, then tracking to the distal interphalangeal joint.

Aetiology

Bacterial infection usually gains entry to the distal interphalangeal (pedal) joint from an interdigital lesion, which then tracks abaxially to discharge above the coronary band. As the distal interphalangeal joint capsule is protected only by skin and a small amount of subcutaneous tissue at its axial margin, it is prone to penetration at this site. Infection of the distal interphalangeal joint rarely arises from an abscessation in the abaxial white line or sole ulceration as commonly occurs in dairy cattle.

Clinical presentation

Affected sheep show severe lameness (**Fig. 9.49**) with marked muscle atrophy of the affected limb. There is general body condition loss due to reduced grazing/feeding. There is marked swelling of the drainage lymph node, which may be four to five times its normal size. The foot is swollen with obvious widening of the interdigital space and a discharging sinus(es) above the coronary band on the abaxial aspect of the hoof wall (**Fig. 9.50**). Rupture of the axial collateral ligament in some cases leads to increased mobility and abaxial deviation of the toe, and eventual dislocation of the third phalanx.

Differential diagnoses

Differential diagnoses include:

- A neglected white line abscess, which has tracked up the wall of the hoof to discharge at the coronary band.
- Severe interdigital infection.

Diagnosis

The combination of widening of the interdigital space and a discharging sinus(es) above the coronary band on the abaxial aspect of the hoof wall is consistent with a diagnosis of septic pedal arthritis. The diagnosis could be confirmed by radiography but this is cost-prohibitive in most practical situations (**Fig. 9.51**). Arthrocentesis is rarely useful because only a small amount of pannus is present within the joint. Injection of sterile saline into the

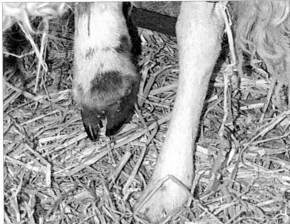

Fig. 9.49 **Sheep with septic pedal arthritis show severe lameness.**

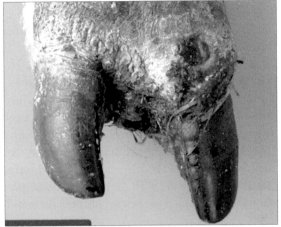

Fig. 9.50 **The foot is swollen with obvious widening of the interdigital space and a discharging sinus above the coronary band of the abaxial wall.**

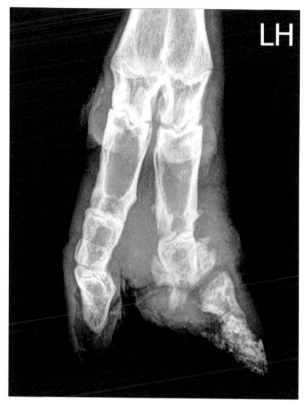

Fig. 9.51 Dorso-plantar radiograph reveals joint sepsis with disarticulation of the distal interphalangeal joint and osteophytosis extending to involve distal P1.

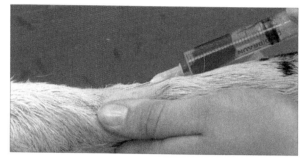

Fig. 9.52 A dose of 5 ml of 2% lignocaine solution (or equivalent) is injected into a superficial vein after application of a rubber tourniquet.

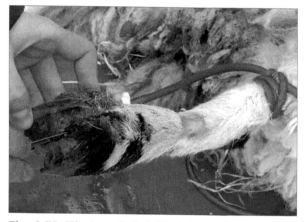

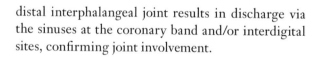

Fig. 9.53 The interdigital skin is incised as close to infected tissue as possible.

distal interphalangeal joint results in discharge via the sinuses at the coronary band and/or interdigital sites, confirming joint involvement.

Treatment

Antibiotic therapy is useless in these cases. Digit amputation under intravenous regional anaesthesia gives excellent results. Intravenous NSAID injection is given prior to amputation. The procedure can be performed in less than 15 minutes and uses the minimum of drugs and dressings, thereby keeping costs reasonable even for commercial-value sheep. A 5 ml dose of 2% lignocaine solution (or equivalent) is injected into a superficial vein after application of a rubber tourniquet either above the hock or below the carpus as appropriate (**Fig. 9.52**). Insertion of the 19 gauge 25 mm needle into the distended superficial

vein releases 5–10 ml of blood under pressure; blood flow then quickly reduces to the occasional drop if the tourniquet is tight enough. Analgesia should be effective within 2 minutes and is tested by pricking the coronary band.

The interdigital skin is incised as close to the infected tissue as possible and the incision extended for the full length of the interdigital space (**Fig. 9.53**). The depth of the incision is approximately 10 mm at the cranial margin extending to 20 mm at the most caudal extent. A length of embryotomy wire is introduced into the incision and the digit removed through the proximal aspect of the second phalanx, and above the discharging sinuses, by rapid sawing action (**Fig. 9.54**). Topical antibiotic spray is applied to the wound. A Melolin dressing is applied to the wound and pressure applied using a large amount of

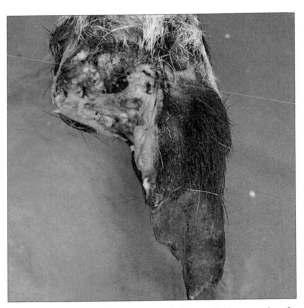

Fig. 9.54 The digit is removed through the proximal aspect of the second phalanx.

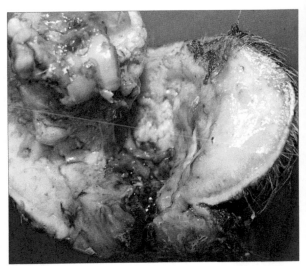

Fig. 9.55 After excision, examination reveals destruction of the articular cartilage on the surface of distal P2, with proliferative and hyperaemic synovial membrane.

cotton wool incorporated into the bandage. A course of parenteral antibiotics is not necessary in most cases. The dressing is removed 2–3 days later and the granulating wound again sprayed with oxytetracycline aerosol. A light protective bandage is applied for a further 2–3 days, by which time the sheep is much less lame. The sheep should then be turned out onto clean pasture, not a muddy field. The long-term prognosis after digit amputation in ewes and rams, unlike dairy cattle, is excellent. Amputation through the distal portion of P1 is recommended in cattle because the proximal portion of P2 has a poor blood supply and may undergo necrosis; however, this author has not encountered any problems with the method described above in sheep. Dissection of the amputated digit reveals extensive synovial proliferation and hypertrophy and variable erosion of articular cartilage (**Fig. 9.55**) depending on chronicity.

Surgical arthrodesis of the infected distal interphalangeal joint has been described but is restricted to valuable sheep because of the higher cost of more veterinary time and the necessity of a radiograph to select suitable cases. Anaesthesia is achieved as described above. The joint space can be accessed through the discharging sinus(es) above the coronary band. The joint surfaces are curetted and the joint then flushed repeatedly with sterile saline. The affected

foot is immobilized in a cast. Alternatively, a 1 cm thick wooden block can be glued to the sole of the normal digit to raise the affected digit off the ground. The toes are then wired together and the foot bandaged. The sheep should be confined indoors. The joint should be radiographed again after 3 weeks to assess progress; there should be considerable osteophytic reaction. Bridging of the joint space should be achieved by 6 weeks.

Management/prevention/control measures

Immediate attention to severe lameness caused by interdigital infections should prevent spread to the distal interphalangeal joint in most cases. Sheep should not be kept in deep muddy fields but moved to dry pasture whenever possible.

Economics

Digit amputation for correction of septic pedal arthritis is an effective procedure in sheep and should be undertaken at the first veterinary examination. Prolonged courses of antibiotics will not achieve a cure in such cases.

Welfare implications

Septic pedal arthritis is a major welfare concern because many cases are neglected unless the affected

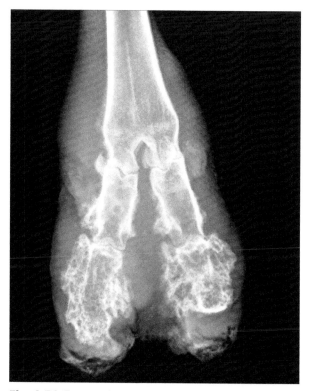

Fig. 9.56 **Dorso-plantar radiograph of the right hind foot of the ram featured in Fig. 9.57. There appears to be ankylosis of the distal interphalangeal joints, although the third phalanges cannot be clearly identified; extensive osteophytosis extends to the proximal joints.**

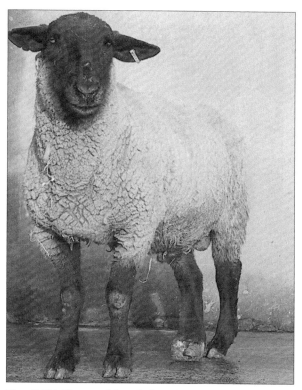

Fig. 9.57 **Sheep with ankylosed joints following untreated septic pedal arthritis (see Fig. 9.56) still show some residual lameness evident by the marked plantigrade stance of the normal left hindlimb in this Suffolk ram.**

sheep is commercially valuable, such as a breeding ram. Ankylosis of the distal interphalangeal joint may eventually result but only after many months of suffering which is unacceptable (**Fig. 9.56**). Sheep with ankylosed joints still show some residual lameness evident by the marked plantigrade stance of the normal contralateral limb (**Fig. 9.57**).

INFECTIOUS POLYARTHRITIS

(syn. joint ill)

Definition/overview

Localization of bacteria within a joint(s), causing an infectious arthritis with moderate to severe lameness, is a major economic problem and welfare concern in all sheep-producing countries (**Figs 9.58–9.60**). The problem is greatly increased when lambs are born indoors under unsanitary conditions, although lameness may not become apparent until several days old, often after turnout to pasture.

The prophylactic or metaphylactic administration of procaine penicillin to all lambs at 24–48 hours old is very effective in the face of a disease outbreak of *Streptococcus dysgalactiae* polyarthritis in the UK, but it raises many concerns about indiscriminate antibiotic usage and this practice is clearly unsustainable.

Aetiology

Bacteraemia in neonatal lambs results from enteroinvasion or entry via the upper respiratory tract, tonsil or, perhaps, an untreated umbilicus. Bacteraemia occurs in lambs kept under poor sanitary conditions with delayed or inadequate colostrum intake. Poor husbandry standards, understaffing and lack of client education of risk factors all contribute to an

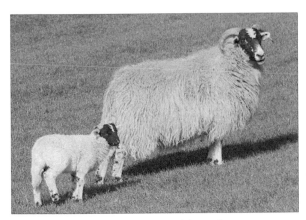

Fig. 9.58 Infectious arthritis with moderate to severe lameness is a major economic problem and welfare concern affecting young lambs; note the severe lameness affecting the right hindlimb of this lamb.

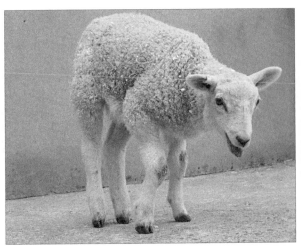

Fig. 9.59 Septic polyarthritis causes severe pain and lameness.

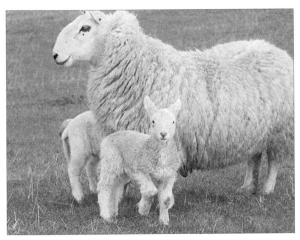

Fig. 9.60 Severe lameness of the right forelimb has caused poor growth compared to this lamb's normal twin, evident as much poorer fleece quality and lower body condition.

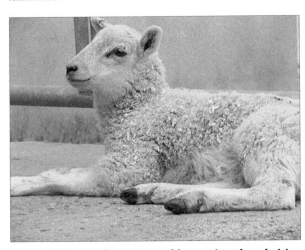

Fig. 9.61 Recumbency caused by septic polyarthritis; *S. dysgalactiae* was isolated from the synovial membrane of affected joints.

increased prevalence of neonatal diseases and compromised sheep health and welfare. Bacteriological surveys have identified *S. dysgalactiae* as the most common isolate from infected joints of young lambs in the UK (>85% of isolates), followed by *Escherichia coli* and *Erysipelothrix rhusiopathiae*.

Clinical presentation
S. dysgalactiae infections are acquired during the first few days of life, with lameness ranging from moderate (4/10) to non-weight-bearing (10/10) present from 5–10 days of age (**Fig. 9.61**). The number of infected joints is highly variable; typically only one joint is affected in approximately 50% of lambs, with two to four joints affected in the remainder. It is not unusual to find both the fetlock and carpal joints affected in the same limb with all other joints normal. Infection of the atlanto-occipital joint causes tetraparesis. The rectal temperature may be marginally elevated but is frequently within the normal range.

Lame lambs spend long periods in sternal recumbency and appear reluctant to follow their dam, often being found sheltering behind walls and hedgerows. Only the toe of the affected limb points the ground when walking. Lambs experience great difficulty walking when two or more limbs are affected and may have a 'crab-like' stance.

The joints most commonly affected, with decreasing frequency, are the carpal, hock, fetlock and stifle joints. The affected joint(s) are hot, painful and initially distended by effusion. The lymph nodes (prescapular or popliteal) are enlarged, although it is not so easy to palpate the popliteal lymph node. Infection causes considerable muscle wastage over the gluteal/shoulder regions. After 2–3 weeks lambs with polyarthritis are much smaller than their co-twin and in very poor body condition (**Fig. 9.60**).

As inflammatory changes progress over several weeks, much of the joint fluid is resorbed and there is considerable thickening of the fibrous joint capsule. Affected joints feel enlarged but firm with much reduced joint excursion. Bony changes with osteo-phyte formation are visible radiographically after 6 weeks in chronically inflamed joints.

Differential diagnoses

A greenstick fracture in a neonatal lamb (see **Fig. 9.13**) can be easily overlooked. Lameness affecting a single limb may result from a foot abscess or interdigital infection. Interdigital dermatitis is very common in young growing lambs and can cause marked lame-ness. Cellulitis following a dog bite or other punc-ture wound is not uncommon. Trauma to joints may cause marked lameness; the stifle is the most com-monly injured joint. Lameness may also result from fracture of a long bone. Unlike calves, osteomyelitis is relatively uncommon in lambs (**Figs 9.62, 9.63**). Growth plate infections are uncommon in lambs but few growing lambs are examined in detail so this condition may be under-diagnosed.

Endocarditis, with associated multiple joint swell-ings, is uncommon in growing lambs, although this condition may be encountered in older lambs with erysipelas. Recumbency can result from spinal cord compression associated with vertebral empyema,

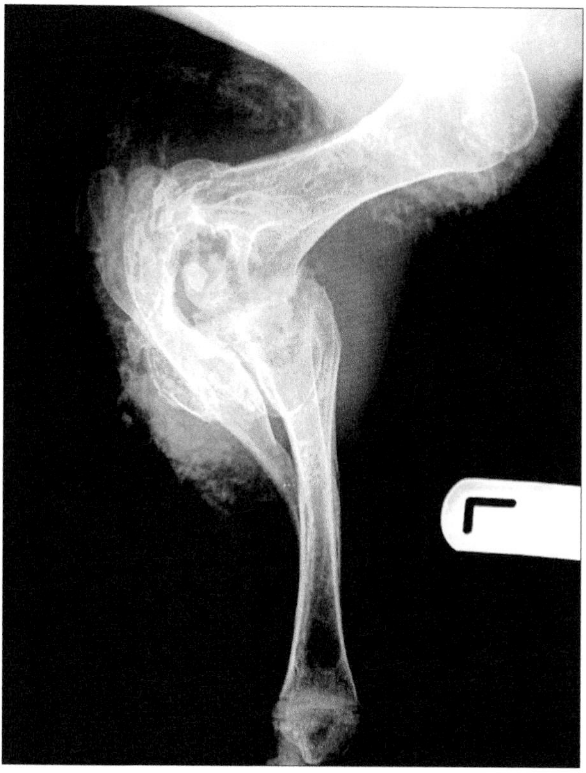

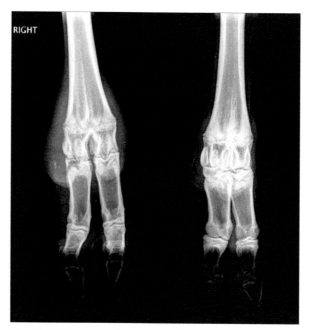

Fig. 9.62 **Lateral view of the left elbow. Osteomyelitis is relatively uncommon in lambs but may be mis-diagnosed as joint ill.**

Fig. 9.63 **Dorso-palmar view. Osteomyelitis affects the lateral digit (proximal growth plate of P1) of the right forelimb.**

which is a common condition of growing lambs from 4 weeks old.

Infection of the atlanto-occipital joint is a common manifestation of *S. dysgalactiae* infection causing sudden onset tetraparesis and recumbency, although these lambs remain bright and alert. These lambs do not always show evidence of other joint infection. Muscular dystrophy causes paresis leading to recumbency. Delayed swayback could be considered in those at-risk flocks that fail to adopt appropriate preventive measures.

Diagnosis

Diagnosis of an infected joint is based on clinical findings, although it may prove difficult to differentiate traumatic lesions from early infective conditions. It has been recommended that all swollen joints affecting lambs less than 1 month old should be considered septic until proven otherwise.

During the acute stages of infection there may be sufficient joint effusion to obtain a sample by needle aspiration. The string of normal viscous joint fluid should extend for at least 2.5 cm when expressed from a syringe before breaking to form droplets. A typical arthrocentesis sample from a septic fetlock joint yields a turbid sample with an elevated protein concentration >18g/l (normal = <3 g/l) and a very high white cell concentration, comprised almost exclusively of neutrophils.

Chronic cases present with marked thickening of the joint capsule, proliferation of synovial membrane and a pannus within the joint. A pannus is a membrane of granulation tissue (fibroblasts and neovascularization) and bone marrow-derived cells (macrophages). Formation of the pannus **(Fig. 9.64)** stimulates the release of interleukin-1, platelet-derived growth factor, prostaglandins and substance P by macrophages, and release of collagenases by fibroblasts, which ultimately cause cartilage destruction and bone erosion. Differentiation of fibrin deposition within a joint and a pannus proves very difficult on gross examination as a pannus is an extension of pathological change within the joint. However, a pannus is more adherent to the synovial membrane and the articular cartilage than fibrin and is less easily peeled off.

Osteophyte formation occurs initially at the insertion of the joint capsule because this area has the greatest blood supply. However, neo-vascularization that occurs within the pannus also stimulates new bone formation, which may progress to ankylosis.

By the time veterinary attention has been sought, lambs have generally been treated with antibiotics for a number of days and are unsuitable for sampling. If the prevalence of polyarthritis is high (>5%) in the flock, swabs of joint fluid, but preferably samples of synovial membrane, should be collected at necropsy from sacrificed lame lambs that have not previously received antibiotic therapy.

Treatment

Sporadic cases of polyarthritis are encountered on most sheep farms but the choice of treatment is most critical when the prevalence exceeds 10–30% of the lamb crop. Procaine penicillin is the drug of choice for polyarthritis in such situations in the UK as *S. dysgalactiae* and *E. rhusiopathiae* are the most common joint pathogens, accounting for over 90% of

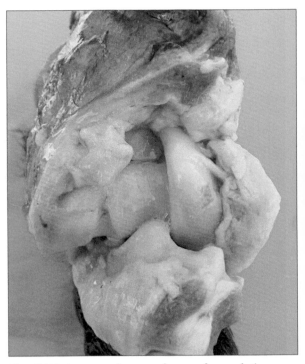

Fig. 9.64 A pannus is a membrane of granulation tissue and bone marrow-derived cells, which ultimately causes cartilage destruction and bone erosion.

positive joint fluid cultures. Penicillin (injected daily for at least 5 consecutive days) commencing at the first signs of lameness effects a good cure rate in many *S. dysgalactiae* infections. However, dead bacteria and white blood cells within the joint may induce further inflammatory changes, including proliferation of the synovial membrane and fibrous thickening of the joint capsule, such that some degree of lameness persists.

While penicillin therapy may render the joints sterile in most cases, some infections are not cleared with the result that progressive and degenerative changes occur within the joint. These physical changes in joint structure are not improved by further antibiotic therapy. Therefore, the prognosis is very poor for lambs that remain lame after at least 5 consecutive days' penicillin therapy, although some temporary improvement may result after another course of antibiotic therapy. Lambs with polyarthritis that continue to show mild to severe lameness after two courses of antibiotic therapy do not grow well. This situation is not uncommon on sheep farms after erysipelas and represents a major welfare concern.

A NSAID can be administered for up to 3 consecutive days to alleviate pain in lambs with polyarthritis. A single injection of dexamethasone should also be carefully considered because such treatment has a dramatic effect in tetraparetic lambs caused by infection of the atlanto-occipital joint.

Within 6–12 hours of intramuscular injection of penicillin and dexamethasone these lambs are often able to walk again (**Figs 9.65, 9.66**). The response to combined penicillin and dexamethasone treatment is much better than antibiotic alone with no greater percentage of relapsed cases. It should also be noted that when treating an outbreak of polyarthritis in lambs there is a >85% chance that the causal organism is *S. dysgalactiae* and fully sensitive to penicillin.

Joint lavage can be attempted to treat a single infected joint in young lambs but this method requires appropriate analgesia and is therefore expensive and time-consuming. High caudal blocks can be used in the case of hindlimb joints, and intravenous alphaxane for general anaesthesia for treatment of a forelimb joint. There is variable response to joint lavage depending on which joint is affected and the duration of infection before treatment. The prognosis for fetlock joint lavage is much better than that for stifle, hock or carpal joints.

A poor response to joint lavage under general anaesthesia is reported in one study, with only one of four adult sheep affected for less than 5 days becoming sound. Necropsy findings of marked synovial membrane hypertrophy and hyperaemia and fibrin/pannus deposition between the articular surfaces readily explains the failure of joint lavage in these sheep.

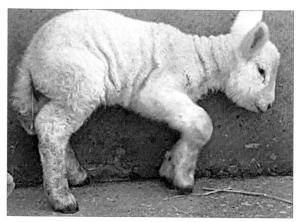

Fig. 9.65 A single injection of dexamethasone should be given in the treatment of early cases of polyarthritis, because such treatment has a dramatic effect in tetraparetic lambs caused by infection of the atlanto-occipital joint (see Fig. 9.66).

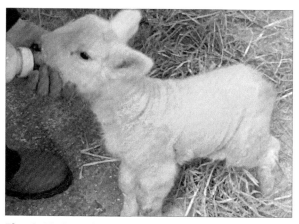

Fig. 9.66 Same lamb as featured in Fig. 9.65 6 hours after dexamethasone and penicillin therapy for *S. dysgalactiae* infection of the atlanto-occipital joint.

The response to antibiotic therapy or joint lavage is hopeless when sheep have been lame for several weeks to many months (**Figs 9.67–9.75**). The true extent of bone destruction is often best demonstrated by boiled out preparations of affected bones (**Figs 9.76–9.79**).

Management/prevention/control measures

Every effort must be taken to reduce the risk of bacteraemia in neonatal lambs by ensuring timely adequate passive antibody transfer and reducing environmental bacterial challenge. However, there

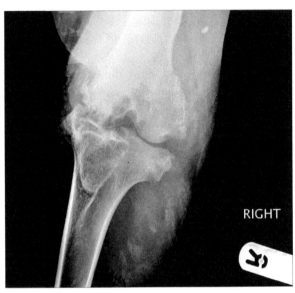

Fig. 9.67 Dorso-plantar view of the right stifle joint shows loss of articular cartilage (see Fig. 9.69).

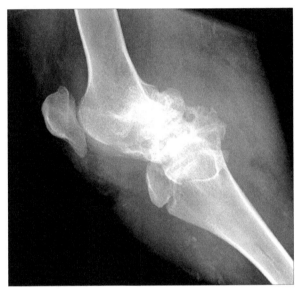

Fig. 9.68 Lateral view of the right stifle joint shows complete loss of articular cartilage and osteophytosis (see Fig. 9.69).

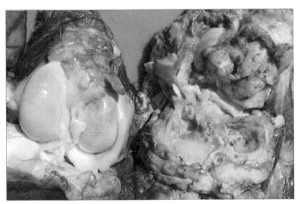

Fig. 9.69 At necropsy, the right stifle joint shows extensive erosion of articular cartilage and synovial hypertrophy; the normal left stifle joint is shown for comparison.

Fig. 9.70 Dorso-palmar view of the left carpus shows osteophytosis and marked widening of the articular space, with loss of articular cartilage of the radio-carpal joint (see normal carpus in Fig. 9.72).

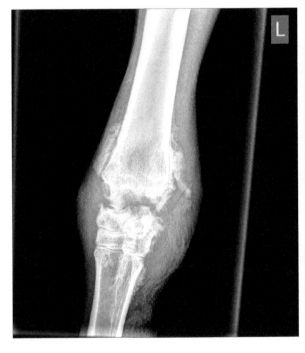

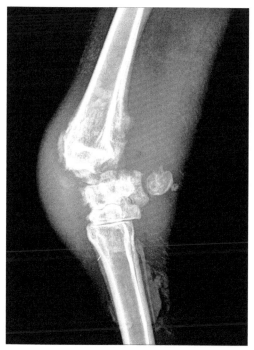

Fig. 9.71 Lateral view of the left carpus shows subluxation, loss of articular cartilage and osteophytosis of the radio-carpal joint.

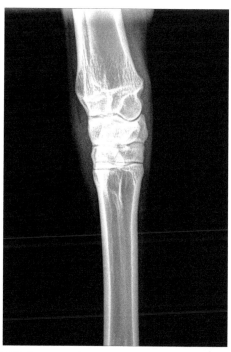

Fig. 9.72 Dorso-palmar view of the normal right carpus.

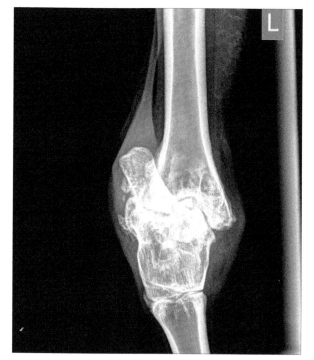

Fig. 9.73 Dorso-plantar view of the left hock shows severe osteoarthritis with fusion of the tarsal bones.

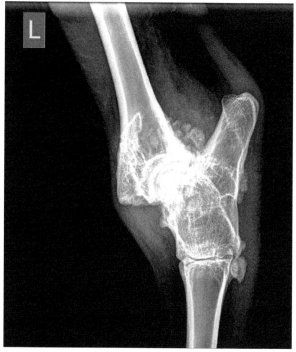

Fig. 9.74 Lateral view of the left hock shows severe osteoarthritis with fusion of the tarsal bones.

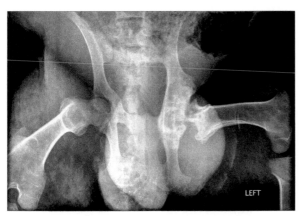

Fig. 9.75 Ventro-dorsal view of the pelvis shows sepsis of the left hip joint extending to involve the ischiatic spine of the ilium.

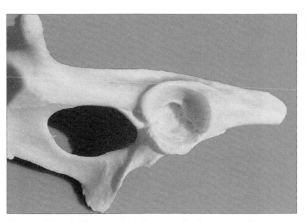

Fig. 9.76 'Boiled out' right acetabulum reveals normal bone structure.

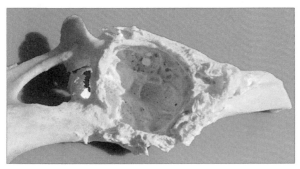

Fig. 9.77 'Boiled out' left acetabulum reveals extensive osteolysis and remodelling.

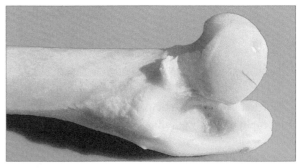

Fig. 9.78 'Boiled out' normal right femur reveals normal bone structure.

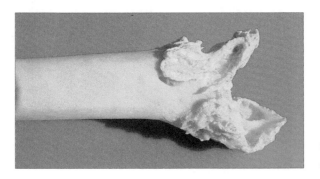

Fig. 9.79 'Boiled out' remodelled left femur reveals extensive osteolysis.

is no evidence that *S. dysgalactiae* polyarthritis is associated with failure of passive transfer. The umbilicus (navel) must be fully immersed in strong veterinary iodine BP within the first 15 minutes of life and repeated at least once 2–4 hours later. Entry of bacteria via ear tags/notches within the first few days of life has been suggested after the prevalence fell markedly after these practices were stopped.

Ewes should lamb on clean pasture where possible. While this can rarely be achieved under UK farming conditions, it is practised in more favourable climates. The source of *S. dysgalactiae* is from a small percentage of carrier ewes. These sheep contaminate the lambing shed, where the bacteria can survive for up to 6 weeks in bedding material such as straw. Unfortunately, most farmers elect to add new straw to the pen after each litter rather than remove all bedding material, disinfect the pen, leave to dry then add clean dry straw before the next ewe and her lambs. Many individual lambing pens are so poorly designed that it can prove impossible to clean them out.

Change of lambing accommodation is rarely an option; turnout to pasture for the remainder of the lambing period has been reported to reduce morbidity markedly.

There are no specific recommendations for the control of *S. dysgalactiae* polyarthritis. A single injection of procaine penicillin to all lambs at 24–48 hours old is very effective in the face of a disease outbreak but must be considered as a last resort after all aspects of lamb management and husbandry practices have been reviewed. The use of prophylactic antibiotic injections to control diseases that can be largely prevented by good husbandry practices will come under ever closer scrutiny by regulatory bodies.

Economics

While antibiotic treatment costs are not high (25–50 pence per 5 day course of procaine penicillin), catching large numbers of young lambs at pasture to administer treatments involves a large amount of staff time.

Lame lambs do not grow well and marketing is delayed by at least several months. Reaction in the drainage lymph nodes may result in condemnation of those lambs that show only mild lameness but have chronic joint swellings caused by fibrosis of the joint capsule.

Welfare implications

Polyarthritis is a major welfare concern in those lambs that do not respond to antibiotic therapy. Lame lambs that do not recover after two treatment courses should be euthanased for welfare reasons. Further antibiotic therapy will not influence the joint pathology that is associated with such chronic infections and affected sheep should be destroyed for welfare reasons.

ERYSIPELAS

Definition/overview

Erysipelothrix rhusiopathiae causes an infective arthritis with high morbidity and moderate to severe lameness, typically affecting growing lambs aged 6 weeks to 4 months. Erysipelas can be effectively controlled in countries where there is a licensed vaccine but it remains a major economic problem and welfare concern in unvaccinated flocks in many sheep-producing countries.

Aetiology

E. rhusiopathiae causes disease in a wide host range including pigs and poultry and is able to survive in the environment for many months. While some texts refer to outbreaks of erysipelas following contamination of surgical castration and docking sites, most farmers now use elastrator rings which do not present such a portal for bacteria. Outbreaks of erysipelas in the UK are more commonly associated with prolonged periods of wet weather leading to contamination of overcrowded shelter areas.

Clinical presentation

There is sudden onset of moderate to severe lameness affecting a large number of growing lambs. Lame lambs spend long periods in sternal recumbency and do not follow their dam. Lambs are often lame on two or more limbs. The joints most commonly affected are the carpal, fetlock (**Fig. 9.80**), hock and stifle joints (**Fig. 9.81**) but there is little joint effusion. As the condition progresses over several weeks to months further inflammatory changes include proliferation of the synovial membrane and fibrous thickening of the joint capsule (**Figs 9.82, 9.83**) such that the joint is swollen and firm; there is little joint effusion. The drainage lymph nodes are enlarged. Erosion of articular cartilage can result in lambs neglected for several months (**Figs 9.84, 9.85**). While crepitus can be appreciated in such severely affected joints, such painful examination of the joint(s) is neither indicated nor necessary; the more gentle the touch, the greater the sensitivity of, and information gained from, such palpation. Vegetative endocarditis is present in a high percentage of growing lambs with erysipelas polyarthritis but is difficult to diagnose because there is usually neither audible murmur nor signs of congestive heart failure.

Differential diagnoses

Interdigital dermatitis is common in this age group of lambs and can present as an outbreak of moderate to severe lameness, but this condition responds dramatically to topical oxytetracycline application.

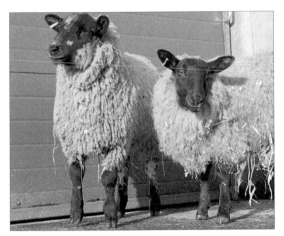

Fig. 9.80 Erysipelas infection causing swelling of the carpal joints and left forelimb fetlock joint (see Fig. 9.82).

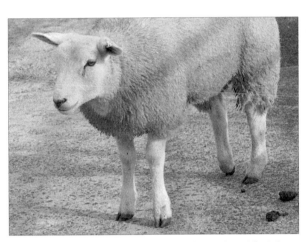

Fig. 9.81 Erysipelas infection of the right stifle joint causes severe lameness (see Fig. 9.83).

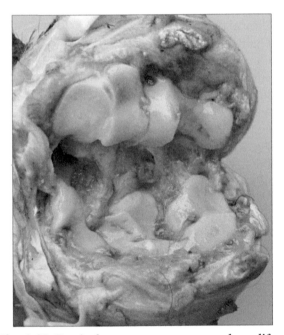

Fig. 9.82 Erysipelas case at necropsy reveals proliferation and hyperaemia of the synovial membrane, with marked thickening of the joint capsule of the right carpus.

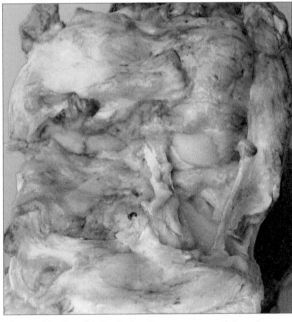

Fig. 9.83 Erysipelas infection causes proliferation and hyperaemia of the synovial membrane with marked thickening of the stifle joint capsule.

Diagnosis

The clinical findings and epidemiology of a large number of severely lame growing lambs with joint lesions showing little effusion, in unvaccinated flocks, is highly suggestive of erysipelas. There is little joint effusion and arthrocentesis often yields more blood from synovial membrane traumatized during attempted aspiration than joint fluid.

The best course of action for diagnostic purposes is to collect synovial membrane at necropsy for bacteriological culture from two or three severely lame lambs that have not received any antibiotic therapy.

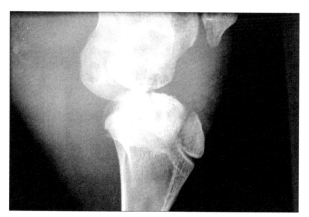

Fig. 9.84 Lateral radiograph of the stifle joint shows erosion of articular cartilage extending into subchondral bone (see Fig. 9.85).

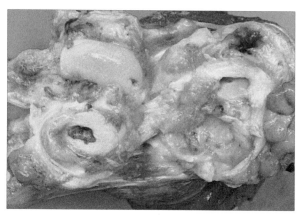

Fig. 9.85 Erysipelas infection has caused erosion of articular cartilage from the surfaces of the femoral condyles extending into subchondral bone.

Serology is not helpful because of the high seroprevalence in clinically normal sheep.

Treatment

Identification and treatment of lame growing lambs presents many practical problems. Penicillin (44,000 IU/kg once daily) for at least 5 consecutive days during the early stages of lameness effects a good cure rate in many lambs suffering from *E. rhusiopathiae* polyarthritis; however, recurrence of lameness is not uncommon 5–10 days after cessation of the original course of antibiotics. Where available, a NSAID should be administered for 3 consecutive days to alleviate pain.

Management/prevention/control measures

There are no reports of the usefulness of metaphylactic antibiotic injection during the early stages of an outbreak of erysipelas polyarthritis in sheep.

Vaccination of ewes in flocks that have a high prevalence of erysipelas in growing lambs achieves very good control of disease following passive antibody transfer. Replacement female breeding stock are vaccinated twice upon introduction into the flock and annually 1 month before lambing.

Economics

Chronically lame lambs do not grow well and cannot be presented at livestock markets, which represents considerable financial loss.

Welfare implications

An outbreak of lameness caused by erysipelas in unvaccinated flocks can result in severe lameness in a large number of growing lambs, with serious welfare concerns. Lame lambs that do not recover after two treatment courses must be euthanased for welfare reasons. Farmers are often reluctant to euthanase 4–5-month-old lame lambs because they believe the lameness will somehow eventually resolve; these lambs therefore suffer chronic lameness for several months before they are eventually destroyed for welfare reasons.

POSTDIPPING LAMENESS

Definition/overview

Postdipping lameness is a severe lameness affecting sheep of all ages but predominantly growing lambs 1–4 days after dipping in contaminated dip solutions.

Aetiology

Postdipping lameness is caused by *Erysipelothrix rhusiopathiae*, which gains entry through traumatized skin from contaminated dip wash.

Clinical presentation

There is severe lameness leading to recumbency in a large number of sheep in the flock within a few days of dipping (**Fig. 9.86**). While 90% of lambs can be affected, the prevalence is more usually around 25%.

Typically, those sheep dipped at the end of the day's work or on the second day's use of dip wash are affected. The coronary band of the affected limb(s) is swollen, hot and painful arising from cellulitis after bacterial entry. Bacteraemia and polyarthritis are uncommon sequelae.

Differential diagnoses
Interdigital dermatitis is common in this age group of lambs and can present as an outbreak of moderate to severe lameness.

Diagnosis
Diagnosis is based on clinical findings and history of recent dipping.

Treatment
Penicillin (44,000 IU/kg once daily) for 5 consecutive days effects a good cure.

Management/prevention/control measures
The disease can be prevented by using an appropriate bacteriostat in the dip wash as specified in the manufacturer's instructions. Dip washes must be discarded at the end of each working day because dangerous levels of bacterial contamination can build up during this time.

Economics
There is the temptation to reuse the same dip wash for a second day but this is unwise. Treatment of large numbers of sheep with postdipping lameness is time-consuming, expensive and unnecessary. An episode of severe lameness adversely affects growth rate with delayed marketing.

Welfare implications
Postdipping lameness causes severe lameness and obvious pain and suffering, which can be readily prevented by appropriate care and attention to standard dipping procedures.

LIMB FRACTURES

Definition/overview
Limb fractures, particularly involving the hindlimbs, are not uncommon in neonatal lambs (**Fig. 9.14**). Correct alignment often cannot be achieved by traction alone and general anaesthesia may be indicated. In hindlimb fractures lumbosacral extradural injection causes paralysis of the hindlimbs, allowing pain-free fracture alignment for casting whilst still maintaining flexion of the hock joint.

Aetiology
Fractures often result during confinement in lambing pens due to the ewe standing on the lamb's limb, falling wooden pen divisions/gates etc. Often the cause of the limb fracture cannot be determined.

Clinical presentation
Long bone fractures present as moderate to severe lameness, with a palpable fracture typically of the third metatarsal bone (**Fig. 9.87**) or third metacarpal bone in growing lambs. Greenstick fractures are not easily palpated and are often overlooked.

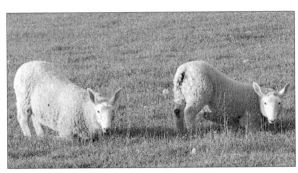

Fig. 9.86 Severe postdipping lameness affects large numbers of sheep within a few days of dipping.

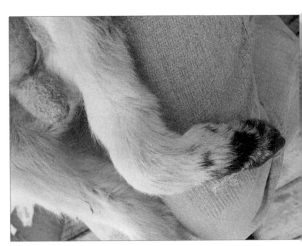

Fig. 9.87 Fractures of the third metatarsal bone are common in neonatal lambs.

Differential diagnoses

Differential diagnoses of moderate to severe lameness include joint trauma and septic joint. Foot abscess and interdigital infections can be readily excluded on clinical examination.

Diagnosis

Radiographic examination is precluded for economic reasons except for potentially valuable pedigree breeding stock. Evaluation of each case is based on detailed palpation and gentle manipulation of the affected limb. Examination is facilitated after administration of appropriate analgesia. Greenstick fractures can only be reliably diagnosed by radiography (**Fig. 9.13**).

Treatment

Fractures should be treated by the application of a plaster or fibreglass cast after appropriate fracture reduction. Correct fracture alignment hastens recovery and return to full function of the limb. Unless the fracture is stabilized, healing will be delayed or not occur with formation of a false joint. Newborn lambs can safely be transported to the veterinary surgery 'packed into a cardboard box'. The cast is extended from the foot to the first joint proximal to the fracture site. Typically, fractures of the third metatarsal bone or third metacarpal bone necessitate immobilization from the hock (**Fig. 9.88**) and carpus distally to incorporate the hoof, respectively.

Splints can also be used to stabilize distal limb fractures. Typically, plastic foam-lined splints are applied to the front and rear of the distal limb and taped in position. Such splints are popular with shepherds as they can be applied quickly in the field without requirement for water, and there is no time wasted waiting for the cast to harden. Once removed, these splints can be cleaned and reused.

Fractures of the humerus and femur cannot be satisfactorily stabilized using a cast; they require internal fixation but farmers are only able to pay for such surgery in the case of pedigree breeding stock. Stabilization resulting from extensive callus formation can occur (**Fig. 9.89**), but the sheep will have been very lame for several months before eventual healing.

Alphaxane or propafol can be safely used to induce short duration general anaesthesia to aid fracture reduction. Excellent analgesia of the hindlimbs can be achieved after lumbosacral extradural injection of 3 mg/kg of 2% lignocaine solution. This regimen allows pain-free clinical examination with more effective fracture reduction and alignment than can be achieved by physical restraint alone, and presents a cheap and readily available alternative to a protocol involving injectable general anaesthetic drugs.

NSAIDs should be administered for 3 consecutive days. As there is always the risk of sepsis in neonatal

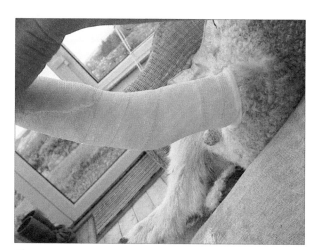

Fig. 9.88 Fractures of the third metatarsal bone necessitate immobilization from the hock distally to incorporate the hoof.

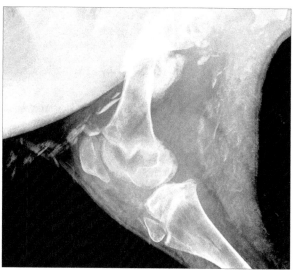

Fig. 9.89 Eventual stabilization of this mid-shaft femoral fracture resulting in extensive callus formation; this sheep had received no veterinary attention.

ruminants, even with closed fractures, a prolonged course of antibiotics, preferably penicillin, should be administered for up to 10 days.

Plaster casts are removed using an oscillating saw after 3 weeks, by which time the fracture site will be stabilized by callus formation. Recasting is not usually necessary but the two halves of the removed cast can be taped together and left supporting the limb for another 2–3 weeks as necessary.

Management/prevention/control measures

Limb fractures occur sporadically in neonatal and growing lambs. Solid partitions rather than post and rail divisions will reduce the risk of broken limbs when sheep are worked through handling facilities.

Economics

The cost of casting materials typically ranges from £3 to £5.

Welfare implications

The correct fracture alignment and fixation achieved by the farmer's veterinary surgeon hastens recovery and return to full function of the limb. Problems with malalignment (**Fig. 9.90**) and pressure sores often result when farmers attempt to stabilize fractures using wooden splints and electrical insulation tape.

OSTEOARTHRITIS IN ADULT SHEEP

Definition/overview

Osteoarthritis in growing lambs commonly follows joint infection; in adults degenerative joint disease more commonly results from serious trauma. In sheep the elbow is the most common site for joint trauma (**Fig. 9.91**), closely followed by the stifle joint (**Fig. 9.92**). In some countries, degenerative joint disease may be caused by visna-maedi virus infection.

The elbow is the ovine joint most commonly affected by osteoarthritis in the UK. Unlike other joints, arthropathy of the elbow joint in adult sheep is characterized by osteophytic reaction and extensive enthesophyte formation involving the lateral ligament (*Lig. collaterale ulnae*) following trauma to the mechanism preventing overextension of the elbow joint.

Aetiology

Trauma is the most common cause of osteoarthritis, which may occur during transport, handling and fighting injuries in rams.

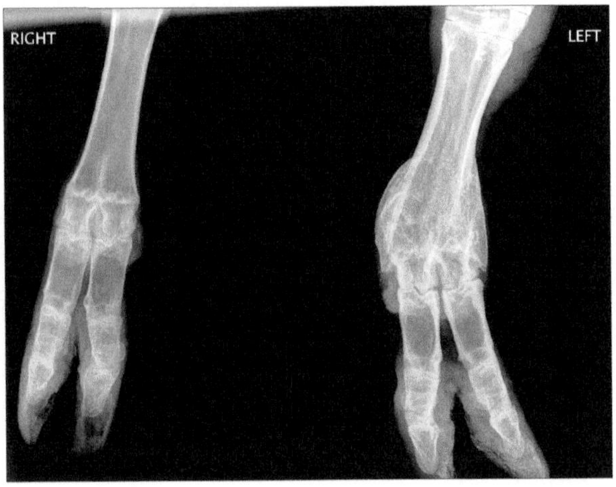

Fig. 9.90 Dorso-palmar radiograph of the left fore fetlock reveals malalignment and excessive callus formation caused by poor fracture reduction.

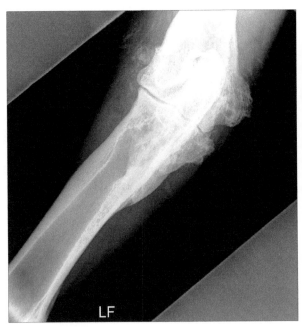

Fig. 9.91 The elbow is the most common site for joint trauma and consequent osteoarthritis.

Enthesitis is a term used to describe changes occurring at the insertion of a muscle, tendon, ligament or articular capsule where recurring concentration of stress provokes inflammation with a strong tendency towards fibrosis and calcification. The elbow joint is a typical ginglymus joint with movements restricted to flexion and extension. The lateral ligament of the elbow is short and strong and, along with tension in the medial collateral ligament and biceps brachii muscle, is largely responsible for limiting the degree of extension of the elbow joint.

Clinical presentation

The clinical presentation of osteoarthritis depends upon the number of joints affected and the duration of the condition. Sheep accommodate joint injury reasonably well which, when coupled with poor supervision, results in advanced changes being present when the sheep is eventually presented for veterinary examination.

Following the initial injury the joint is hot, painful and distended due to effusion. Over the course of several weeks there is muscle atrophy over the affected limb(s) and palpable thickening of the joint due to fibrous tissue reaction. There is reduced joint excursion (flexion) caused by the fibrous tissue reaction such that the sheep may drag the dorsal surface of the hoof along the ground, causing excessive wear at the toe. Elsewhere in the foot, reduced wear of the normal weight-bearing surfaces (abaxial wall) results in horn overgrowth. Affected sheep spend long periods in sternal recumbency. Reduced grazing leads to a gradual loss of body condition.

Stifle arthritis: Trauma to the stifle joint often results in severe lameness caused by damage to the cruciate ligament(s) and other joint support structures. Affected sheep typically present 6–8/10 lame. The stifle and hock joints are often more flexed than usual with only the toe touching the ground (**Figs 9.93, 9.94**). Careful palpation reveals

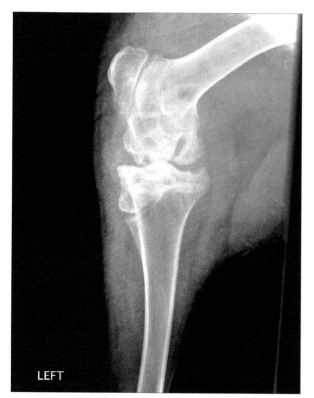

LEFT

Fig. 9.92 Osteoarthritis also commonly follows trauma to the stifle joint (see Figs 9.93, 9.94).

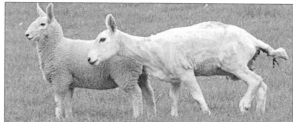

Fig. 9.93 The stifle and hock joints are more flexed than usual, with only the toe touching the ground in this case.

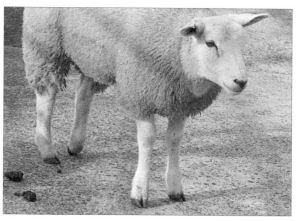

Fig. 9.94 Severe lameness resulting from trauma to the stifle joint; the toe just touches the ground but bears little weight.

marked thickening of the stifle joint capsule, more easily detected at its distal insertion over the tibial crest where the normal sharp triangular contour feels rounded. Initially, there may be joint effusion but there is scant joint fluid in advanced cases.

Elbow arthritis: Sheep with elbow arthritis are typically 2–5 years old with either unilateral, or more commonly bilateral, forelimb lameness of 3 months' duration or longer (**Fig. 9.95**). Rams are more commonly presented for veterinary examination but this may simply reflect their higher economic value. Elbow arthritis is also commonly seen in old pet sheep, presumably because of their longer life span as they are rarely bred, and their excessive body condition.

Affected sheep are in poorer bodily condition than other sheep in the group. They spend long periods in sternal recumbency, with extension of the shoulder and carpal joints such that the forelimbs are positioned in front of the animal rather than alongside the chest with these joints flexed. Affected sheep experience considerable difficulty rising. Varying intervals are spent with weight borne by the flexed carpal joints before finally standing. Skin abrasions over the carpal joints, with chronic skin trauma causing callus formation and changes in hair colour (**Fig. 9.95**), indicate that the sheep has spent several months grazing on its knees.

When standing, sheep with unilateral lesions hold the affected forelimb in rigid extension and positioned more caudally and slightly abducted. There is considerable muscle wastage over the scapula, with a prominent spine and acromion compared with the contralateral limb. Sheep with bilateral lesions adopt a characteristic stance with the hindlimbs positioned well forward underneath the body (**Figs 9.96, 9.97**). The head is not held upright as normal but level with the thoraco-lumbar vertebral column (**Fig. 9.96**). This head posture with the neck flexed makes the neck appear shorter than normal because the head is held in towards the shoulders (**Fig. 9.97**). The sheep are reluctant to walk and display a characteristic stilted forelimb gait with marked abduction of affected forelimbs. Affected sheep experience great difficulty turning and this is achieved only by pivoting on their hindlimbs.

There is no enlargement of the prescapular lymph node(s). Affected elbow joints are grossly swollen but the joint capsule does not feel thickened and there is no joint effusion. The joint swelling is caused by considerable enthesophytic reaction on the lateral aspect of the elbow. This extends distally from the attachment of the lateral ligament immediately proximal to the lateral epicondyle of the humerus and proximally from the lateral tuberosity of the radius.

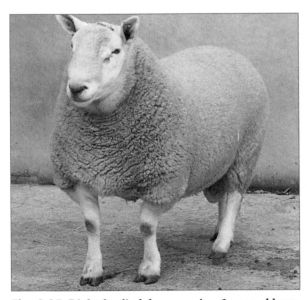

Fig. 9.95 Right forelimb lameness in a 2-year-old ram caused by elbow arthritis. Hair discolouration over the knees reveals that this ram often grazes on its knees.

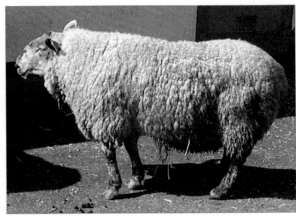

Fig. 9.96 Sheep with bilateral elbow arthritis lesions adopt a characteristic stance with the hindlimbs positioned well forward underneath the body to bear weight.

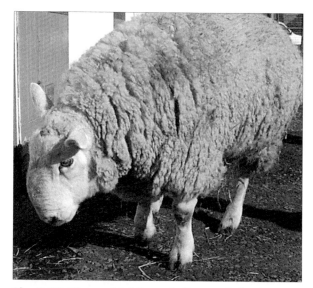

Fig. 9.97 Sheep with bilateral elbow arthritis lesions have a lowered head carriage.

Careful palpation of the cranio-lateral aspect of the affected elbow joints at the level of the articular surfaces in some cases reveals a 10–15 mm wide depression between the advancing edges of enthesophyte proliferation. In advanced cases, with an estimated duration of several years, fusion of these advancing bony margins has occurred, effectively achieving ankylosis of the elbow joint.

Measurement across the affected elbow joints with McLintock callipers reveals an increased width of 10–30 mm compared with readings for sound sheep of equivalent age, breed and sex. Typically, measurements range from 40–50 mm for normal adult Blackface and Greyface ewes and 50–65 mm for Suffolk rams. Joint excursion is severely restricted to 15–30° in many affected elbow joints.

Differential diagnoses

Footrot and white line abscesses are the major causes of lameness in adult sheep. Joint infections in adult sheep are relatively uncommon except for infections of the interdigital area, which extend into a distal interphalangeal joint. Occasionally, puncture wounds may penetrate into a joint. Joint infection following bacteraemia is uncommon. Endocarditis can present with severe lameness and multiple joint effusions.

Diagnosis

In most situations, diagnosis of osteoarthritis is based upon careful clinical examination with gentle palpation of the affected joint(s), appreciating that these joints are painful. Palpation is aimed at determining the extent of any effusion and thickening of the joint capsule.

In general, palpable joint effusion, joint laxity and no appreciable thickening of the joint capsule is consistent with a recent injury. Reduced joint excursion, absence of palpable joint effusion but obvious thickening of the joint capsule (3–5 mm) is consistent with injury of some weeks' to months' duration. Detection of crepitus is not a necessary part of the joint examination and such manipulation only serves to increase allodynia and aggravate any existing significant lesion.

Arthrocentesis: Arthrocentesis is rarely undertaken in cases of degenerative joint disease because there is scant joint fluid. The technique is painful unless the joint is distended.

Ultrasonography: Ultrasonography using a 7.5–10 MHz linear scanner with stand-off is useful to measure the extent and nature of any joint effusion and the thickness of the joint capsule. The contralateral joint, if normal, can be scanned for direct comparison.

Radiography: Dorso-palmar/plantar and latero-medial radiographs of affected joints identify soft tissue swelling and new bone formation. Erosion of articular cartilage can be identified by reduction in the joint space. Radiographic examination is limited by cost to valuable breeding sheep.

Elbow arthritis: Radiographic examination using a dorso-lateral, palmero-medial oblique view of the elbow joint in the standing sheep reveals osteophyte formation and pronounced enthesophyte formation proximal to the lateral epicondyle of the humerus and immediately distal to the lateral tuberosity of the radius involving the lateral ligament. The gap between the leading edges of enthesophyte formation is clearly visible in the radiograph of the affected elbow joints (**Fig. 9.98**) but may extend to ankylosis (**Fig. 9.99**). A latero-medial radiograph of the affected elbow joint provides little additional information and is not needed for diagnostic purposes (**Fig. 9.100**).

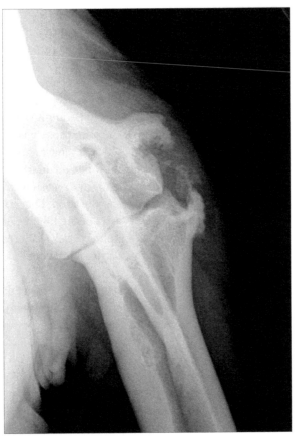

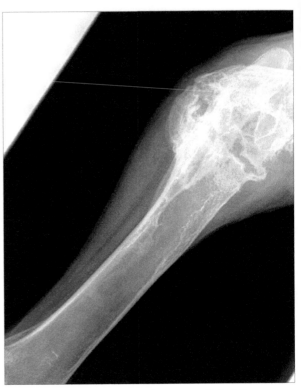

Fig. 9.99 Dorso-lateral, palmero-medial oblique radiograph of the elbow reveals complete ankylosis of the elbow joint, caused by fusion of enthesophyte formation involving the lateral ligament.

Fig. 9.98 Radiographic examination of an affected elbow joint in a standing sheep using a dorso-lateral, palmero-medial oblique view reveals considerable enthesophyte formation.

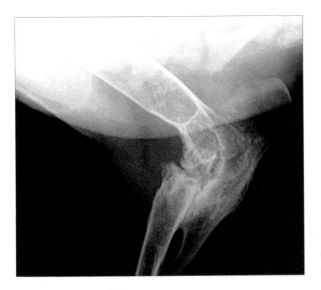

Fig. 9.100 A latero-medial radiograph of an affected elbow joint provides little additional information and may underestimate enthesophyte deposition.

Ultrasonographic examination of the lateral aspect of affected elbow joints does not reveal any joint effusion. At the cranio-lateral extent of the bony swelling there is often sudden disruption to the broad hyperechoic line representing bone surface which, by its width of 10–20 mm and absence of fluid, does not represent the elbow joint. These margins of the hyperechoic line observed during ultrasonographic examination correspond to the typical enthesophytic reaction noted during radiographic examination.

Gross postmortem examination of affected elbow joints reveals erosion of articular cartilage and extensive osteophyte formation (**Fig. 9.101**). Enthesophyte formation is best demonstrated by 'boiled out' preparations.

Treatment

There is no effective treatment for elbow arthritis and affected sheep should be culled for welfare reasons. Chondroprotective agents, such as chondroitin sulphate or polysulphated glycosaminoglycan, are useful in other species for degenerative joint disease but have not been used in sheep. It is probable that these agents would be less effective in sheep because of the more advanced pathological state when presented for diagnosis and treatment.

In acute cases, NSAIDs should be administered for 3–5 days. The sheep should be isolated and confined to a small pen. Long-term pain relief can be attempted by daily administration of 10 mg/kg phenylbutazone but such use is strictly 'off-label' and treated sheep must not enter the food chain.

Management/prevention/control measures

Joint injuries occur sporadically during handling and transport. Greater care and patience could be exercised when handling stock. Care must be taken to reduce fighting when introducing new rams into established groups. The rapid growth and excessive body condition in ram lambs and shearlings demanded for sale purposes may predispose to elbow ligament damage. However, the apparent sex predisposition encountered in this author's practice may be considerably influenced by economic factors, with rams costing a great deal more than ewes. Trauma to the elbow joint may result during management procedures such as shearing and foot-trimming, which involve casting the sheep.

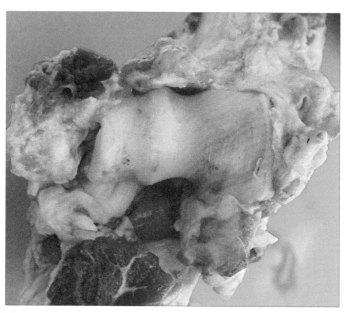

Fig. 9.101 Gross postmortem examination of an affected elbow joint shows erosion of articular cartilage and extensive enthesophytosis on the left of the image.

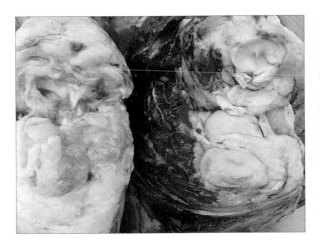

Fig. 9.102 Osteoarthritis of this stifle joint (left) represents a serious welfare concern because of the chronicity and severity of the lesion, indicated by the proliferative synovial membrane obscuring the articular surfaces.

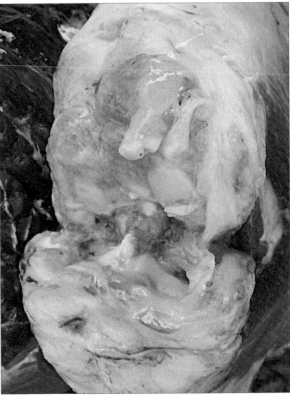

Fig. 9.103 Necropsy reveals hyperaemia and proliferation of the synovial membrane in a stifle joint with osteoarthritis.

Economics

Elbow arthritis necessitates culling of severely affected sheep thereby shortening the sheep's productive lifespan. This financial loss is greater when culling rams rather than ewes.

Welfare implications

Arthritis of the elbow and stifle joints represents a considerable welfare concern because of the chronicity and severity of the lesions (**Figs 9.102, 9.103**).

CLINICAL EXAMINATION

Infections of the urinary system are rare in sheep and mostly commonly follow urethral surgery to correct an obstruction. Urolithiasis in male sheep is common whenever inappropriate rations are fed, leading to calculus formation.

Normal urination in male sheep produces a steady flow lasting around 15–30 seconds (**Fig. 10.1**). Tenesmus producing only drops of blood-tinged urine is highly abnormal and must be investigated immediately. Blockage to the free flow of urine leads to bladder distension and abdominal pain, expressed by frequent tail swishing and long periods in sternal recumbency (**Fig. 10.2**). Frequent vocalization is common in lambs suffering from urolithiasis, while bruxism is more common in adults.

Examination of the preputial hairs reveals the presence of a small number of calculi in many normal male sheep and is not a reliable indicator of urolithiasis. The penis can readily be exteriorized in sexually mature males to allow examination of the glans and vermiform appendage (**Fig. 10.3**). The ram is seated on its rump and the penis is held through the sheath and the sigmoid flexure extended at the same time as retracting the prepuce. A gauze swab is then wrapped around the penis just proximal to the glans.

Urinalysis

Sheep rarely develop ascending urinary tract infections; bacteraemic spread to the kidneys does occur but causes significant problems in very few cases (**Fig. 10.4**). Catheterization of the bladder is possible in females but is rarely indicated. Urine specific gravity ranges from 1.015–1.045 in normal sheep, with pH values of 7.4–8.0. Urine should be checked for the presence of sediment, in particular struvite crystals. Glucose, ketones, protein, blood and bilirubin should be absent from urine. Because ultrasonography provides instant results with respect to urolithiasis diagnosis and gross bladder infection, urinalysis is rarely necessary.

Biochemistry

Serum creatinine and blood urea nitrogen (BUN) concentrations are commonly used to determine renal function. Due to its distribution throughout

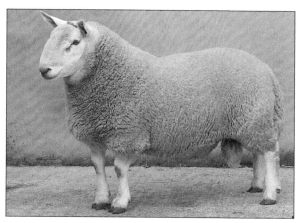

Fig. 10.1 Normal urination in male sheep produces a steady flow lasting at least 10–15 seconds.

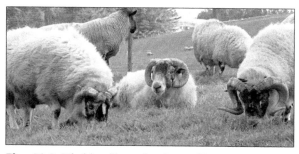

Fig. 10.2 Bladder distension is manifest as abdominal pain with long periods in sternal recumbency.

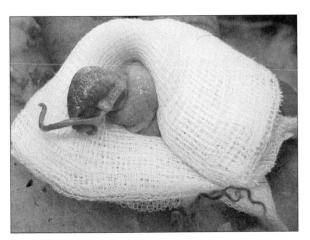

Fig. 10.3 Exteriorization of the penis enabling examination of the glans and vermiform appendage.

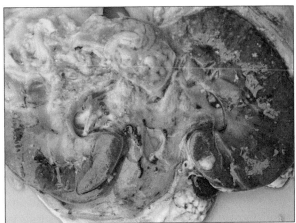

Fig. 10.4 Bacteraemia with significant infection of the kidney is very uncommon in sheep.

the body, the BUN concentration may fall more slowly than serum creatinine following return to more normal renal function; therefore, creatinine concentration affords the more accurate prognosis. Under certain grazing conditions the high dietary nitrogen content may be reflected in an elevated BUN concentration but this rarely exceeds twice the normal level.

Bacteriology

Bacteriology of a urine sample is rarely undertaken because of the rare occurrence of primary urinary tract infections. Those infections that do arise post urethrostomy surgery are caused by *Corynebacterium renale*.

Bacteraemic spread to the parenchymatous organs from a septic focus elsewhere may result in bacterial shedding into the urine from a renal infarct, but such secondary lesions rarely compromise renal function.

Ultrasonography

Ultrasonography has great practical application in the field investigation of urolithiasis in male sheep. Bladder distension, uroperitoneum and subcutaneous urine accumulation after urethral rupture can readily be determined using both linear array and sector scanners. Examination of the right kidney can be undertaken with a sector scanner. There is no requirement to scan the left kidney because hydronephrosis secondary to urethral obstruction affects both kidneys.

Radiography

Unlike in dogs and cats, radiography is rarely used to gather further information on the urinary tract in sheep. Radiography is costly, presents numerous safety concerns and is not readily portable for on-farm use and it adds little additional information to that gathered by ultrasonography.

Renal biopsy

While theoretically it is possible to undertake ultrasound-guided renal biopsy, this technique is not indicated in sheep as they rarely develop glomerulonephritis or similar conditions.

UROLITHIASIS

Definition/overview

Partial or complete urethral obstruction is a common condition of intensively-reared entire male and castrated lambs fed incorrectly formulated rations, and occurs occasionally in mature rams. Urolithiasis rarely affects pasture-fed lambs and is not recorded in ewes.

Early recognition of clinical signs by the farmer and prompt veterinary treatment are essential to ensure a satisfactory outcome, because irreversible hydronephrosis from urinary back pressure can result within 5–10 days of onset of clinical signs (**Figs 10.5, 10.6**). Early diagnosis is also important to allow rapid implementation of control measures and reduce the occurrence of future cases.

Aetiology

The most common cause of urolithiasis in male sheep is magnesium ammonium phosphate hexahydrate (struvite) calculi associated with feeding concentrate rations high in phosphate (>0.6%) and magnesium (>0.2%). Proteins within the bladder combine with these minerals to form calculi, which lodge within the urethra just proximal to the sigmoid flexure or within the vermiform appendage.

Clinical presentation

The early clinical signs of urinary tract obstruction in male sheep include separation from others in the group with long periods spent in sternal recumbency and 'dog-sitting'. There is frequent tail swishing and foot stomping, especially in lambs. Affected sheep have a wide stance with the hindlimbs held well back, and they stretch frequently (**Fig. 10.7**). Affected sheep are inappetent and have an anxious, painful expression; there is frequent curling of the upper lip (**Fig. 10.8**). There is frequent tenesmus accompanied by painful bleating (lambs), and teeth grinding (adults). The mucous membranes are congested and the heart and respiratory rates are increased. Nil or only a few drops of blood-tinged urine are voided rather than a clear continuous flow. The preputial

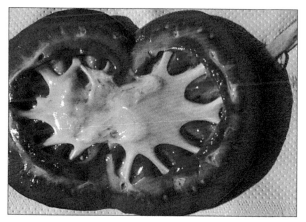

Fig. 10.5 Necropsy reveals severe hydronephrosis from high urinary back pressure that can result within 7–10 days of onset of clinical signs.

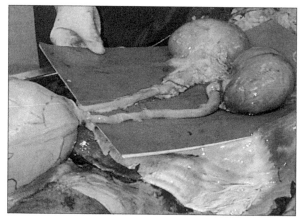

Fig. 10.6 Necropsy reveals that high urinary tract back pressure has caused hydroureters and hydronephrosis.

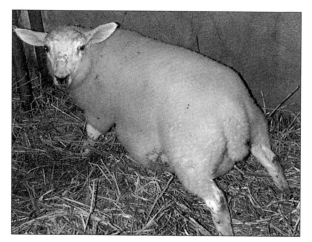

Fig. 10.7 Lambs with urethral obstruction have a wide stance with the hindlimbs held well back and they stretch frequently.

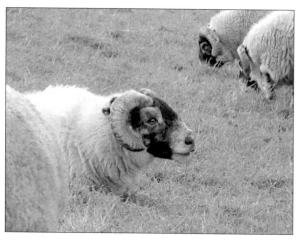

Fig. 10.8 Sheep with urethral obstruction are inappetent and have an anxious, painful expression with frequent curling of the upper lip.

hairs are often dry compared to a moist/wet appearance in normal sheep. Calculi are frequently present on the preputial hairs of normal male sheep and are not indicative of urolithiasis.

High pressure may result in urine leakage across the taut bladder wall, leading to uroperitoneum in growing lambs (**Fig. 10.9**). This is uncommon in adult sheep unless neglected. Rupture of the urethra/penis may occur in sheep neglected for several days with resultant subcutaneous swelling up to 6–10 cm deep extending along the prepuce (**Fig. 10.10**) and involving the scrotum (**Fig. 10.11**). Large sharply-demarcated areas of purple skin develop along

the ventrum overlying this subcutaneous urine accumulation (**Fig. 10.10**). The discoloured skin becomes cold and, with associated necrotic muscle, will slough after 10–14 days if the animal survives.

Rather than rupture of the bladder wall, high urinary back pressure within the bladder causes hydroureters and bilateral hydronephrosis (**Fig. 10.12**), which may be detected ultrasonographically in the right kidney after 5–7 days.

Differential diagnoses

The differential diagnosis list can be restricted by a thorough clinical examination.

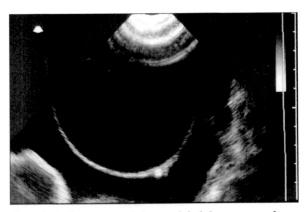

Fig. 10.9 Sonogram of the caudal abdomen reveals extensive fluid within the abdominal cavity (5 MHz sector scanner). Note the bladder wall is intact.

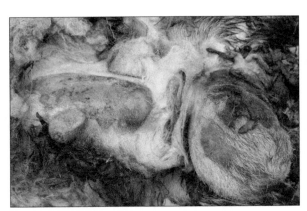

Fig. 10.10 Rupture of the urethra/penis where subcutaneous urine extends up to 10 cm deep along the prepuce with necrosis of overlying skin.

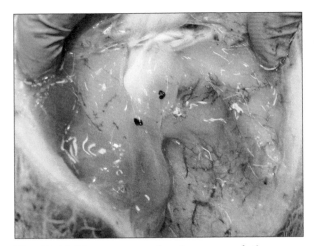

Fig. 10.11 Necropsy reveals urine accumulation within the scrotum.

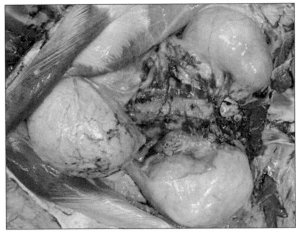

Fig. 10.12 Necropsy reveals that high urinary back pressure has caused hydroureters and bilateral hydronephrosis.

Transabdominal ultrasonography readily identifies the massively-distended urinary bladder (**Figs 10.13–10.15**) and hydronephrosis of the right kidney (**Figs 10.16–10.19**).

The initial colic signs in young growing lambs can be mistaken for abomasal/small intestinal volvulus, but these conditions cause marked abdominal distension and profound toxaemia with rapid deterioration. Coccidiosis and intussusception, and possibly nematodirosis, in lambs cause frequent tenesmus and abdominal pain.

In rams, the clinical signs are frequently less pronounced with the ram presented as inappetent, lethargic and spending long periods in sternal recumbency. Many infectious diseases can present with similar clinical signs including painful foot lesions, chronic respiratory disease/pleurisy and peritonitis.

Diagnosis

Excision of vermiform appendage: Partial/complete urethral obstruction in mature rams most commonly occurs at the vermiform appendage. The granular calculus can be felt within the vermiform appendage. The diagnosis is confirmed following excision of the vermiform appendage, which produces a free flow of urine when the ram is released. The portion of the vermiform appendage distal to the calculus is frequently discoloured and often necrotic. While urination after excision of the vermiform appendage confirms the diagnosis of urethral obstruction, it is not possible to establish an accurate prognosis based upon clinical

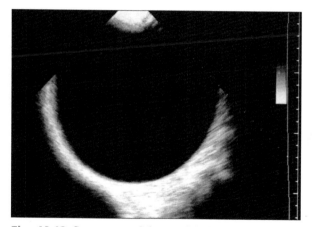

Fig. 10.13 Sonogram of the caudal abdomen reveals bladder distension extending to 14 cm diameter (5 MHz sector scanner).

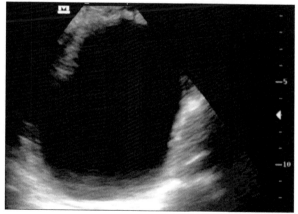

Fig. 10.14 Sonogram of the caudal abdomen reveals bladder distension extending to 12 cm diameter (5 MHz sector scanner).

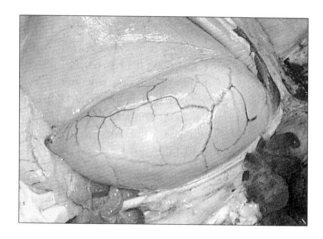

Fig. 10.15 Confirmation of bladder distension and absence of uroperitoneum revealed at necropsy.

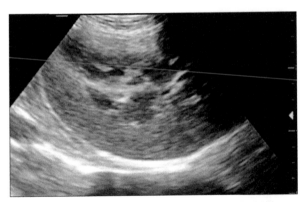

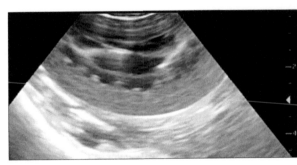

Fig. 10.17 Sonogram shows mild hydronephrosis of the right kidney; the renal pelvis is distended with urine (5 MHz sector scanner).

Fig. 10.16 Sonogram shows the normal right kidney with the hyperechoic line representing the kidney capsule clearly identified (5 MHz sector scanner).

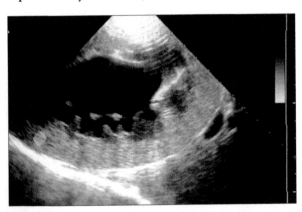

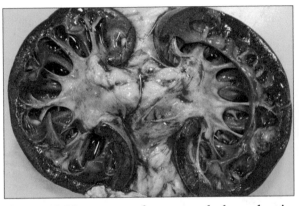

Fig. 10.18 Sonogram shows severe hydronephrosis of the right kidney; the renal pelvis, represented by the large anechoic central area, is greatly distended with urine (5 MHz sector scanner).

Fig. 10.19 Necropsy confirms severe hydronephrosis of the right kidney (see Fig. 10.18).

examination alone. Often farmers are unsure how long the sheep has been ill and may underestimate the duration of illness.

Laboratory tests: Marked serum elevations of BUN and creatinine concentrations occur as a result of partial or complete urethral obstruction; however, such increases are not pathognomonic and there are no recognized threshold concentrations. For example, in abdominal catastrophes such as intestinal volvulus, BUN and creatinine concentrations can be increased five- to 10-fold.

Concentrations of BUN and creatinine can be increased up to 30–60 mmol/l (normal range = 2.2–6.6 mmol/l) and >1000 μmol/l (normal range = 40–150 μmol/l) respectively in male sheep with

urolithiasis of less than 2 days' duration that recover after excision of the vermiform appendage. Such concentrations are not significantly different from those in sheep with a more prolonged urethral obstruction which has resulted in severe hydronephrosis. Rams in the latter category fail to recover irrespective of the treatment regimen.

Ultrasonographic examination: Diagnostic quality images of the bladder can readily be obtained using a 5.0 MHz sector transducer connected to a real-time, B-mode ultrasound machine. Many farm animal practices own a 5.0 MHz linear array scanner. This is used for early pregnancy diagnosis in cattle but can also be used to examine the abdomen in sheep, although the depth of field is limited to 10 cm.

Examination using a 5.0 MHz linear array scanner will readily identify uroperitoneum and distended bladder. However, the true size of the bladder may not be measured because it may extend to 20 cm in diameter. The bladder in normal male sheep is contained within the pelvis; therefore, the presence of the bladder extending for up to 10 cm or more beyond the pelvic brim is abnormal. Determination of the actual size of the bladder is of secondary importance.

Ultrasonographic examination of the bladder and caudal abdomen are undertaken in the standing animal using either a 5.0 MHz linear array or sector scanner. The right inguinal region immediately cranial to the pelvis is cleaned using a mild detergent solution diluted in warm tap water to remove superficial grease and debris. Ultrasound gel is liberally applied to the wet skin to ensure good contact. The transducer head is firmly held at a right angle against the abdominal wall. There is scant peritoneal fluid in normal sheep and this cannot be visualized during ultrasonographic examination.

The distended bladder is clearly visible as an anechoic (black) area bordered by a hyperechoic (bright white) line where the diameter may exceed 18 cm (**Figs 10.13, 10.14**). Urine within the abdominal cavity appears as an anechoic area; the walls of abdominal viscera appear as broad hyperechoic lines/circles displaced dorsally by the urine. Fibrin tags can sometimes be visualized within the uroperitoneum as hyperechoic filaments within the anechoic fluid.

Bladder distension is a very useful indicator of partial or complete urethral obstruction and it can be determined within minutes of the on-farm ultrasonographic examination. The distended bladder is typically 6–8 cm in diameter in 20–40 kg growing lambs increasing to 16–20 cm in mature rams.

The distended bladder and clinical findings confirm the diagnosis of urethral obstruction. Prognosis is determined by the duration of the obstruction resulting in hydronephrosis (**Figs 10.16–10.19**). Examination of the right kidney can be undertaken using a 5.0 MHz sector transducer. The concave nature of the right sublumbar fossa may preclude use of a 5.0 MHz linear transducer. The right kidney is juxtaposed to the caudal pole of the liver underlying the dorsal aspect of the right sublumbar fossa. Advanced hydronephrosis is identified by the increased renal pelvis which

is represented by the anechoic (fluid-filled) centre of the kidney and reduced renal cortex (**Fig. 10.18**). It is not possible to scan the left kidney in sheep but such examination is unnecessary because the urinary tract obstruction is distal to the ureter; therefore, the condition is bilateral.

Treatment

In mature rams the blockage is commonly relieved when the penis is extruded and vermiform appendage excised during the clinical examination, with production of a free flow of urine. Subsequent acidification of the urine by daily drenching with ammonium chloride is seldom undertaken and appears not to be necessary as recurrence is uncommon. It is very unusual to encounter large numbers of calculi within the bladder (**Fig. 10.20**). Antibiotic therapy is not indicated after excision of the vermiform appendage.

Subischial urethrostomy: Surgical correction of urolithiasis caused by blockage proximal to the sigmoid flexure involves a subischial urethrostomy under caudal block; this is not a simple procedure, however. There are a number of important factors

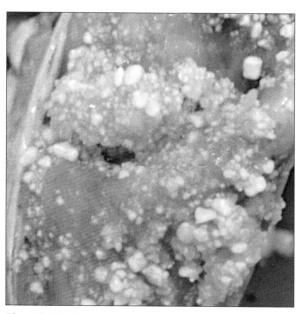

Fig. 10.20 Necropsy of a yearling male sheep that was euthanased for urolithiasis and hydronephrosis; it is very unusual to encounter such large numbers of calculi within the bladder.

to consider prior to this salvage procedure: firstly the welfare of the sheep, especially if there are considerable accumulations of urine subcutaneously (see **Figs 10.10, 10.11**); secondly, the likely interval to slaughter; and finally, the cost of surgery relative to carcase value. It must be remembered that drainage lymph nodes, such as the deep inguinal lymph nodes, could remain reactive for many weeks, resulting in condemnation of the carcase hindquarters at slaughter. Ascending infection of the sectioned urethra after surgery frequently causes cystitis/pyelonephritis with clinical signs apparent around 4–6 weeks following surgery. It is this author's recommendation that this surgical procedure is not undertaken and the sheep is humanely destroyed as soon as the condition has been confirmed on clinical examination.

Tube cystotomy: A subischial urethrostomy would not be appropriate in a breeding ram, where a tube cystotomy should be performed to maintain integrity of the male reproductive tract. This surgical procedure should only be undertaken when there are no ultrasonographic findings indicating advanced hydronephrosis (**Fig. 10.18**). A Foley catheter is sutured into the bladder via a paramedian laporotomy incision performed under either general anaesthesia or sedation and a high extradural block. It is reported that there is no requirement to attempt to dissolve the calculus and that urethral patency is restored after 4–6 weeks. This can be checked by temporarily closing the catheter.

Urethral rupture: Rupture of the urethra results in subcutaneous urine accumulation involving the prepuce and extending caudally along the ventral abdomen to involve the scrotum. It is not uncommon for urine to collect to a depth of 6–8 cm. Surgery should be considered carefully in these rams because considerable sloughing of necrotic skin and muscle occurs even if surgery is successful. The multi-pocketed sonographic appearance of the subcutaneous swelling would suggest that urine drainage would be poor even using multiple skin stab incisions into these areas.

Management/prevention/control measures

Correct ration formulation with appropriate mineral supplementation is the basis for prevention of urolithiasis in intensively reared sheep. Urine acidifiers, such as ammonium chloride, are commonly added to rations. Sodium chloride has been added to rations to promote water intake. Provision of roughage promotes saliva production and water intake. Fresh clean water must always be available and frequent checks must be made for frozen pipes in subzero temperatures.

Economics

Excision of the vermiform appendage soon after obstruction has occurred affords an excellent prognosis in adult rams and involves little expense. However, surgical correction of urolithiasis by subischial urethrostomy is a salvage procedure that is not warranted for either welfare or financial reasons. Tube cystotomy is possible in valuable breeding rams but must be undertaken before the development of significant hydronephrosis.

Welfare implications

With the exception of simple blockages relieved after excision of the vermiform appendage, all commercial value sheep with urolithiasis should be euthanased for welfare reasons at first presentation.

Further complications of urethral obstruction and build-up of pressure within the urinary tract include rupture of the kidney (**Figs 10.21, 10.22**).

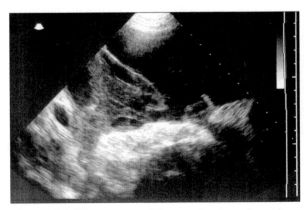

Fig. 10.21 Ultrasonographic examination of a male sheep with bladder distension failed to identify the right kidney. Instead there were large hyperechoic structures within an anechoic area consistent with a blood clot (see Fig. 10.22).

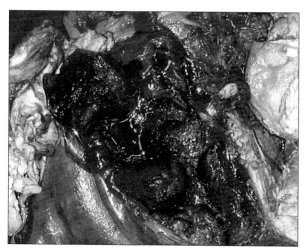

Fig. 10.22 Necropsy reveals considerable haemorrhage in the region of the right kidney.

PELVIC NERVE DYSFUNCTION

Definition/overview

Marked urinary bladder distension, hydroureters and severe bilateral hydronephrosis have been identified ultrasonographically consistent with a diagnosis of obstructive urolithiasis, but these rams were observed to urinate. However, the flow rate of urine was estimated to be less than normal and the duration was reduced to around 5–10 seconds when around 15–30 seconds is considered normal. This presentation has also been reported in ewes (**Fig. 10.23**), with normal tone of the tail and rectum and normal perineal and pelvic limb reflexes. A presumptive diagnosis of pelvic nerve dysfunction causing detrusor atony and bladder distension with secondary pressure-induced hydronephrosis was suggested but unproven. Detailed dissection at necropsy found no evidence of urethral obstruction in male sheep. This condition may be much more common than reported because few cases of suspected urolithiasis are subjected to detailed necropsy.

Aetiology

The cause of pelvic nerve dysfunction remains unproven.

Clinical presentation

The flow of urine in affected sheep is approximately one-half the normal flow rate and the duration is reduced to 5–10 seconds when a steady flow of around 15–30 seconds is considered normal. Urine then drips from the prepuce for 10–20 seconds after urination in affected rams. There is normal tone of the tail and rectum and normal perineal and pelvic limb reflexes, ruling out cauda equina syndrome and a lesion of the thoraco-lumbar spinal cord, respectively. Urinary bladder distension and marked hydronephrosis causing enlargement of the right kidney have been identified ultrasonographically. In two rams there was also 4–8 cm of fluid surrounding the right kidney, bridged by fine hyperechoic filaments consistent with fibrin tags (**Figs 10.24–10.29**), presumably caused by urine leakage.

Careful dissection of the entire urethra in rams has found no evidence of obstructive urolithiasis; there were no calculi in the bladder. Passage of a continuous flow of urine in rams, albeit at a reduced rate and duration, makes a specific diagnosis problematic on clinical examination alone. The report of a similar presentation in ewes would suggest that partial urethral obstruction is an unlikely aetiology. During urine voiding the detrusor muscle receives its innervation from the parasympathetic nervous system via the pelvic nerve; thus pelvic nerve dysfunction remains the most likely cause of this urinary system pathology.

Differential diagnoses

Partial urolithiasis.

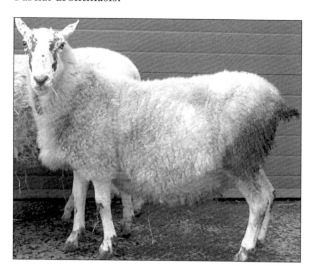

Fig. 10.23 Urine staining of the tail and perineum of an adult ewe attributed to pelvic nerve paralysis.

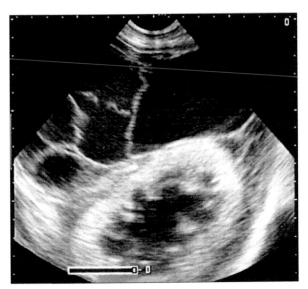

Fig. 10.24 Sonogram of the right kidney of a ram diagnosed with pelvic nerve paralysis. The right kidney shows changes consistent with severe hydronephrosis and is separated from the body wall by 8 cm of fluid containing fine hyperechoic tags (5 MHz sector scanner). (See Fig. 10.25.)

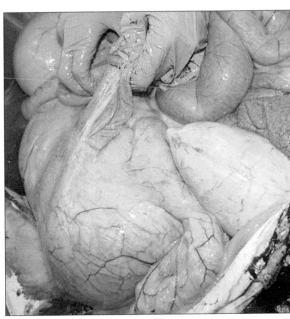

Fig. 10.25 Necropsy reveals bladder distension and a large swelling surrounding the right kidney.

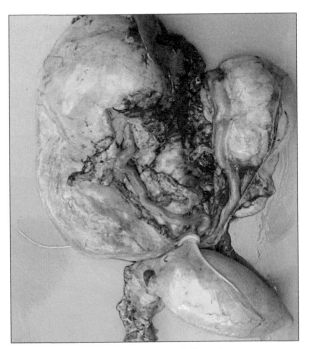

Fig. 10.26 Further dissection of the urinary tract (Fig. 10.25) reveals hydroureters and a normal-sized left kidney.

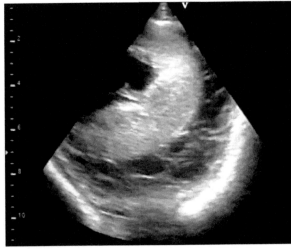

Fig. 10.27 Ultrasound examination reveals up to 4 cm of fluid surrounding the right kidney, bridged by hyperechoic filaments beneath a 1 cm thick capsule (5 MHz sector scanner).

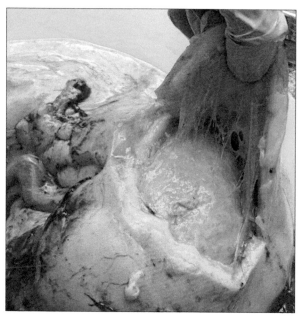

Fig. 10.28 Necropsy reveals fibrin tags beneath a thick capsule; much of the fluid has drained away.

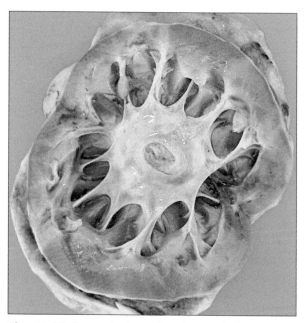

Fig. 10.29 Severe hydronephrosis revealed at necropsy (see Fig. 10.24).

Diagnosis

Passage of a continuous flow of urine, albeit at a reduced rate, rules out obstructive urolithiasis. Potential causes of pelvic nerve dysfunction, such as protozoal myelitis, should be investigated.

Treatment

Until the aetiology has been confirmed there is no recommended treatment other than euthanasia for welfare reasons.

Management/prevention/control measures

There are no prevention/control measures.

ULCERATIVE POSTHITIS

(syn. sheath rot)

Definition/overview

An ulcerative condition of the sheath commonly associated with high dietary protein intake. Affected sheep often have concurrent lameness. Long periods spent in sternal recumbency may exacerbate the sheath infection.

Aetiology

The condition is caused by *Corynebacterium renale*, which contains the enzyme urease. Urease is capable of breaking down urea in the urine to release ammonia, which is caustic to the epithelium of the prepuce.

Clinical presentation

There is a strong ammoniacal smell from the stained fleece around the prepuce. Typically, the prepuce is swollen and oedematous, with a necrotic circumferential lesion about 1 cm wide at the skin/prepuce margin (**Fig. 10.30**). The lesion is often covered by scab material and bleeds profusely if the scab is removed. Secondary cutaneous myiasis may occur in neglected cases.

Differential diagnoses

Urolithiasis.

Diagnosis

The diagnosis is based upon the clinical signs and rapid response to antibiotic therapy.

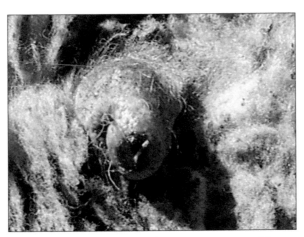

Fig. 10.30 Swollen and oedematous prepuce with a necrotic circumferential lesion about 1 cm wide at the skin/prepuce margin is typical of sheath rot.

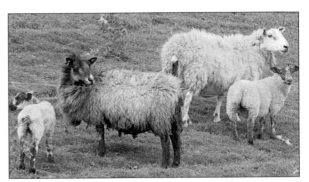

Fig. 10.31 Nephrosis causes chronic weight loss leading to emaciation (left) compared with a lamb of the same age.

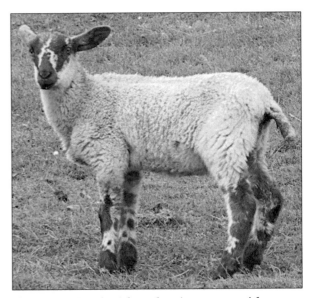

Fig. 10.32 Lamb with nephrosis presents with severe weight loss, poor coat and depression.

Treatment

Ulcerative posthitis can be treated with daily intramuscular penicillin injections for 5 or more consecutive days. Topical antiseptics can be applied to the lesions. Reducing the protein content in the diet is not possible when rams are at pasture; any concentrate supplementation should have a low protein content. Any lameness should be treated promptly to prevent prolonged sternal recumbency and urine scalding and also to reduce the risk of infectious posthitis. Phimosis is uncommon following infectious posthitis. The farmer should be advised to remove the wool around the prepuce to reduce the risk of contamination leading to cutaneous myiasis.

Management/prevention/control measures

Appropriate nutrition and prompt attention to lameness should prevent this condition.

NEPHROSIS

Definition/overview

Nephrosis occurs sporadically in growing lambs up to 4 months old, often appearing after an outbreak of coccidiosis or nematodirosis.

Aetiology

A toxic insult is considered the probable aetiology.

Clinical presentation

Affected lambs are very depressed and do not suck. They appear thirsty as they frequently stand with their heads over a water trough but drink little. The rectal temperature is normal but the lambs appear gaunt with little abdominal content and they rapidly become emaciated (**Figs 10.31, 10.32**).

Differential diagnoses

The important differential diagnoses include coccidiosis, nematodirosis and starvation. Bacterial infections including hepatic necrobacillosis, chronic suppurative pneumonia, chronic peritonitis and infected urachus can also present with many of the clinical signs listed above.

Diagnosis

The diagnosis is based upon the clinical findings and biochemical results of hypoalbuminaemia and markedly elevated BUN concentrations. Necropsy reveals very swollen pale kidneys (**Fig. 10.33**).

Treatment

There is no treatment and affected lambs should be euthanased for welfare reasons.

Management/prevention/control measures

The condition occurs sporadically and there are no recognized control measures.

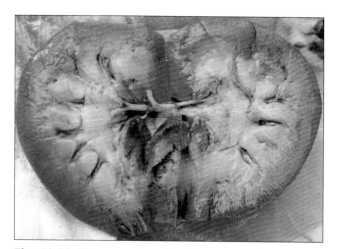

Fig. 10.33 Necropsy of nephrosis cases reveals very swollen, pale kidneys.

CLINICAL EXAMINATION

Diseases of the skin are important because wool yield and quality are adversely affected and wool is the major product of the sheep industry in some countries (**Figs 11.1, 11.2**), including Australia.

Generalized infections and infestations can lead to debility and possibly death. Focal bacterial infections of the skin are common in sheep and may become generalized under favourable climatic conditions such as prolonged wet weather after shearing. Viral infections of the muco-cutaneous junctions are common in young lambs but may also affect adults. Ectoparasite infestations are very common in sheep, causing severe economic losses and raising serious welfare concerns. Some ectoparasites are also vectors for bacterial, rickettsial and viral infections, which may cause serious disease outbreaks. Therefore, the skin should not be considered in isolation and

reference will be made to diseases of other organ systems (e.g. louping-ill, which is transmitted by ticks).

CONTAGIOUS PUSTULAR DERMATITIS

(syn. orf, scabby mouth, contagious ecthyma)

Definition/overview

Contagious pustular dermatitis (CPD) virus most commonly results in proliferative lesions following trauma of the coronary band and muco-cutaneous junction of the mouth and is particularly severe in artificially-reared lambs less than 2 months old. Outbreaks of CPD may occur within 10–14 days of change onto pastures containing thistles, gorse or stubble (**Fig. 11.3**), which cause superficial trauma to the lips and feet. CPD has a worldwide distribution and is a major disease problem in many countries. CPD is a zoonosis.

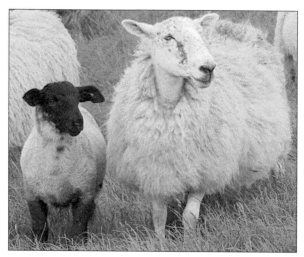

Fig. 11.1 Wool is the major product of the sheep industry in some countries but is largely worthless in European countries.

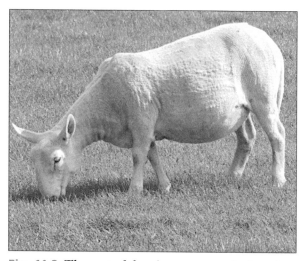

Fig. 11.2 The cost of shearing now exceeds the value of wool in many countries.

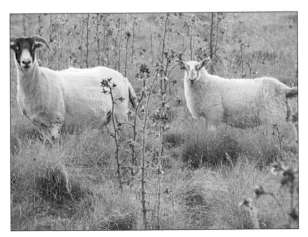

Fig. 11.3 Outbreaks of contagious pustular dermatitis (CPD) may occur within 10–14 days of change onto pastures containing thistles, gorse or stubble.

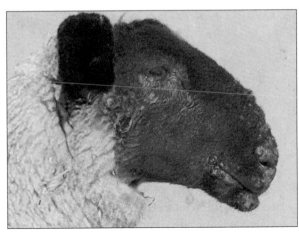

Fig. 11.4 CPD virus most commonly results in proliferative lesions at the muco-cutaneous junction of the mouth.

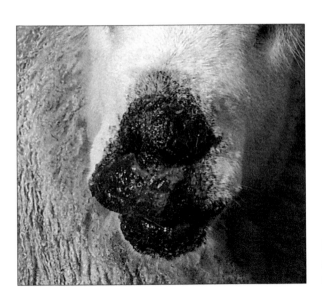

Fig. 11.5 Proliferative lesions of CPD at the muco-cutaneous junction of the mouth extend onto the muzzle.

Aetiology

The cause is a pox virus (genus Parapoxvirus), which can remain infective in dried scabs for many months.

Clinical presentation

CPD virus most commonly results in proliferative lesions at the muco-cutaneous junction of the mouth (**Figs 11.4, 11.5**) and coronary band. It is particularly severe in artificially-reared lambs less than 2 months old. Morbidity can be high but mortality in uncomplicated cases is low. Lesions persist for some 2–4 weeks then slowly regress. Disease in the flock generally persists for 6–8 weeks.

Initial papule and vesicle stages are rarely observed. Scabs progressing to large granulomatous structures, which bleed profusely following trauma, are the more common presentation. Large scabs are often present at the commisures of the lips and along the gum margins surrounding the incisor teeth. Much less commonly, lesions may involve the hard palate and tongue.

In the UK, CPD virus rapidly spreads within a group of orphan lambs sharing the same feeding equipment. In sucking lambs lesions frequently develop on the medial aspect of the ewe's teats, due to trauma by the lamb's incisor teeth. This permits entry of the virus. These teat lesions are painful and the ewe will typically not allow the lambs to suck. Mastitis, occasionally gangrenous in nature, may follow the development of such teat lesions.

CPD virus and *Staphylococcus aureus* may act synergistically to cause severe facial dermatitis, which appears as sharply-demarcated areas extending 8 cm from the muzzle and involving the lower lip, with scab material also palpable within the hairs extending for a further 2–3 cm from the periphery of the visible lesions (**Fig. 11.6**). The skin is oedematous with serous exudation and superficial pus accumulation, which may become desiccated forming hard scabs separated by deep fissures (**Fig. 11.6**). There is a deep bed of granulation tissue underneath the scab material. Exuberant granulation tissue and overlying scab material can narrow the nostrils in severely affected lambs, causing dyspnoea with stertor and abdominal breathing.

CPD virus and *Dermatophilus congolensis* may act synergistically to produce large granulomatous masses extending 4–8 cm proximally from the coronary band; this is often referred to as 'strawberry footrot' (**Fig. 11.7**). These lesions bleed profusely when traumatized. Typically, the strawberry footrot lesion only affects one limb. They are more commonly seen in weaned lambs recently moved on to stubble. While lesions are severe in individual lambs, the morbidity is generally low. Healing takes many months and lesions may not completely resolve. Slaughter is delayed because of marked enlargement of the drainage lymph node(s).

Differential diagnoses

The very early stages of CPD with papule and vesicle formation could be mistaken for foot and mouth disease (FMD) but the CPD lesions affect the lambs' mouths only and are not seen around the coronary band. Furthermore, not all CPD lesions would be at this early vesicular stage and more typical proliferative crusting lesions would also be present. Sheep affected with FMD are febrile, inappetent and often severely lame for a brief period with vesicles in the interdigital skin and around the coronary band.

Facial dermatitis in growing lambs can be caused by *S. aureus*, *D. congolensis* and photosensitization. *S. aureus* infection of the skin of the head typically causes oedematous and painful eyelids and adjacent skin with rapid hair loss (periorbital eczema). *D. congolensis* infection of haired skin typically results in multiple, small superficial pustules but rarely causes significant skin lesions except in debilitated lambs.

Sheep pox should also be included in the differential diagnoses in countries where this infection is endemic.

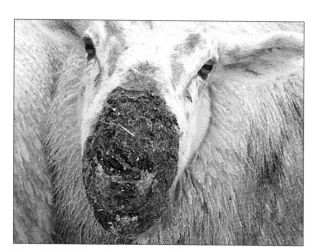

Fig. 11.6 **CPD virus and *Staphylococcus aureus* may act synergistically to cause severe facial dermatitis.**

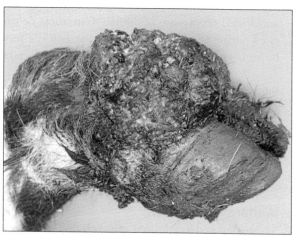

Fig. 11.7 **CPD virus and *Dermatophilus congolensis* may act synergistically to produce large granulomatous masses referred to as 'strawberry footrot'.**

Diagnosis

The diagnosis is based upon finding large proliferative lesions around the lips and nostrils of growing lambs. Virus can be demonstrated by direct electron microscopy of fresh lesions.

Treatment

Treatment is largely unsuccessful except for lambs with superficial secondary bacterial infection of scabs and associated oedema, which show a good response to intramuscular procaine penicillin injections for 5–7 consecutive days.

There is some evidence that levamisole (2.5 mg/kg injected subcutaneously every 3–4 days) speeds up remission of lesions.

Management/prevention/control measures

Disease is introduced into a flock by carrier sheep with no obvious skin lesions. Infection can remain viable in dry scab material in buildings for many months and is the likely reason for persistence of infection from year to year on the same premises. Thorough cleaning and disinfection of lambing accommodation may, therefore, help to break the usual annual appearance of disease.

Control following scarification with a live vaccine proves difficult to quantify but is routinely undertaken in many flocks in the UK. Vaccine must never be used in a clean flock. Vaccination is by scarification of the inner thigh in lambs and the axillary region in ewes. The timing of vaccination is approximately 6 weeks before the anticipated occurrence of disease. Care must be exercised during handling the live vaccine as it is affected by high temperatures and inactivated by disinfectants.

Economics

CPD is a significant problem in orphan lambs and other ill-thriven lambs. CPD is rarely a major problem in well-fed, well-thriven stock. The cost of vaccination is around 20 pence per dose but is time-consuming and there is the risk of accidental human infection.

Welfare implications

Severe oral and foot lesions cause obvious discomfort and are associated with weight loss and poor body condition. Every effort should be undertaken to rear orphan lambs using automated feeders.

DERMATOPHILOSIS

(syn. lumpy wool, mycotic dermatitis, rain scald)

Definition/overview

Dermatophilosis is a common skin infection of sheep worldwide. Dermatophilosis is of minor significance in the UK but is a major concern in sheep economies that rely upon fine wool production.

Aetiology

The disease is caused by *Dermatophilus congolensis*. Transmission of infection requires wet conditions and close contact (e.g. during gathering). Prolonged moist skin allows penetration of the bacterium and establishment of infection. It is reported that under certain circumstances infection can cause a severe suppurative inflammation of the skin.

Clinical presentation

In the UK dermatophilosis is encountered along the dorsum in short-wool breeds such as the Suffolk and Border Leicester, where it causes serum exudation and scab formation at the base of the wool fibres, which then slowly grows out. Dermatophilosis is usually encountered in summers when there has been prolonged wet weather after shearing. The lesions rarely develop clinical significance, being restricted to a small number of well-circumscribed scabs up to 5 cm in diameter, which eventually lift off exposing superficial skin infection. Such damaged skin regrows pigmented wool, which appears unsightly in sale rams. Occasionally, such scabs attract blowfly strike. Discrete 3–5 mm diameter 'bottle-brush' lesions are often found around the muzzle (**Fig. 11.8**), the bridge of the nose and on the margins of the ears (**Fig. 11.9**) of poorly-conditioned sheep but they are of no clinical significance, being more an indication of debility rather than the cause.

In New Zealand it is reported that young lambs may suffer extensive skin lesions of dermatophilosis with loss of fleece protection, which may result in death during adverse weather. In addition, lumpy wool lesions attract blowflies leading to cutaneous myiasis. Such severe infections are rarely encountered in the UK. In Australia lumpy wool causes shearing difficulties and downgrading of fine wool.

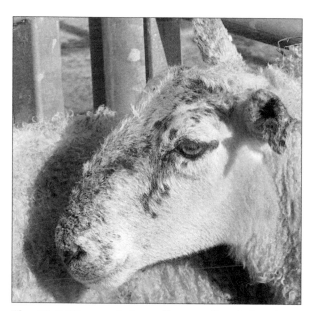

Fig. 11.8 Discrete 3–5 mm diameter 'bottle-brush' lesions of dermatophilosis are often found around the muzzle and along the bridge of the nose.

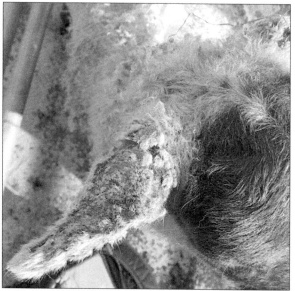

Fig. 11.9 Discrete 3–5 mm diameter 'bottle-brush' lesions of dermatophilosis are often found on the margin of the ears.

Differential diagnoses

Dermatophilosis lesions along the dorsum are readily differentiated from psoroptic mange on clinical examination. Dermatophilosis lesions on the face and muzzle should be distinguished from ringworm.

Diagnosis

The diagnosis of dermatophilosis is based upon clinical examination and, if necessary, stained smears from the underside of scabs plucked from the fleece, which reveal coccoid bacteria.

Treatment

Treatment is rarely indicated in the UK but rams intended for sale are sometimes treated to prevent skin lesions regrowing black wool, which is considered a cosmetic defect at sale. Procaine penicillin injected intramuscularly for 3 consecutive days effects a cure but it may take several weeks for the scabs to be shed from the growing fleece.

Management/prevention/control measures

A variety of dip solutions has been used in New Zealand and Australia to prevent dermatophilosis following shearing, including 1% potassium aluminium sulphate spray or dip solution. Dermatophilosis is rarely a disease of well-fed sheep; severe disease occurs only in sheep debilitated from another cause.

Economics

Effective control strategies, including antibiotic therapy and sprays/dips, limit production losses in those countries producing fine wools. Dermatophilosis is not an economic concern in the UK.

Welfare implications

Dermatophilosis does not present welfare concerns in the UK unless secondary cutaneous myiasis occurs.

CASEOUS LYMPHADENITIS

Definition/overview

Caseous lymphadenitis (CLA) is a chronic contagious disease of sheep, goats and cattle with the incidence of disease increasing with age. The epidemiology of CLA varies between countries, from little within flock transmission in the UK to epizootic proportions in flocks in Australia and the USA.

Aetiology

CLA is caused by *Corynebacterium pseudotuberculosis*. Transmission occurs either directly between sheep during close confinement or indirectly via shearing equipment contaminated with fomites from sheep with lung lesions or discharging skin lesions. Shearing cuts are believed to be the major portal of entry, although it is reported that the organism can also penetrate intact skin. Fighting causing skin lesions to the head facilitates disease transmission between rams in the UK (**Fig. 11.10**). The prevalence of infection increases with age and in sheep under intensive management conditions.

Clinical presentation

The disease is characterized by suppurative necrotizing inflammation of superficial lymph nodes particularly the parotid, submandibular, popliteal, precrural and prescapular lymph nodes. This form of the disease is often referred to as the cutaneous or superficial form of CLA. Spread of infection to the mediastinal (**Fig. 11.11**) and bronchial lymph nodes and internal viscera, including lungs, spleen, kidneys and liver, constitutes the visceral or internal form of CLA. Sheep with the superficial form of CLA may show no clinical signs of illness unless enlargement of the abscess causes compression of the pharynx or larynx and impairs function.

In Australia shearing wounds lead to infection of the prescapular and precrural lymph nodes, with <1% of lesions affecting lymph nodes of the head region. Carcase lymph nodes may be 15 cm in diameter and are characterized by the lamellar ('onion-ring') appearance of affected lymph nodes containing yellow-green viscous pus, which may become inspissated with a toothpaste-like consistency. Conversely, CLA in the UK is characterized by abscessation of the parotid (**Fig. 11.10**) and submandibular lymph nodes.

The visceral form of CLA is commonly associated with the 'thin ewe syndrome' with lesions in the lungs, mediastinum, liver and kidneys. Less common sites are the vertebral column, udder and scrotum. Large lung and mediastinal lesions may result in dyspnoea and this form of the disease is common in the USA, where affected sheep are referred to as 'lungers'. Spread of infection to cause significant visceral lesions is rare in the UK.

Differential diagnoses

Flock history may be important in forming a provisional diagnosis. The characteristic location of superficial lesions within drainage lymph nodes differentiates CLA infection from abscesses and cellulitis lesions. Skin tumours and lymphosarcoma are rare in sheep.

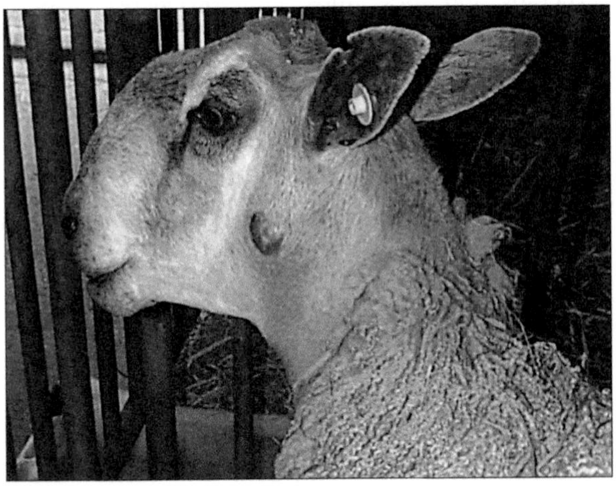

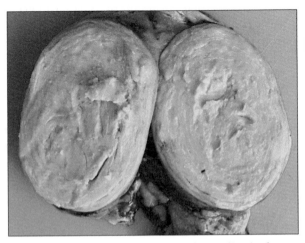

Fig. 11.10 Fighting causing skin lesions to the head facilitates caseous lymphadenitis (CLA) transmission between rams causing infection of the drainage parotid lymph nodes.

Fig. 11.11 Spread of infection to the mediastinal lymph nodes constitutes the visceral or internal form of CLA.

Definitive diagnosis of the cutaneous form of CLA is based on careful clinical examination of suspected cases and culture of *C. pseudotuberculosis* from discharging lymph nodes. The differential diagnoses list should also include actinobacillosis and tuberculosis.

Common differential diagnoses for the visceral form of CLA affecting the chest include chronic suppurative pneumonia, pleural or mediastinal abscesses and ovine pulmonary adenocarcinoma (OPA).

In more general terms, common causes of chronic weight loss in adult sheep include restricted nutrition, poor dentition, chronic parasitism, paratuberculosis, visna-maedi virus infection, chronic suppurative processes and tumours of the gastrointestinal tract.

Diagnosis

CLA lesions in the liver and superficial lesions involving the visceral pleura may be imaged using ultrasonography, and within the lung and mediastinum by radiography. Liver-specific enzymes will only identify the occurrence of a hepatic insult, not the cause, and may not be significantly elevated in cases of liver abscessation. Samples for bacteriology can be collected at necropsy from suspicious lesions.

There is a humoral response to the *C. pseudotuberculosis* exotoxin and this forms the basis for serological testing. A seropositive result indicates exposure to the exotoxin and may indicate active infection; however, severely debilitated animals may yield a false-negative result (low sensitivity). Vaccinated animals will be seropositive and this may lead to an erroneous conclusion, especially in purchased sheep with an undeclared vaccination history.

The diagnosis is confirmed at necropsy with culture of *C. pseudotuberculosis*.

Treatment

Despite the sensitivity of *C. pseudotuberculosis* to a number of antibiotics *in vitro*, therapy is unsuccessful due to the intracellular site of the bacteria and the fibrous capsule surrounding the lesions. Lancing lesions only results in contamination of the environment, increasing the potential for disease spread. Abscesses frequently recur after drainage and lavage with antiseptics.

Management/prevention/control measures

Disease prevention in clean flocks can be maintained by effective biosecurity measures. In such programmes the role of shearing equipment and handling facilities (e.g. mobile plunge dippers and feeders) as vectors for disease must be carefully considered. However, disease risks are highest from purchased animals, which must be inspected before purchase and quarantined for at least 2 months. Replacement breeding stock must be purchased from disease-free flocks whenever possible. Alternatively, unvaccinated sheep should be purchased and serological testing undertaken before admission of seronegative stock to the flock.

In endemically infected flocks the control programme must involve reducing exposure to contaminated fomites, culling sheep with unexplained weight loss and vaccination. Young animals should be raised separately from older infected animals. Shearing equipment, particularly the combs and blades, must be regularly disinfected, especially after contact with a discharging lesion. Sheep should be shorn in age groups, youngest first, and those with skin lesions must be shorn last. Skin wounds inflicted during shearing should be treated with topical iodine spray. Shower dipping for ectoparasite control and keeping sheep under cover for 1 hour or more after shearing increased the likelihood of high CLA incidence in Western Australia flocks.

Commercial vaccines have reduced the incidence of CLA within a flock but do not prevent all new infections nor cure sheep already infected. Commercial vaccines are used in many countries with a high CLA prevalence, such as the USA and Australia, but they are not used in many countries within Europe. All commercial vaccines contain the phospholipase D (PLD) toxoid and some also contain killed whole bacterial cells. Clostridial antigens may also be included in the vaccine. Care must be exercised not to challenge heavily pregnant sheep with too many vaccine antigens at the same time, as reduced feed intake may precipitate ovine pregnancy toxaemia.

Eradication of CLA is difficult and involves culling all infected sheep from vaccinated flocks. Thereafter, once clinical disease is at a low level, vaccination can be stopped and unvaccinated seropositive animals removed. In unvaccinated flocks all seropositive animals must be culled and testing repeated until disease is eliminated.

Economics

Economic losses arise from poor performance, including reduced milk and wool production, weight loss, carcase condemnation and restricted trade.

Welfare implications

The superficial form of CLA may increase the risk of cutaneous myiasis. The visceral form of disease can result in debility and emaciated sheep should be destroyed for welfare reasons during routine flock inspections.

PHOTOSENSITIZATION

(syn. yellowses, plochteach, alveld, facial eczema)

Definition/overview

Photosensitization occurs sporadically in countries worldwide but severe outbreaks are occasionally reported in southern hemisphere countries and in Norway. Typically, lambs 2–6 months old are affected during the summer months. In New Zealand and areas of Australia and South Africa, facial eczema is one of the most important diseases of sheep.

Aetiology

In sheep, photosensitization occurs either as a primary condition or secondary to hepatotoxic damage resulting in retention of the photosensitizing agent phylloerythrin.

Primary photosensitization follows ingestion of photodynamic agents (e.g. hypericin from St. John's Wort [*Hypericum perforatum*]). In Norway ingestion of bog asphodel (*Narthecium ossifragum*) is reported to cause photosensitization in large numbers of lambs.

In New Zealand facial eczema is caused by ingestion of the toxin sporidesmin, which is produced by the saprophytic fungus *Pithomyces chartarum*, which proliferates in vegetation during the autumn months. Sporidesmin is absorbed and accumulates in the liver and bile where metabolic changes result in the release of free radicals, with consequent damage to the biliary tree and reduced excretion of phylloerythrin. The clinical signs depend on the amount of sporidesmin ingested and the amount and intensity of direct sunlight.

Clinical presentation

Typical cases of ovine photosensitization occur in white-faced breeds (**Fig. 11.12**). Initially, affected animals are dull and attempt to seek shade. Lambs are often separated from their dam. The ears in particular are affected and become swollen, oedematous and droopy. The face, eyelids, lips and lower limbs may also become oedematous (**Fig. 11.13**). The vulva

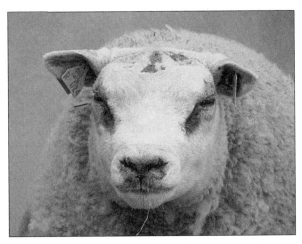

Fig. 11.12 Photosensitization typically occurs in predominantly white-faced breeds.

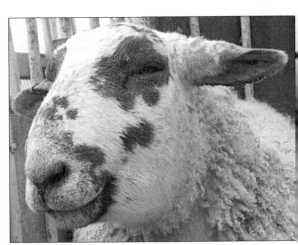

Fig. 11.13 Photosensitization causes oedema of the ears, face, eyelids and lips.

may be affected in those sheep where unnecessarily short tail docking is still practised. There is frequent head shaking and there is often self trauma to the head by rubbing against fence posts or kicking at the head. Affected skin oozes serum, with development of superficial secondary bacterial infection in some cases. Necrosis of the ear tips may develop within a few days which gives them a 'curled-up' appearance. There is loss of hair over the affected skin areas within 7–10 days (**Fig. 11.14** was taken 7 days after **Fig. 11.12**).

The response to protection from sunlight and corticosteroid and antibiotic therapy is generally good.

In New Zealand it is reported that recovered sheep may develop cirrhosis which may not be evident clinically until periods of increased metabolic demand such as late gestation.

Differential diagnoses
- Bighead.
- Cellulitis (e.g. from dog bite).
- Submandibular oedema associated with many protein-losing conditions including haemonchosis and fasciolosis and, much less commonly, paratuberculosis.

Diagnosis
Diagnosis is based upon the clinical signs and exposure to plants known to cause primary or hepatogenous photosensitization. In secondary photosensitization enzyme concentrations indicating both acute (aspartate transaminase, AST) and chronic (gamma-glutamyl transferase, GGT) hepatocellular damage are elevated.

Treatment
Affected sheep must be removed from pasture and confined in dark buildings to prevent further exposure to sunlight. Corticosteroids are helpful during the early stages to reduce the associated oedema. Other symptomatic treatments include topical antibiotic powders and fly control preparations.

Management/prevention/control measures
Primary photosensitization occurs sporadically and the cause is often not determined. It would be prudent to avoid those pastures where outbreaks of photosensitization have occurred in previous years.

There is considerable variation in breed susceptibility to photosensitization, and in New Zealand the individual variation within a breed is used to commercial advantage in breeding programmes. Growth of *P. chartarum* in New Zealand has well-recognized weather influences, and spore counting on pasture is employed to recognize high-risk grazings. Challenge with small doses of sporedesmin, combined with monitoring serum GGT concentration, has been used to identify more resistant rams.

Economics
Facial eczema is a major commercial concern in New Zealand. Economic loss from sporadic cases is very low in northern Europe.

Welfare implications
Affected sheep must be housed and given symptomatic treatment as necessary.

PERIORBITAL ECZEMA

Definition/overview
Periorbital eczema is a common skin condition in the UK, often resulting when sheep have too little space allowance at feed troughs. The cornea is unaffected.

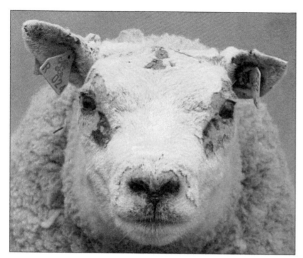

Fig. 11.14 The hair overlying the photosensitization areas is lost; the ears are sloughed in severe cases.

Aetiology

Trauma to skin allows entry of *Staphylococcus aureus*, which causes severe local infection.

Clinical presentation

Affected sheep have markedly swollen eyelids, which may close the palpebral fissure and effectively block vision. The eyelids are oedematous and painful. Ewes with both eyes affected are blind, wander aimlessly and frequently become caught in fences. Sheep with healing lesions have sharply-demarcated hair loss extending for 2–3 cm around the eyes.

Differential diagnoses

- Photosensitization.
- Infectious keratoconjunctivitis (pink eye).
- Anterior uveitis.

Diagnosis

Diagnosis is based upon the clinical signs and rapid response to antibiotic therapy.

Treatment

Suprisingly, a single intramuscular injection of procaine penicillin affects a rapid response within 24 hours. Ewes with impaired vision in both eyes should be housed to ensure adequate feeding and prevent death by misadventure.

Management/prevention/control measures

Periorbital eczema can be prevented by appropriate space requirements at the troughs (450 mm per sheep). An alternative regimen involves feeding the grain ration as cobs on a clean area of pasture using a 'snacker'.

Economics

Periorbital eczema is not a major economic concern to the sheep industry unless blindness leads to losses from misadventure or increased susceptibility to ovine pregnancy toxaemia because of reduced feeding patterns.

Welfare implications

The condition is obviously painful and must be treated promptly.

CUTANEOUS MYIASIS

(syn. fly strike, blowfly)

Definition/overview

Cutaneous myiasis lesions may range from centimetre diameter areas of skin hyperaemia with a small number of maggots (**Fig. 11.15**) to extensive areas of traumatized/devitalized skin causing death of the sheep (**Figs 11.16, 11.17**). Cutaneous myiasis causes major economic losses worldwide and is a serious welfare concern.

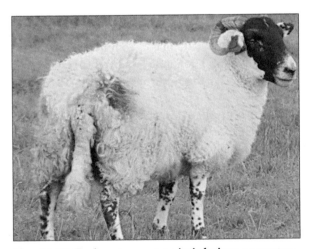

Fig. 11.15 Early cutaneous myiasis lesions present as small areas of discolored wool around the perineum provoking frequent nibbling by the sheep.

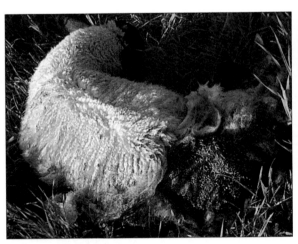

Fig. 11.16 Neglected case of cutaneous myiasis where extensive areas of traumatized/devitalized skin may cause death of the sheep.

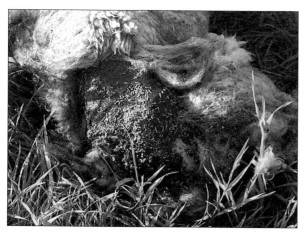

Fig. 11.17 The extensive areas of traumatized/ devitalized skin cause toxaemia and possibly death of the sheep.

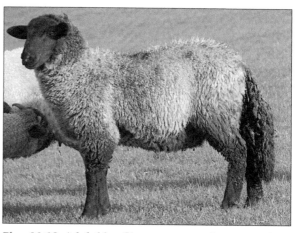

Fig. 11.18 Adult blowflies are attracted to areas of faecal staining surrounding the perineum.

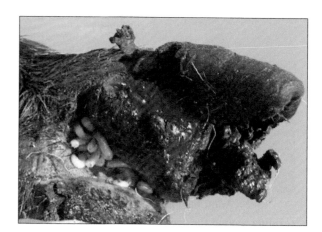

Fig. 11.19 Adult blowflies are attracted to footrot lesions with exposed corium/exuberant granulation tissue.

Aetiology

Cutaneous myiasis is caused by the larval stages of Dipteran flies. In the UK three species parasitize sheep: *Lucilia sericata*, which is the most important, *Phormia terraenovae* and *Calliphora erythrocephala*. The obligate blowfly *L. sericata* is the important species in southern hemisphere countries. Eggs are deposited on soiled areas of the fleece or adjacent to traumatized skin. The larvae attack the skin surface with a combination of anterior hooks and proteolytic enzymes.

Clinical presentation

Fly strike more commonly affects growing lambs but on occasion ewes and rams can be infested. Fly strike is most common during hot humid weather with little wind. The severity of cutaneous myiasis depends upon numerous factors including flock husbandry, the degree of supervision and diligence of the shepherd. Lesions may range from centimetre diameter areas of skin hyperaemia with a small number of maggots when detected during the first days of infestation, to extensive areas of traumatized/ devitalized skin covering up to one-third of the skin area and causing death of the sheep.

Adult flies are attracted to areas of faecal staining surrounding the perineum (**Fig. 11.18**) and, less commonly, footrot lesions with exposed corium/exuberant granulation tissue (**Fig. 11.19**), dermatophilosis lesions on the skin (**Fig. 11.20**) and urine scalding around the prepuce (**Fig. 11.21**). Granulating wounds in growing lambs caused by rubber ring castration and tail docking

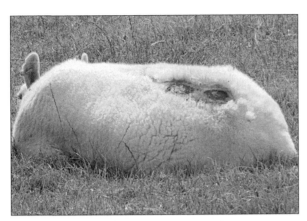

Fig. 11.20 Adult blowflies are attracted to dermatophilosis lesions on the skin.

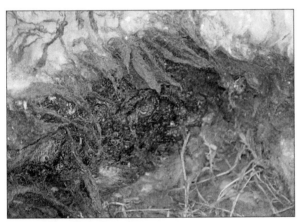

Fig. 11.21 Adult blowflies are attracted to urine scalding around the prepuce.

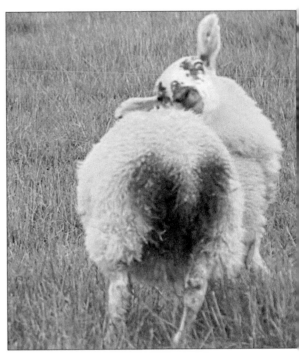

Fig. 11.22 During the early stages of cutaneous myiasis affected sheep frequently turn their head and attempt to nibble at the affected area.

also attract blowflies. Occasionally, head wounds in rams acquired during fighting become infested with maggots. Frequent head shaking and lowered head carriage is common in the latter situation.

During the early stages affected sheep frequently turn their head and attempt to nibble at the affected area, usually the tail head (**Fig. 11.22**). Grazing behaviour is disrupted as sheep nibble at pasture for 5–10 seconds then suddenly trot away with frequent tail swishing before recommencing grazing. This cycle of abnormal behaviour is repeated many times. The fleece surrounding the lesion becomes wet and discoloured. As the infestation progresses the sheep may rub against fences and hedges, causing a ragged appearance with fleece loss.

In severe infestations the sheep are depressed, do not graze and become isolated from the flock (**Fig. 11.23**). Large numbers of adult flies are seen on the fleece with maggots on the blackened skin once the surrounding fleece has been lifted clear. There is an associated putrid smell. Clinical examination reveals toxic mucous membranes and dehydration. Severely affected sheep have a drawn-up appearance due to poor rumen fill, and have lost considerable condition. Death soon follows in such severely affected sheep (**Fig. 11.24**). Recovered skin lesions grow black wool (**Fig. 11.25**).

Differential diagnoses
Clinical inspection eliminates other possible diagnoses.

Diagnosis
The diagnosis is confirmed by gathering and close inspection of the skin.

Treatment
Affected sheep can be treated by plunge dipping using a synthetic pyrethroid or organophosphate

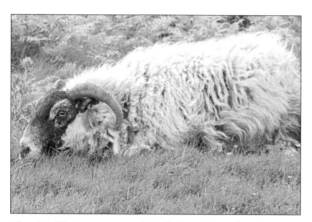

Fig. 11.23 In severe myiasis infestations the sheep are depressed, do not graze and become isolated from the flock.

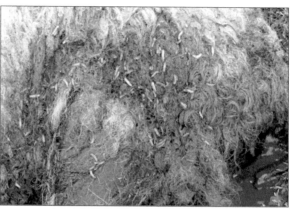

Fig. 11.24 Damage to the skin caused by the feeding patterns of the maggots allows absorption of toxins and ammonia which may cause death in neglected cases.

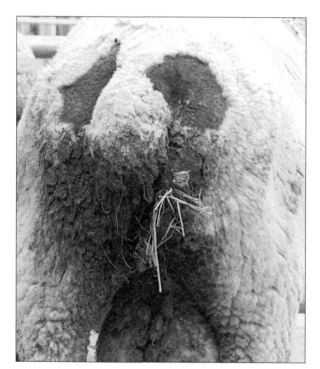

Fig. 11.26 Sheep suffering from cutaneous myiasis can be treated by plunge dipping.

Fig. 11.25 Healed cutaneous myiasis lesions grow black wool.

preparation (**Fig. 11.26**), but it is more usual to treat infested sheep with dip wash applied directly to the struck area after first clipping away overlying wool. Antibiotics and a non-steroidal anti-inflammatory drug (NSAID) are indicated in more severely affected individual sheep, which must be housed to prevent irritation by headflies.

Management/prevention/control measures

Before preventive measures using various chemicals are considered, much can be done to reduce the attraction of blowflies. In the UK a grazing programme to prevent the massive build-up of infective helminth larvae on permanent pasture during July and August (mid-summer rise) reduces diarrhoea caused by high parasite burdens. In sheep flocks in the UK it should be possible to turn weaned lambs on to silage or hay aftermaths to reduce further such larval challenge and diarrhoea during the fly season.

In the absence of a clean grazing system, control of parasitic gastroenteritis relies on targeted anthelmintic treatments, which should be part of the veterinary-supervised flock health programme. Where faecal staining of the perineum occurs, this wool must be removed ('dagging' or 'crutching' [**Figs. 11.27, 11.28**]).

In adult sheep prompt removal of the fleece and any faecal contamination by shearing during late May/June in the UK (**Fig. 11.29**) removes this attraction well before the peak of the blowfly season.

All sheep carcases must be disposed of immediately as they provide a site for rapid fly multiplication (**Fig. 11.30**); this is a legal requirement in many countries.

Human health concerns and environmental controls have reduced the use of organophosphorus dips, which provide good protection against blowfly strike for up to 6 weeks. Dimpylate (diazinon) and propetamphos are effective against blowfly strike and the data sheet instructions must be read carefully

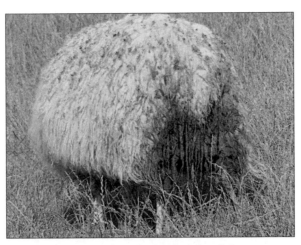

Fig. 11.27 Perineal wool with faecal staining must be removed using shears to reduce the attraction for blowflies.

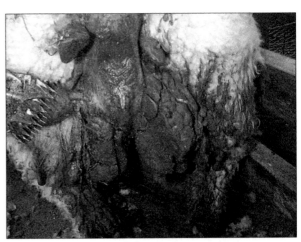

Fig. 11.28 Removal of faeces from the perineum and tail using shears helps prevent cutaneous myiasis.

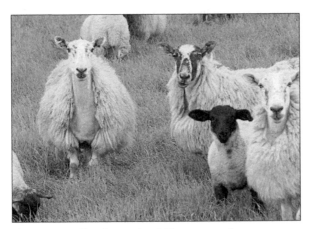

Fig. 11.29 The fleece should be removed as soon as possible to reduce the risk of blowfly strike.

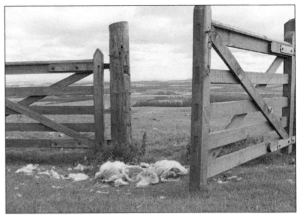

Fig. 11.30 All sheep carcases must be disposed of immediately as they provide a site for rapid fly multiplication.

before use, with particular attention paid to the protection of operators. In some countries proficiency tests with proof of competence are necessary before farmers can use organophosphate dips. These compounds are strongly lipophilic and replenishment of dips is important to maintain effective concentrations within the bath. The synthetic pyrethroids, including high-cis cypermethrin, have a much higher human safety margin than the organophosphorus compounds and persist in the fleece for up to 8 weeks.

While plunge dips are commonly used in the UK, shower dips are more popular in New Zealand. Specific recommendations for shower times in relation to the interval since shearing must be followed. Jetting wands can be used as an alternative to plunge or shower dipping to apply dip wash to the target areas. The wand is combed through the fleece applying the correct volume of dip wash at skin level. The advantages of jetting wands are that they apply clean dip wash to the target areas and use less concentrate dip, therefore reducing costs, but the process is time-consuming and hard work.

While topical application of high-cis cypermethrin pour-on preparations provides protection against fly strike, these preparations persist for only 6–8 weeks and require reapplication in most situations. Cyromazine applied before the risk period is effective against blowfly strike for up to 10 weeks after topical application. Dicyclanil affords 16 weeks' full body protection against cutaneous myiasis. Dicyclanil acts specifically on larvae, interfering with moulting and pupation and therefore preventing larval development. No resistance has been reported to these insect growth regulators, which are very safe; however, they are considerably more expensive than other control measures and this may limit their use. Meat withholding times may limit their application in some lamb production systems.

Flytraps have been developed in Australia but have limited application in Europe.

Economics

Cutaneous myiasis is a major economic concern worldwide with considerable prevention and treatment costs. Pour-on products containing high-cis cypermethrin to prevent blowfly strike typically cost 25–50 pence for growing lambs and adult sheep, respectively. Insect growth regulators are approximately twice the cost of these pour-on products.

Welfare implications

Cutaneous myiasis is a serious welfare concern and all husbandry and chemical control measures must be taken.

HEADFLY

Definition/overview

In the UK, headfly can present a major problem during the summer months, particularly in horned sheep (**Fig. 11.31**) grazed near woodland.

Aetiology

The muscid fly *Hydrotea irritans* causes considerable irritation by feeding around the horn base, which may result in self-trauma by the sheep. Flies may also feed on lachrymal secretions.

Clinical presentation

Grazing patterns are disturbed (**Figs 11.32, 11.33**) and affected sheep often isolate themselves and

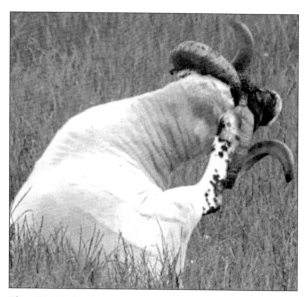

Fig. 11.31 In the UK headfly can present a major problem during the summer months, particularly in horned sheep.

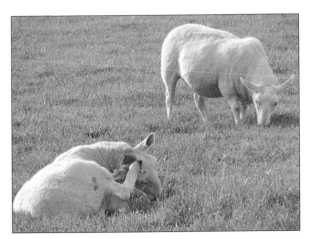

Fig. 11.32 Disturbed grazing due to headflies causes rapid loss of body condition (see Fig. 11.33).

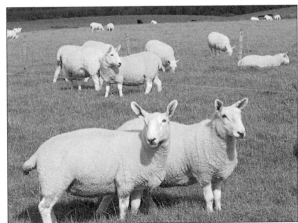

Fig. 11.33 Sheep with headfly lesions are not grazing in this group.

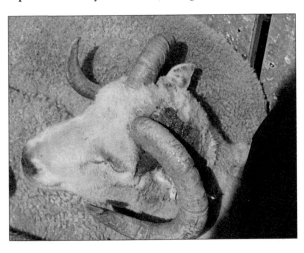

Fig. 11.34 Kicking at the head can greatly exacerbate damage caused by headflies to the horn base.

remain in shade where available. They may stand with the head held lowered with frequent head shaking and ear movements. Alternatively, sheep adopt a submissive posture in sternal recumbency with the neck extended and the head held on the ground. Kicking at the head often greatly exacerbates damage caused by headflies to the horn base (**Fig. 11.34**), and such action may also traumatize the skin of the neck and ears. Head rubbing also causes considerable self-trauma. Bleeding and serum exudation attracts other flies and aggravates the problem. There is rapid loss of body condition in severely affected sheep.

Differential diagnoses

Inspection confirms the cause of the skin trauma around the horn base and head.

Diagnosis

The diagnosis is confirmed by gathering the sheep and close inspection of the skin.

Treatment

Housing is essential for sheep with large skin lesions to allow time for complete healing. Parenteral antibiotic administration may be indicated if there is localized infection but this is unusual. Topical emollients and antibiotic preparations are not usually necessary and skin wounds heal well provided that flies are denied access to these areas, which is best achieved by housing.

Management/prevention/control measures

Control of headfly proves more difficult once a lesion is present on the head; prevention is much more important than cure. Pour-on fly control preparations, such as high-cis cypermethrin or deltamethrin, must be applied before the anticipated headfly season and especially to horned sheep. Such treatments should be repeated every 3–4 weeks during the fly season or as directed by the data sheet instructions.

Economics

Lesions resulting from headfly activity in mid-summer cause sheep great distress and result in considerable weight loss and poor lactation, with consequent poor lamb weaning weights. Disruption to grazing continuing throughout the late summer leads to poor condition of lambs at sale and ewes at the prebreeding check, which may result in premature culling.

Pour-on products to prevent headfly strike typically cost 25–50 pence for growing lambs and adult sheep, respectively.

Welfare implications

Headfly lesions present a serious welfare issue because they cause great distress to affected sheep (**Figs 11.31–11.35**). Lesions may become large because horned hill breeds often graze extensive pastures and are infrequently shepherded. It is essential that horned sheep, especially lambs, are handled correctly and never caught by the horns. Damage or loss of a horn during handling readily attracts headflies causing a major problem from self-inflicted trauma.

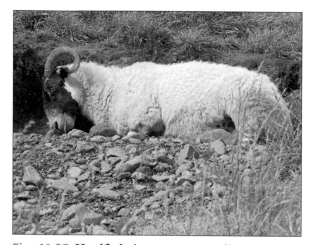

Fig. 11.35 Headfly lesions cause great distress and are a major welfare concern of affected sheep.

LICE

Definition/overview

Infestations with lice probably affect all sheep-producing countries but cause production concerns only in Australia and New Zealand, where the body louse *Bovicola ovis* reduces fleece quality. Louse populations are highest in sheep in poor body condition kept in unhygienic conditions rather than the reverse situation where lice cause debility. Recent evidence suggests that moderate louse infestations may not cause significant production loss in the UK.

Aetiology

Three species of louse infest sheep: the chewing louse *Bovicola ovis*, and the blood sucking lice *Linognathus ovillus* and *Linognathus pedalis*. Infestation with *B. ovis* may cause disrupted feeding patterns, fleece damage/loss and self-inflicted trauma. Spread occurs by close contact more quickly in hot climates than in temperate climates, with increases in population size during cooler weather. The entire life cycle, comprising egg, three nymph stages and adults, is spent on the sheep. The slow reproductive capacity of *B. ovis* results in a gradual build-up of louse numbers over several months. Shearing removes many lice and exposes the remaining population to desiccation, with rain further reducing numbers.

Clinical presentation

Many louse infestations are asymptomatic but heavy infestations during cooler weather cause irritation, leading to rubbing against fences (**Fig. 11.36**) and fleece damage (**Fig. 11.37**). Sheep may nibble at their fleece overlying the dorsal midline and flanks causing wool plucks (**Fig. 11.38**). Lice congregate in colonies on the fleece; therefore, a minimum of 10 to 20 fleece partings to a depth of 10 cm should be examined per sheep, with a minimum of 10 sheep examined per group. An average count of more than five lice per fleece parting is generally considered a heavy infestation with *B. ovis*.

Differential diagnoses

The important differential diagnosis for flock problems of pruritus and fleece loss is psoroptic mange (sheep scab). Other differential diagnoses include cutaneous myiasis and scrapie in individual sheep.

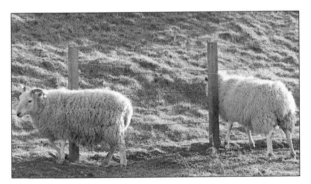

Fig. 11.36 Heavy louse infestations during cooler weather months cause irritation leading to rubbing against fences.

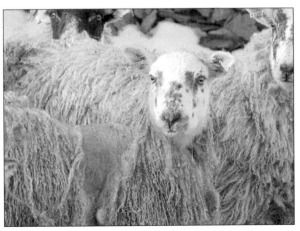

Fig. 11.37 Fleece damage results from heavy louse infestation.

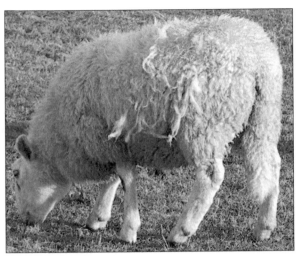

Fig. 11.38 Sheep with heavy louse infestations often nibble at their fleece overlying the dorsal midline and flanks, causing wool plucks.

Diagnosis

Careful inspection of the fleece using a magnifying glass will identify significant *B. ovis* populations. Further investigation involves microscopic examination of fleece samples.

Treatment

Infested sheep can be readily treated by plunge dipping in a synthetic pyrethroid or organophosphate preparation. Use of plunge dipping for other reasons, such as control of sheep scab, cutaneous myiasis and headfly problems, also effectively eliminates any louse infestation.

Management/prevention/control measures

Reliance on systemic endectocides rather than plunge dipping to control sheep scab has resulted in a huge upsurge of louse infestations in sheep flocks in the UK. Maintenance of a closed flock and effective biosecurity measures will prevent introduction of louse infestations.

Use of plunge dipping for the control of sheep scab and other skin infestations will eliminate louse infestations. Louse infestations can also be controlled by the topical application of high-cis cypermethrin or deltamethrin after shearing.

Economics

Louse infestations do not present a significant financial concern except in countries such as Australia, where wool rather than meat is the more significant ovine product.

Welfare implications

Heavy louse infestations cause irritation and disrupted grazing patterns and therefore warrant treatment for welfare reasons. The cause of any underlying debilitating condition/disease should be investigated and corrected.

SHEEP SCAB

(syn. psoroptic mange)

Definition/overview

Sheep scab is found in many sheep-producing areas of the world with the notable exceptions of North America, Australia and New Zealand, where the infestation was eradicated in the 1890s. If left untreated, infestations cause rapid loss of body condition, debility and possibly death in severe cases, although there appears to be considerable breed susceptibility.

Sheep scab was rarely seen in the UK until withdrawal of compulsory dipping in 1989. Thereafter, sheep scab became widespread affecting up to 10% of flocks, causing serious welfare concerns. Industry initiatives have proved largely unsuccessful in the UK and sheep scab was made a notifiable disease in Scotland in 2011 (Sheep Scab [Scotland] Amendment Order 2011).

Aetiology

Sheep scab is caused by *Psoroptes ovis*. Sheep scab mites can be transmitted by direct contact when sheep are gathered and held tightly together, such as during sales, or indirectly from contact with infested material on fence posts or vehicles used for animal transport.

Clinical presentation

In the UK disease is typically encountered during the autumn/winter months from September to April. During the early stages of infestation some sheep in the group have disturbed grazing patterns and are observed kicking at their flanks with their hind feet and/or rubbing themselves against fence posts (**Figs 11.39–11.41**), which leads to a dirty ragged appearance to the fleece and loss of wool. There is serum exudation, which gives the fleece overlying the skin lesions a moist yellow appearance (**Figs 11.42, 11.43**). Some infested sheep show few clinical signs.

The skin lesions are most commonly observed on the flanks and over the back of the sheep but may extend to involve the whole body in neglected cases (**Fig. 11.43**). As the condition progresses over several

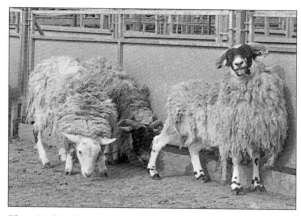

Fig. 11.39 Severe irritation caused by sheep scab.

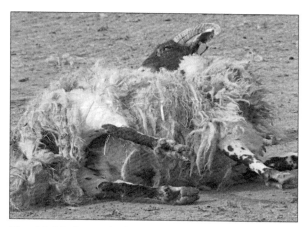

Fig. 11.40 Severe irritation caused by sheep scab with affected sheep nibbling at their fleece causing wool loss.

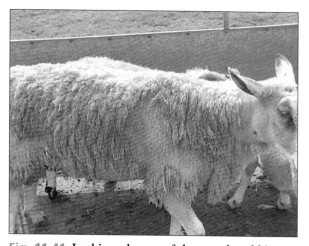

Fig. 11.41 In this early case of sheep scab, rubbing over the shoulder has caused damage to the fleece.

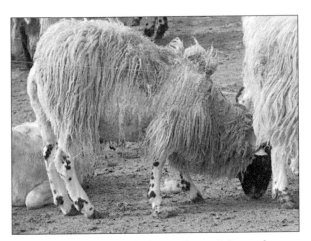

Fig. 11.42 Serum exudation at the periphery of the sheep scab lesion gives the fleece a moist yellow appearance.

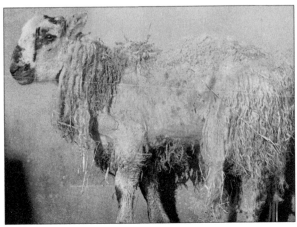

Fig. 11.43 After about 8 weeks' infestation there has been almost complete fleece loss with active infestation continuing at the periphery.

weeks the sheep appear increasingly uncomfortable and nibble at their flanks and rub themselves against the pen divisions with greater frequency, causing excoriation. Some ewes appear in considerable distress and kick at themselves with their hind feet. The fleece is wet, sticky, yellow and frequently contaminated with dirt from the hind feet. It may prove difficult to part the wool fibres overlying the lesions due to serum exudation, which has formed a thick layer within the fleece.

Typically after about 8 weeks' infestation the hair loss on the flanks may extend to 20 cm in diameter, surrounded by an area of hyperaemia and serum exudation at the periphery (**Fig. 11.43**). The skin is thrown into thickened corrugations in many advanced cases. There is often marked enlargement of the drainage lymph nodes, the prescapular lymph nodes being the easiest to palpate. By this stage, infested sheep have lost considerable body condition and are frequently emaciated; death may result in neglected sheep.

Cutaneous stimulation during handling procedures may precipitate seizure activity which lasts for 2–5 minutes before animals recover fully. This is particularly distressing for the sheep, which should be treated immediately with dexamethasone (see treatment below).

Eventually, once the whole body has been infested and fleece lost, there is no longer an active periphery of the lesion and the sheep may recover without treatment, although the healing process may only start some 4–6 months after initial infestation. The fleece begins to grow and mite isolations may be restricted to cryptic sites such as the external auditory canal, inguinal area and infraorbital fossae.

It is sometimes reported that aural haematomata are encountered in flocks with chronic sheep scab but these lesions have largely been attributed to reaction with *P. cuniculi* infestation.

Differential diagnoses
- Louse infestation.
- Keds.
- Severe dermatophilosis.
- Cutaneous myiasis.
- Severe photosensitization.
- Scrapie should be considered in individual sheep showing emaciation, seizure activity and fleece loss.

Diagnosis
Skin scrapings taken using a scalpel held at a right angle to the skin surface at the periphery of active lesions demonstrate large numbers of mites under ×100 magnification. Prior digestion in potassium hydroxide is not usually necessary. Liquid paraffin can first be applied to the skin to aid collection of the scrapings. Lice can be visualized on careful examination of the fleece/skin; however, both lice and sheep scab can infest the same sheep.

Treatment

Systemic endectocides: avermectins and milbemycins:
The avermectins, ivermectin and doramectin, and the milbemycins, including moxidectin, have a wide range of activity against immature and mature arthropods and nematode species when administered by injection. One injection of doramectin is effective against sheep scab mite infestation but two injections of ivermectin 1 week apart are needed for scab treatment. Two injections of moxidectin 1%, 10 days apart are needed for scab treatment.

Ivermectin provides no significant residual protection against reinfestation from a contaminated environment; therefore, it is essential that sheep are not returned to the same pastures/buildings for at least 17 days post treatment. Although doramectin and moxidectin do have residual action against reinfestation, it would be prudent to apply this rule to all systemic endectocide treatments. Subcutaneous injection of moxidectin 2% at the base of the ear provides 60 days' protection against sheep scab.

Plunge dips: Dips containing dimpylate (diazinon), flumethrin and propetamphos treat and prevent sheep scab, while dips containing high-cis cypermethrin are effective for treatment only if used a second time after 14 days. Treatment for sheep scab necessitates that sheep are immersed in the dip wash for 60 seconds with the head submerged twice. Sheep dipped in high-cis cypermethrin must not be returned to infested pastures after dipping because of the limited residual action against scab mites.

In addition to scab treatment, severely affected animals should be treated with dexamethasone injected intramuscularly in an attempt to reduce the anaphylactic reaction occasionally encountered in severely infested sheep.

Following treatment sheep may still appear distressed and nibble at their flanks for a couple of days. Thereafter, they appear more settled with no rubbing or scratching noted. Two weeks after treatment the skin appears normal and the fleeces less 'sticky'. Regrowth of the fleece is often apparent after 2–3 weeks, with black pigmentation in those areas where there had been considerable skin trauma.

Management/prevention/control measures

Effective ring fencing with proper treatment of all sheep moved onto the farm are essential measures to prevent introduction of sheep scab. Biosecurity is no less important for many other infections/infestations and an effective veterinary health programme is essential for all sheep farms.

In the UK the compulsory dipping regulations proved their worth for many years in the control of sheep scab. Their removal in 1989 demonstrated that some sectors of the sheep industry were not capable of implementing even the most rudimentary disease control measures.

There are individual reports of mite resistance to flumethrin and propetamphos in the UK, but no reports of avermectin or milbemycin resistance. Potential mite resistance problems only serve to emphasize the urgent need to eradicate this problem.

Economics

Sheep scab is a major economic concern in the UK and many other countries, despite the existence of a wide range of highly effective treatment and control strategies. Financial losses result from damage/loss of wool, poor growth, weight loss in significant infestations and possible death of neglected cases. Lambs born to ewes with significant scab lesions have lower birthweight and experience increased neonatal mortality.

Welfare implications

Sheep scab is one of the most important welfare concerns affecting the UK sheep industry. Infested sheep show obvious discomfort even with early infestations, leading to self excoriation/trauma when the condition remains neglected. Seizure activity, while temporary, is particularly distressing for the sheep. Damage to the fleece with eventual loss renders the sheep highly susceptible to adverse weather conditions until significant wool regrowth occurs.

IN-GROWING HORNS

In-growing horns can cause problems in some breeds (**Figs 11.44, 11.45**) and present as a common welfare issue in law courts. A conservative approach is sometimes adopted (**Fig. 11.46**) to avoid haemorrhage and possible sensitive areas nearer the horn base.

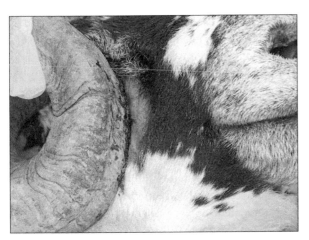

Fig. 11.44 In-growing horns in certain breeds can cause damage to the cheeks.

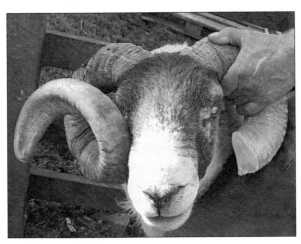

Fig. 11.45 Timely removal of the horn tip before damage to the cheek occurs; this action will prove necessary again in about 12 months.

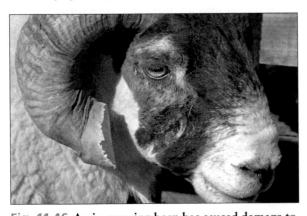

Fig. 11.46 An in-growing horn has caused damage to the cheek; a conservative approach was used as much more of the horn could have been removed.

SQUAMOUS CELL CARCINOMAS

Definition/overview

Ovine squamous cell carcinomas (SCCs) are reported commonly affecting 3–6-year-old sheep in many subtropical countries world-wide, especially Australia. These tumours are very uncommon in northern Europe.

Aetiology

SCCs occur following exposure of areas of epidermis to prolonged ultraviolet radiation. The frequency of these tumours increases at high altitudes.

Clinical presentation

Numerous tumours occur at one or more sites including the eyelids, the dorsal surface of the ears, the muzzle, and the musculo-cutaneous junctions of the vulva and anus and sites of Mules' operation (mutilation). The proliferative lesions are readily traumatized and become secondarily infected. Metastases to drainage lymph nodes do occur but can be difficult to appreciate during the clinical examination because bacterial infection of lesions will also increase local lymph nodes. Flystrike of lesions is very common.

Differential diagnoses

Ocular lesions should be differentiated from periorbital eczema. Lesions around the face/muzzle should be distinguished from cutaneous pustular dermatitis although the age prevalence differs significantly.

Diagnosis

The diagnosis is based on clinical examination and elimination of other common differential diagnoses. The epidemiology of ovine SCC will probably be well known on the farm.

Treatment

Treatment in the first instance is symptomatic, with antibiotic therapy to limit bacterial involvement and removal of maggots in fly strike lesions. Surgical removal is not an option for commercial value sheep which must be culled for welfare reasons.

Management/prevention/control measures

Provision of shade is not a practical option on extensive grazing systems. Ewes must have sufficient tail length to at least cover the vulva. There is no justification for Mules' operation (mutilation).

Economics

Culling of ewes with significant lesions will increase the replacement rate.

Welfare implications

Superficial bacterial infection of tumours will cause pain and discomfort but could be treated with antibiotics. Of greater concern is the risk of cutaneous myiasis. Culling of ewes with early tumour lesions should reduce the risk of such complications.

WOOL SLIP

Wool slip occurs sporadically in sheep (**Fig. 11.47**) and most commonly starts 2-4 weeks after recovery from ovine pregnancy toxaemia, infectious causes of abortion/metritis and other serious diseases. There is no inflammation of the skin and no pruritus (**Fig. 11.48**). Surprisingly, the sheep are typically in very good body condition at presentation (**Fig. 11.47**) despite recent serious illness. There is no treatment and the new fleece is normal in appearance, although there will be no requirement for shearing that year.

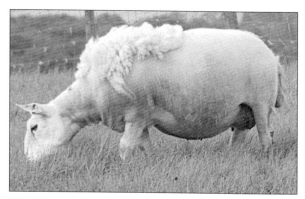

Fig. 11.47 Wool slip may occur 2–4 weeks after recovery from ovine pregnancy toxaemia or illness associated with abortion/metritis.

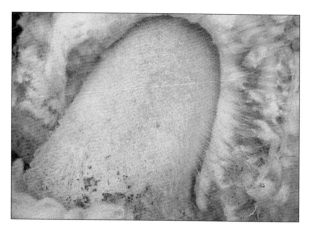

Fig. 11.48 Wool slip presents with no inflammation of the skin or pruritus.

OVINE INFECTIOUS KERATOCONJUNCTIVITIS

(syn. contagious ophthalmia, 'pink eye')

Definition/overview

In the UK, ovine infectious keratoconjunctivitis (IKC) is often associated with high winds and driving snow during the winter months, which gives rise to the colloquial term 'snow blindness' (**Figs 12.1, 12.2**). Large numbers of sheep can be affected during these weather conditions. Competition at feed troughs also increases the rate of spread of this infection. IKC is more commonly seen in adults, presumably because some of the risk factors, such as severe winter weather, do not apply to growing lambs during the summer months. IKC is seen in sheep worldwide.

Aetiology

Chlamydia psittaci and *Mycoplasma conjunctivae* are the only organisms that have been associated with the disease. While disease in the UK is associated with high winds and snow, in New Zealand IKC is associated with dust and indirect spread by flies. Surface trauma caused by feeding big bales may also be a risk factor in the UK (**Fig. 12.3**).

Clinical presentation

The condition can be either unilateral or bilateral. Most cases are selected for treatment on the basis of obvious epiphora with tear staining of the face (**Figs 12.4, 12.5**). On closer examination of the affected eye(s) there is marked conjunctivitis with injected tortuous scleral vessels and hyperaemic conjunctivae. There is marked photophobia with blepharospasm when sheep are exposed to bright sunlight (**Fig. 12.5**). More advanced cases show keratitis and, possibly, corneal ulceration, which is readily identified after application of fluorescein-impregnated strips to the surface of the eye. By this stage lymphoid hyperplasia gives the bulbar conjunctiva and third

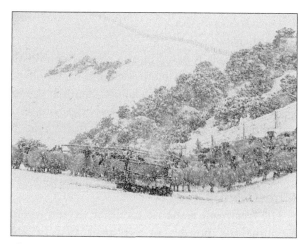

Fig. 12.1 In the UK ovine infectious keratoconjunctivitis (IKC) is associated with high winds and driving snow during the winter months.

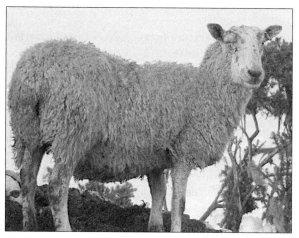

Fig. 12.2 IKC with blepharospasm and purulent ocular discharge affects the right eye after a snowstorm.

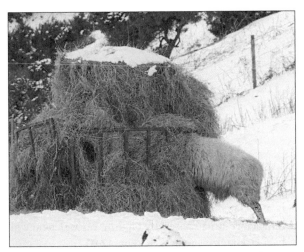

Fig. 12.3 Superficial trauma to the eye caused by feeding big bales may also be a risk factor for IKC.

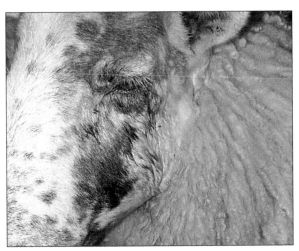

Fig. 12.4 Most sheep with IKC are selected for treatment on the basis of obvious epiphora with tear staining of the face.

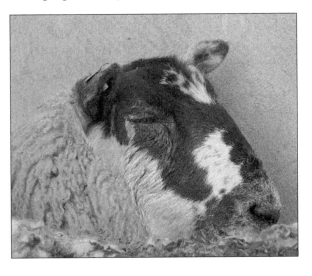

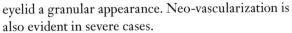

Fig. 12.5 Epiphora with tear staining of the face and blepharospasm affects this sheep.

eyelid a granular appearance. Neo-vascularization is also evident in severe cases.

Spontaneous recovery starts in most cases 3–5 days after clinical signs are first observed, and is complete 2 weeks later. In severe cases, ulceration may progress to rupture of the anterior chamber but this is uncommon.

Sheep may die from misadventure if the condition causes temporary blindness. During late pregnancy in multigravid ewes, pregnancy toxaemia may result as a consequence of blindness and inability to find sufficient food.

Differential diagnoses
Differential diagnoses include foreign bodies within the conjunctival sac, ovine iritis and periorbital eczema.

Diagnosis
The diagnosis is based on the clinical examination and response to antibiotic therapy. Bacteriological isolation is rarely undertaken. Conjunctival swabs should be taken from early clinical cases with serous not purulent ocular discharge, noting that the bacteria are fragile and transport media are required before sample despatch to the laboratory.

Treatment
The treatment response to either oxytetracycline ophthalmic powder or ointment is very good within 24 hours. A single intramuscular injection of long-acting oxytetracycline is economically justifiable and very effective in sheep, and

is the treatment method of choice. Twice daily topical antibiotic therapy is recommended but cannot always be accomplished under farm conditions because of other commitments on staff time. Subconjunctival antibiotic injection can be difficult to achieve in sheep because the conjunctivae are very inflamed and painful, and restraint is not easy with only one operator. This technique has no advantage over intramuscular injection except the lower unit cost because of the smaller antibiotic volume.

Blind sheep should be housed with ready access to food and water. Sheep must be approached carefully, to avoid panic and possible injury.

In severe outbreaks involving heavily pregnant ewes, metaphylactic injection of all at-risk sheep with a single intramuscular injection of long-acting oxytetracycline could be considered. Immunity following infection is poor, and lesions recur within weeks in many sheep.

Management/prevention/control measures

Provision of care can prove very time-consuming because sheep are often grazing large areas and may have strayed from the main group and are difficult to find in stormy weather conditions. While affected sheep should be housed with ready access to food and water, it may prove difficult to move these sheep from remote hill pastures. Provision of shelter from storms is good husbandry practice on hill pastures. Adequate trough space and feeding concentrates on the ground may help to limit spread of infection throughout a group.

Outbreaks of IKC may occur after the introduction of purchased stock; therefore, whenever possible, all new stock should be managed separately as one group away from the main flock.

Economics

Secondary losses may result from misadventure and pregnancy toxaemia.

Welfare implications

Temporary bilateral blindness must be very traumatic and sheep should be managed quietly indoors in small groups with ready access to food and water. Individual penning causes considerable distress to blind sheep as evidenced by their frequent vocalization. Pens should have solid walls as horned sheep may become entangled in wire fences.

ANTERIOR UVEITIS

(syn. ovine iritis)

Definition/overview

Anterior uveitis, also referred to as ovine iritis, probably follows conjunctival infection with *Listeria monocytogenes*. It occasionally occurs in sheep of all ages being fed on big-bale grass silage. There are no reports of sheep developing signs of meningoencephalitis following primary listerial infection of the anterior chamber of the eye.

Aetiology

Anterior uveitis probably follows conjunctival infection with *L. monocytogenes*.

Clinical presentation

The initial presenting signs are blepharospasm, photophobia, miosis and iridocyclitis, either unilaterally or bilaterally. The iris may be thrown into a series of radial folds extending from the ciliary border to the pupillary edge. Within 2–3 days more severe inflammatory changes develop, with bluish-white corneal opacity (**Figs 12.6, 12.7**) starting at the limbic border and spreading centripetally. Focal aggregations of fibrin accumulate in the anterior chamber attached to the inner surface of the cornea, and are seen as accumulations of white material beneath the cornea. Regression of ocular lesions takes 4–6 weeks without treatment.

Differential diagnoses

Differential diagnoses include foreign bodies within the conjunctival sac, keratoconjunctivitis and periorbital eczema.

Diagnosis

Diagnosis is based on clinical signs and history of silage feeding. The significance of isolation of *L. monocytogenes* from conjunctival swabs is equivocal.

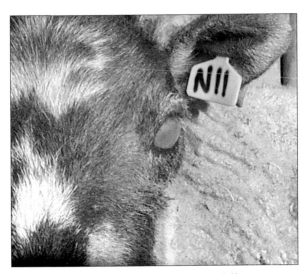

Fig. 12.6 Bluish-white corneal opacity follows anterior uveitis caused by *L. monocytogenes*.

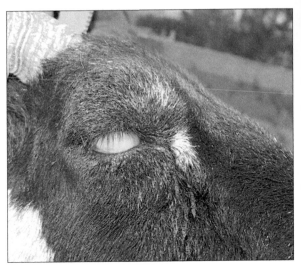

Fig. 12.7 Severe inflammatory changes have developed with bluish-white corneal opacity.

Treatment

There is a marked response to a combined sub-conjunctival injection of oxytetracycline and dexamethasone (1 mg). The dose of dexamethasone is not sufficient to effect abortion. Without treatment, regression of ocular lesions takes several weeks.

Management/prevention/control measures

It proves difficult to feed big-bale silage in another way to sheep. Attention to detail when baling and wrapping silage, and ensuring appropriate fermentation conditions, should limit contamination with *L. monocytogenes*. However, exposure to air for many days before the large bale is eventually eaten provides an ideal environment for *L. monocytogenes* multiplication.

Economics

Anterior uveitis is not a major concern as ocular lesions regress spontaneously over several weeks. As a consequence, many farmers elect not to treat sheep with anterior uveitis.

Welfare implications

While ocular lesions do regress spontaneously over some weeks, there is a dramatic response to combined subconjunctival injection of oxytetracycline and dexamethasone.

ENTROPION

Definition/overview

Entropion is a very common hereditary problem of certain breeds and their cross-bred progeny. In the UK entropion affects many newborn lambs of the Border Leicester breed and their progeny. The problem is also often seen in Suffolk-sired lambs and may affect almost all progeny of a particular ram.

Aetiology

Entropion is an inherited condition probably transmitted as a dominant allele. This form of entropion is sometimes referred to primary entropion and is very much more common than secondary entropion, which may develop in association with dehydration and loss of retrobulbar fat in debilitating diseases.

Clinical presentation

With primary entropion, inversion of the lower eyelid is either present at birth (**Fig. 12.8**) or appears soon afterwards (**Fig. 12.9**). The condition is frequently bilateral. There is epiphora, blepharospasm and photophobia. The ocular discharge quickly becomes purulent. Direct contact between the eyelashes and cornea causes a severe keratitis with ulceration

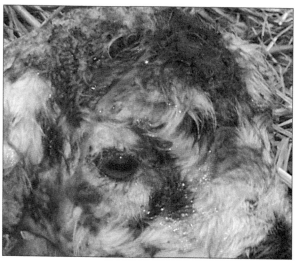

Fig. 12.8 Newborn lamb presents with turned-in lower eyelid of the right eye.

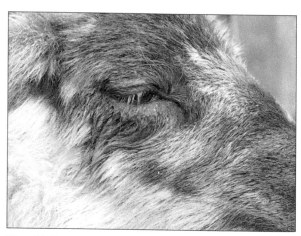

Fig. 12.9 Neonatal lamb presents with turned-in lower eyelid of the right eye and ocular discharge.

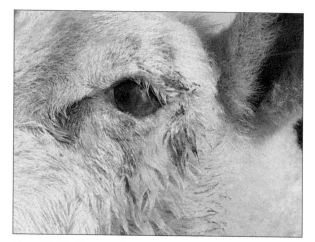

Fig. 12.10 Contact between the lower eyelashes and cornea causes a severe keratitis with ulceration.

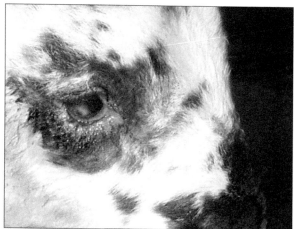

Fig. 12.11 Contact between the lower eyelashes and cornea causes a severe keratitis with ulceration.

(Figs 12.10, 12.11) in more advanced cases with consequent blindness. Hypopyon and possible rupture of the cornea with prolapse of the lens develop in neglected lambs (Fig. 12.12).

Differential diagnoses
- IKC.
- Anterior uveitis.
- Hypopyon following bacteraemia.

Diagnosis

The diagnosis is made during the routine supervision of all newborn lambs and, at regular intervals within the first few days of life, of those lambs with epiphora (Fig. 12.13).

Treatment

In simple cases of entropion of short duration the lower eyelid is everted. An ophthalmic ointment containing an antibiotic is then applied to the cornea to control potential secondary bacterial infection. In addition, such an oily presentation lubricates movement of the lower eyelid, thus reducing the likelihood of inversion.

If eyelid inversion recurs after rolling out the lower eyelid, subcutaneous injection of 0.5 ml of

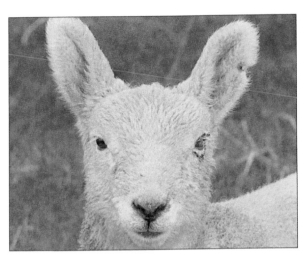

Fig. 12.12 Hypopyon (left eye) has developed in this lamb as a consequence of delayed treatment.

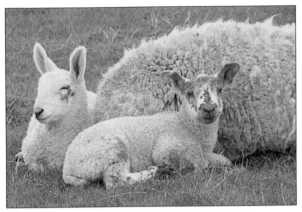

Fig. 12.13 Regular inspection readily identifies potential entropion cases (blepharospasm and ocular discharge) within the first few days of life.

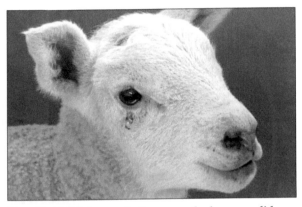

Fig. 12.14 Thin metal clips evert the lower eyelid thus correcting the entropion.

antibiotic, often procaine penicillin, is injected into the lower eyelid. The lamb is held securely and a 21 gauge 15 mm needle introduced through the skin of the lower eyelid parallel to, and approximately 10 mm below, the palpebral fissure. This volume of antibiotic physically everts the lower eyelids and forms a depot to control possible secondary bacterial infection. This technique is effective in almost all cases of primary entropion.

Thin metal clips (Eales clips) can also be used to evert the lower eyelid (**Fig. 12.14**). This method has the advantage that the clips can be quickly inserted by one person.

Excision of an elliptical strip of skin under local anaesthesia and drawing the cut edges together with sutures can be used to evert the lower eyelid but is rarely necessary.

Management/prevention/control measures
Entropion is managed by regular inspection of neonatal lambs and prompt correction. The genetic component of entropion should be carefully investigated and when the condition can be attributed to certain ram(s), they should be culled; in reality this rarely happens. Many farmers accept entropion as a 'breed characteristic'.

Welfare implications
Keratitis is a very painful condition, especially when the condition is not correctly treated (**Fig. 12.12**). The high morbidity rate adds to welfare concerns.

OVINE SQUAMOUS CELL CARCINOMA

Definition/overview
Ovine squamous cell carcinoma is reported commonly affecting older sheep in many subtropical countries worldwide, especially Australia. These tumours are rare in northern Europe.

Aetiology
Ovine squamous cell carcinoma occurs following prolonged exposure of areas of epidermis to ultraviolet radiation. The frequency of these tumours increases at higher altitudes.

Clinical presentation

Tumours may arise at several sites including the eye-lids, the dorsal surface of the ears, the muzzle and the muco-cutaneous junctions of the vulva and anus, and sites of Mules' mutilation. The proliferative lesions are readily traumatized and become secondarily infected. Metastases to drainage lymph nodes occur but can be difficult to appreciate because bacterial infection of the lesions also increases local lymph node size. Fly strike of lesions is very common.

Differential diagnoses

Ocular lesions should be differentiated from perior-bital eczema. Lesions around the face/muzzle should be distinguished from cutaneous pustular dermatitis, although age prevalence differs significantly.

Diagnosis

The diagnosis is based on clinical examination and elimination of other common differential diagnoses. The epidemiology of ovine squamous cell carcinoma is likely to be well known on the farm.

Treatment

Treatment in the first instance is symptomatic, with antibiotic therapy to limit bacterial involvement and removal of maggots in struck lesions. Surgical removal is not an option for commercial value sheep which must, therefore, be culled for welfare reasons.

Management/prevention/control measures

Provision of shade is not a practical option on extensive grazing systems.

Economics

Culling of ewes with significant lesions will increase the replacement rate.

Welfare implications

Culling of ewes with early tumour lesions should reduce the risk of secondary complications.

MICROPHTHALMIA

Microphthalmia is an autosomal recessive condition recognized in certain breeds, such as the Texel (**Fig. 12.15**). It can occur at a high prevalence following the introduction of a new ram. Affected lambs should be euthanased for welfare reasons. The carrier ram should be identified and culled or used for cross-breeding purposes only.

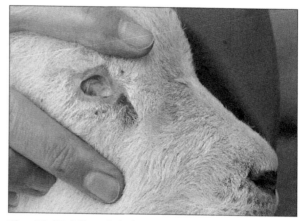

Fig. 12.15 Microphthalmia is an autosomal recessive condition recognized in certain breeds, such as the Texel.

CLINICAL EXAMINATION

The mammary system has two distinct glands, supported by the median suspensory ligament, each with its own teat, nerve and blood supplies and lymphatic drainage. The supramammary lymph nodes are only detected by deep palpation and their enlargement is often masked by oedema and swelling of the infected gland. Except for the first few weeks of lactation, it may prove difficult to express more than a few millilitres of milk from the normal glands because of frequent sucking by the lambs.

Clinical examination of the mammary gland involves palpation for the presence of heat, pain and swelling, and examination of secretions. The normal gland is firm, without obvious swellings and pain, although the ewe may fidget during gland palpation. Inspection of the teats involves casting the ewe onto her hindquarters. Palpation of the gland and examination of mammary secretions are the most informative aspect of clinical examination. Gland secretions can be submitted for somatic cell counts and standard bacteriological culture and antibiotic sensitivity after aseptic collection, but such examinations are restricted to sheep kept for milk production and rarely undertaken in sheep used for meat production.

Ultrasonography

Ultrasound examination of the udder can be undertaken using either 5 MHz linear array or sector scanners to differentiate soft tissue structures such as deep-seated abscesses (**Fig. 13.1**). However, ultrasonography adds little additional information to that gathered by careful palpation. Tumours of the mammary gland in sheep are rare.

Biopsy

Mammary gland biopsy is rarely undertaken.

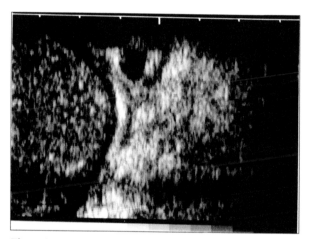

Fig. 13.1 Sonogram of the mammary gland showing a well-encapsulated abscess approximately 5 cm from the probe head, positioned to the right of the image (5 MHz linear scanner).

MASTITIS

Mastitis is a major disease problem in all intensive sheep production systems worldwide. The clinical manifestations of mastitis in ewes range from peracute gangrenous mastitis with severe illness and toxaemia to chronic mastitis and abscess formation without premonitory signs. Severe illness during the first month of lactation may result in death of the lamb(s) unless they are fed supplementary milk. Chronic mastitis is an important cause of culling in meat-producing sheep and reduced lactation in milking sheep.

Clinical cases of mastitis in sheep occur sporadically and most are predisposed by teat lesions. Unlike in dairy cattle, the California mastitis test is infrequently used to detect increases in bulk milk somatic cell counts, although it may have some application in dairy sheep. Similarly, individual somatic cell counts are not commonly used in sheep to detect and treat subclinical mastitis.

Gangrenous mastitis

Definition/overview

Gangrenous mastitis occurs sporadically during the first 8 weeks of lactation, often preceded by trauma to and/or superficial infection of the teat(s).

Aetiology

Gangrenous mastitis, caused by either *Mannheimia haemolytica* or *Staphylococcus aureus*, occurs sporadically during the first 2 months of lactation and is associated with poor milk supply related to ewe under-nutrition and over-vigorous sucking by the lambs. Many sheep farmers believe that gangrenous mastitis is associated with cold weather but this may simply be an association with reduced grass growth during a cold spell and poorer nutrient supply. The condition is more commonly reported in ewes nursing triplets rather than twins, and is rarely seen in ewes rearing singletons. Gangrenous mastitis often follows staphylococcal skin lesions (**Fig. 13.2**) or contagious pustular dermatitis (CPD) infection on the ewe's teat.

M. haemolytica is present in the oropharynx of young lambs and can be isolated from the teat skin of lactating ewes. As few as 10 colony-forming units of *M. haemolytica* can produce mastitis; therefore, these sites present a constant risk of intramammary infection. *S. aureus* can be isolated from the healthy teat skin of many ewes but especially those with teat skin lesions such as abrasions and CPD infection.

Clinical presentation

The condition is sudden in onset, ewes being healthy 12 hours previously. Affected ewes are separated from the remainder of the flock and show no interest or concern over their lambs. They are profoundly dull and have a gaunt appearance with sunken sublumbar fossae due to a poor appetite (**Fig. 13.3**). Affected ewes drag the hindlimb ipsilateral to the gangrenous quarter. The udder is visibly swollen and the skin is discoloured, first red but quickly turning purple, then black (**Fig. 13.4**). The lambs are hungry and attempt to suck but the ewe will not stand and walks away. Clinical examination reveals toxic mucous membranes and injected scleral vessels. The rectal temperature is elevated, often >41.0°C. The pulse is greatly increased, often exceeding 120 beats per minute. The respiratory rate is also increased. There are no ruminal sounds. Examination of the udder reveals marked swelling of one gland, with sharply demarcated purple/black discoloration extending along the ventral abdominal wall caused by thrombus formation. While only one gland is affected, the discoloration often extends over two-thirds or more of the udder skin. There is marked subcutaneous oedema of the affected gland (**Fig. 13.5**), extending cranially

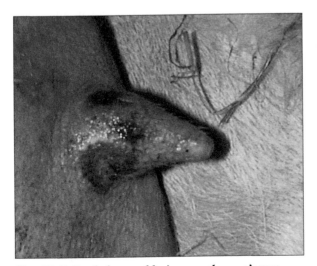

Fig. 13.2 Staphylococcal lesions on the ewe's teat often precede gangrenous mastitis.

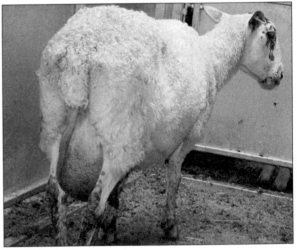

Fig. 13.3 This ewe with gangrenous mastitis is profoundly dull and has a gaunt appearance, with sunken sublumbar fossae due to a poor appetite.

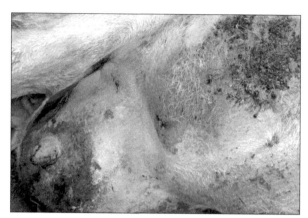

Fig. 13.4 With gangrenous mastitis, the udder is visibly swollen and red but quickly turns purple, then black, tracking along the ventral abdomen due to thrombus formation within the mammary vein.

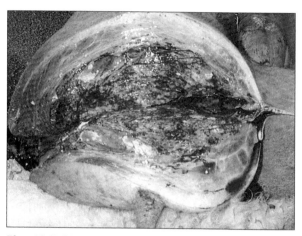

Fig. 13.5 Necropsy of gangrenous mastitis reveals marked subcutaneous oedema of the affected mammary gland.

along the ventral abdomen. The gangrenous areas of skin on the udder and ventral abdomen are cold. There are almost invariably traumatic lesions on the medial aspect of the teats caused by the lambs' incisor teeth. These superficial lesions may be infected with either *S. aureus* or CPD virus. Expression of the associated oedematous teat is resented by the ewe and releases a very small quantity (10–20 ml) of yellow/red serum-like fluid.

Differential diagnoses

Clinical examination reveals the extent of the udder infection. The severe mechanical lameness observed during the early stages of gangrenous mastitis must not be mistaken for a toe abscess or joint injury.

Diagnosis

Diagnosis is confirmed during clinical examination, although bacteriological examination is necessary to determine the causal organism.

Treatment

Affected ewes should be housed and lambs offered supplementary feeding. While intravenous antibiotic and non-steroidal anti-inflammatory drug (NSAID) injections will assist the ewe's survival of the initial phase of profound toxaemia, the long-term future for these ewes is hopeless and they should be euthanased before they suffer any further.

Management/prevention/control measures

With some notable breed exceptions, ewes must not be expected to rear triplets under commercial farming conditions. Appropriate ewe body condition score at lambing time and an appropriate level of nutrition during lactation should prevent teat skin abrasions caused by over-vigorous sucking by hungry twin lambs. Outbreaks of CPD in lambs may precede gangrenous mastitis in ewes, but it should be noted that CPD is most severe in poor lambs on a low plane of nutrition. Staphylococcal teat skin infections have been associated with outbreaks of gangrenous mastitis in housed sheep. Prompt treatment of these teat skin lesions with procaine penicillin and topical antibiotic, plus supplementary lamb feeding, has prevented further cases of gangrenous mastitis.

Economics

Gangrenous mastitis is a sporadic cause of ewe loss, rarely exceeding 2% of sheep at risk. Loss of lambs may also occur in those ewes affected within the first month of lactation. In the UK, for example, 100 ewes could be fed an extra 250 g of barley per head per day (3 MJ per head per day) for 6 weeks for the cost of loss of one ewe with twin lambs at foot. While extra feeding may not prevent all cases of gangrenous mastitis, there are other benefits from supplementary feeding, e.g. improved lactation and lamb growth rate. Supplementary feeding will also help restore ewe body condition so that they are in good condition when lambs are weaned. Sale of lambs at or before weaning eliminates diseases associated with this stressful period (e.g. systemic pasteurellosis) and avoids the mid-summer challenge from nematode larvae on pasture, cutaneous myiasis and headflies.

Welfare implications

Gangrenous mastitis is a major welfare concern in lactating ewes and is a subject that requires urgent review. Despite antibiotic and supportive therapy during the per-acute phase of disease, affected sheep endure an initial phase of profound toxaemia, with resultant marked loss of body condition. After several weeks the gangrenous udder tissue sloughs (**Fig. 13.6**), leaving a large granulating wound with superficial bacterial infection. The granulation tissue continues to proliferate over the coming months (**Fig. 13.7**) and affected ewes cannot be presented at market. They are also unsuitable for breeding stock. There is no market for such sheep and affected ewes should be euthanased during the per-acute phase of disease once the diagnosis of gangrenous mastitis has been established. It is not uncommon for bacteraemia from the infected udder to cause lung abscesses/pleurisy, endocarditis and renal infarcts (**Figs 13.8–13.10**).

Acute mastitis
Definition/overview

Acute mastitis occurs sporadically in grazing sheep and causes systemic illness but does not extend to gangrene of mammary tissue. Acute mastitis is a major concern in southern European countries with large populations of milking sheep.

Aetiology

A wide range of bacteria, including *Streptococcus* spp., *Staphylococcus* spp. and *Escherichia coli*, can gain entry through the streak canal and cause acute mastitis.

Clinical presentation

The initial clinical signs are broadly similar, although less severe, than those for gangrenous mastitis. Affected ewes are separated from the remainder of the flock and are depressed and have a gaunt appearance. The rectal temperature is elevated. There is marked swelling and oedema of the affected gland (**Fig. 13.11**) but this rarely extends cranially along the ventral abdomen. There may be traumatic lesions on the medial aspect of the teats caused by the lambs' incisor teeth. The udder secretion varies from 'normal' milk containing large white clots to serum-like, depending on the causal organism.

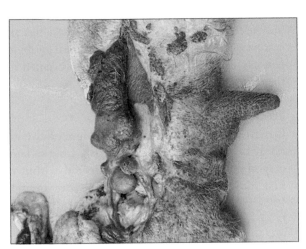

Fig. 13.6 Necropsy findings several weeks after onset of gangrenous mastitis; the necrotic udder tissue has sloughed leaving a large granulating wound with superficial bacterial infection.

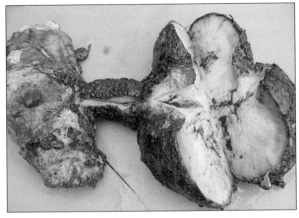

Fig. 13.7 Necropsy findings several months after onset of gangrenous mastitis; fibrous tissue has formed from remnants of the affected mammary gland.

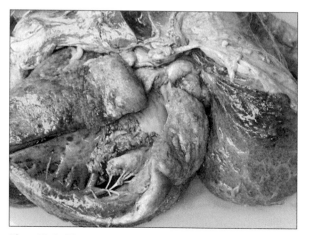

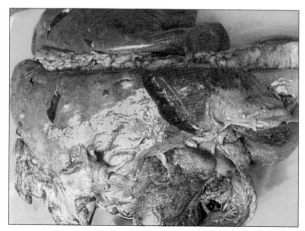

Fig. 13.8 Necropsy findings several months after onset of gangrenous mastitis; the lung abscesses/pleurisy have probably arisen due to bacteraemia from infection at the sloughed udder site.

Fig. 13.9 Necropsy findings several months after onset of gangrenous mastitis; the endocarditis lesion has probably arisen from infection at the sloughed udder site.

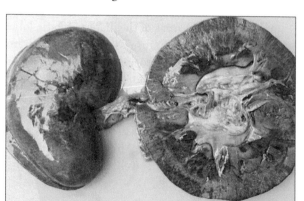

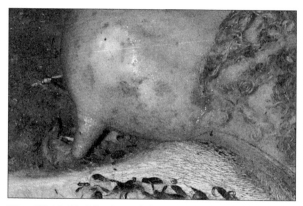

Fig. 13.10 Necropsy findings several months after onset of gangrenous mastitis; renal infarcts which have probably arisen from infection at the sloughed udder site.

Fig. 13.11 Reddening of the skin with pitting oedema of a mastitic gland.

Differential diagnoses

The major differential diagnosis of sudden onset illness in grazing sheep is acute respiratory disease caused by *Pasteurella* (*Mannheimia*) species.

Diagnosis

Diagnosis is confirmed during clinical examination, although bacteriological examination is necessary to determine the causal organism.

Treatment

Treatment involves parenteral antibiotic therapy, typically oxytetracycline or penicillin, with an equivalent intramammary preparation, although there may not be a licensed intramammary formulation in many countries. Tilmicosin is licensed for the treatment of ovine mastitis in many countries; it has the advantages of activity against mycoplasmas and a single injection formulation. Regular stripping of the mastitic gland will remove toxins. A NSAID will assist treatment of the toxaemia.

Management/prevention/control measures

The sporadic nature of the condition in grazing meat-producing sheep makes prevention difficult. In milk-producing sheep, control is aimed at hygiene during the milking process and maintenance of the milking plant with regular servicing. Sampling of mastitis cases and bacteriological culture will give some indication of the important epidemiological factors contributing to a high disease incidence in milking sheep.

Economics

Acute mastitis is a major problem of milking sheep in many countries. In meat breeds, losses result from reduced lamb growth rate due to reduced milk supply and the increased culling rate subsequent to the development of chronic mastitis in these ewes.

Welfare implications

There is a considerable body of evidence indicating significant pain associated with both acute and chronic mastitis in cattle. The administration of a NSAID during the acute phase should reduce pain in sheep with mastitis, and it may reduce pain as the condition becomes more chronic.

Chronic mastitis

Definition/overview

Chronic mastitis develops from an acute episode of disease during lactation; few new mammary infections become established following weaning. Chronic mastitis is a major cause of culling in both meat-producing and milk-producing sheep.

Aetiology

Incomplete resolution of acute mastitis results in the establishment of chronic infection, which manifests as abscess formation within the mammary parenchyma. *Trueperella pyogenes* is almost invariably cultured from udder abscesses, although it may not have been the original pathogen.

Clinical presentation

The teat is often thickened with a fibrous cord blocking the streak canal. Abscesses range in both number and diameter within the udder. Some abscesses may be detected at weaning but they are often masked at this time by milk within the udder. The best time to detect chronic mastitis is the prebreeding check undertaken some 2–3 months after weaning, when mammary gland involution makes palpation much more accurate. Deep-seated abscesses have a fibrous capsule, which may extend to several centimetres thick, with a core of green viscous pus. Superficial abscesses have a thin wall, often only a few millimetres thick, which may rupture and discharge pus. Development and growth of abscesses with proliferation of surrounding fibrous tissue leads to gross enlargement of the associated gland and udder over 3–6 months (**Figs 13.12–13.14**), and this can measure up to 20 cm in diameter in neglected sheep.

Chronic mastitis cases not detected during the prebreeding check are subsequently identified post lambing, when the first sign is a hungry lamb(s). The teat of the affected gland is thickened and no milk, or only a small amount of inspissated pus, can be expressed from the teat.

Bacteraemic spread to the lungs is not uncommon and results in numerous abscesses, typically distributed in the dorsal areas of the diaphragmatic lobe(s). These abscesses rarely result in signs of respiratory disease but contribute to general malaise in some sheep. Bacteraemic spread from the udder to the endocardium and joints is much less common.

Differential diagnoses

It may prove difficult to differentiate whether a small, deep-seated, firm swelling in the udder is an

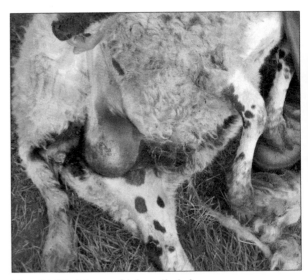

Fig. 13.12 A large thick-walled abscess causes gross enlargement of a mammary gland readily palpable at the prebreeding check.

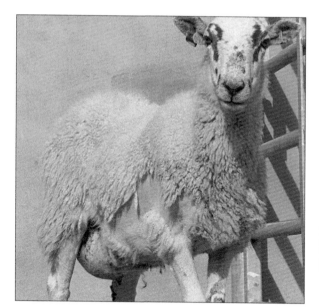

Fig. 13.13 Marked enlargement of the right mammary gland detected at the prebreeding check.

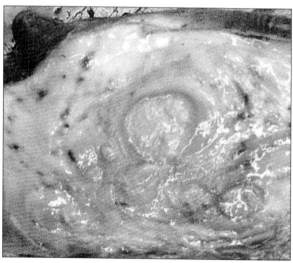

Fig. 13.14 Necropsy reveals well-encapsulated abscesses and proliferation of fibrous tissue within the affected mammary gland.

abscess or simply involuted mammary tissue. Visna-maedi virus infection can result in chronic fibrosis of the mammary gland, although this manifestation of infection varies between countries, and is uncommon in the UK.

Diagnosis

Diagnosis of a mammary abscess, particularly a deep-seated lesion, can be confirmed by ultrasonographic examination and/or fine needle aspirate.

Treatment

Encouraging results have been reported for the treatment of mild cases of chronic mastitis using tilmicosin (s/c) at weaning. Treatment of chronic mastitis that has progressed to abscessation within the gland is not usually undertaken because of the hopeless prognosis and associated loss of normal mammary tissue and lactogenesis.

Management/prevention/control measures

Ewes with chronic mastitis and abscesses (Fig. 13.14) should be culled following identification at weaning or at the prebreeding check.

There are no licensed long-acting intramammary antibiotic preparations in many countries, although preparations for cattle are used 'off-label' at weaning to control/prevent chronic mastitis. Care must be exercised with intramammary infusion in sheep because iatrogenic infections are common when the procedure is undertaken in wet or unhygienic conditions. Appropriate teat disinfection before antibiotic infusion is essential. The intramammary syringe nozzle is held against the teat orifice; it must not be forced into the streak canal. Sheep are often turned out onto poor-quality grazing after weaning (Fig. 13.15) or grazed at very high stocking densities (Fig. 13.16) to speed up udder involution, but there is little evidence that these management practices work.

Economics

Chronic mastitis is an important cause of premature culling in sheep flocks worldwide and as such represents an important economic loss, although there are few recent reliable data. Carcase condemnation may result if there is reaction in the deep inguinal lymph nodes draining the udder. Chronic mastitis also results in reduced lactation and subsequent lower growth rate in lambs.

The use of tilmicosin in all ewes at weaning to treat existing subclinical udder infections and

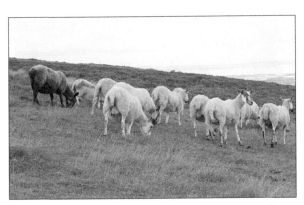

Fig. 13.15 There is little evidence that poor-quality grazing post weaning reduces mastitis.

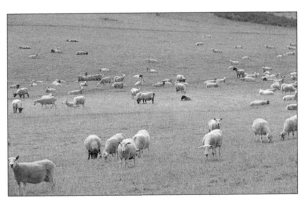

Fig. 13.16 Farmers may graze sheep at very high stocking densities in an attempt to reduce milk production and speed up udder involution.

prevent postweaning mastitis works well but may be restricted to valuable milking sheep and pedigree meat breed ewes.

Welfare implications

Udder abscessation is painful and presents a welfare concern when there are numerous large abscesses, although the extent of the surrounding fibrous capsule may limit the impact of external stimuli such as hindlimb movements.

Teat lesions

In gangrenous and acute mastitis cases there are almost invariably traumatic lesions to the skin on the medial aspect of the teats caused by the lambs' incisor teeth. They are more common in ewes nursing triplets and may, in part, explain the much higher incidence of mastitis in these ewes. These superficial skin lesions may become infected with *S. aureus*, or with CPD virus if it is present in the flock at that time.

Treatment of staphylococcal teat lesions may become necessary and a good response is achieved with procaine penicillin (44,000 IU/kg i/m for 3–5 consecutive days) and topical antibiotic cream/aerosol spray. Supplementary feeding of lambs may be necessary but few nursing lambs will suck from a bottle and teat; therefore, concentrates may offer a better and easier option.

CONTAGIOUS AGALACTIA

Definition/overview

Contagious agalactia affects sheep and goats in many parts of the world, particularly in southern Europe and the Middle East. The disease is not recognized in the UK, Australia and New Zealand.

Aetiology

Contagious agalactia is caused by *Mycoplasma agalactiae* but the role of other mycoplasmas is under discussion.

Clinical presentation

Affected sheep are dull, inappetent and pyrexic. Abortion may result in pregnant sheep in the flock. There is severe bilateral mastitis in lactating ewes, with clots present in the much reduced udder secretions. Nursing lambs are hungry, have a gaunt appearance and die if not given appropriate supplementary feeding. Commonly, there is marked lameness resulting from involvement of the carpal and hock joints, characterized by considerable joint effusion. There may be epiphora and blepharospasm associated with keratoconjunctivitis.

Diagnosis

Diagnosis is based on the clinical findings in a large number of sheep and isolation of *M. agalactiae* from mammary secretions and arthrocentesis samples.

Treatment

Tylosin and tilmicosin are especially effective *in vitro* against mycoplasmas but they may not be licensed for use in sheep in some countries. Problems arise with achieving sufficient antibiotic penetration into joints. Even prolonged antibiotic therapy is unlikely to effect a cure in sheep with numerous infected joints.

Management/prevention/control measures

Vaccines appear to afford little protection against contagious agalactia.

Economics

Contagious agalactia can result in serious financial loss due to the refractory nature of the condition and consequent high culling rate.

Welfare implications

The prognosis for polyarthritis associated with *M. agalactiae* infection is poor and affected sheep should be euthanased.

VISNA-MAEDI VIRUS

Definition/overview

The clinical manifestations of visna-maedi virus (VMV) infection vary considerably between countries. In the USA, VMV infection is more commonly referred to as ovine progressive pneumonia when affecting the lungs and 'hardbag' when affecting the mammary gland. Such pathology is rarely identified in the UK, where maedi and visna are the more common clinical presentations of VMV infection.

Aetiology

Infection with VMV may cause a lymphocytic mastitis ('hardbag'), as well as joint, brain (visna) and lung (maedi) lesions.

Clinical presentation

Reports describe an indurative mastitis without changes in the milk. The udder is smaller and more fibrous than normal but this proves difficult to detect in the lactating ewe and is better appreciated during the prebreeding check some 2–3 months after weaning. The shepherd is alerted to these ewes by the unexplained poor growth rate of their lambs.

Differential diagnoses

Chronic mastitis of bacterial origin causes more focal swellings, often resulting in abscessation, which can be identified during ultrasonographic examination.

Diagnosis

Sheep infected with VMV can be detected serologically by complement fixation test (CFT) or enzyme-linked immunosorbent assay (ELISA).

Treatment

There is no treatment and affected sheep should be culled.

Management/prevention/control measures

Control measures depend on the flock VMV seroprevalence and other factors (see Chapter 7 Respiratory System).

Economics

It is reported that indurative mastitis caused by VMV infection is a major cause of starvation of lambs in western range flocks in the USA.

Welfare implications

Indurative mastitis is not painful but concerns arise when lambs die of starvation caused by poor lactation.

CHAPTER 14

TRACE ELEMENT DEFICIENCIES AND METABOLIC DISORDERS

THE clinical signs associated with trace element deficiency in sheep are often insidious in onset and usually present as poorly grown lambs during late summer/early autumn with few specific clinical features (**Fig. 14.1**). There is considerable interplay between chronic parasitism, malnutrition and trace element deficiencies such that it may not be possible, or desirable, to ascertain which is the most important condition (**Fig. 14.2**). The problem of diagnosing trace element deficiency is further compounded when purchased sheep are presented as poorly grown.

The trace element deficiency states generally considered are: cobalt, copper, vitamin E and selenium, and iodine although in certain areas of the world manganese, iron and zinc may be limiting elements.

COBALT DEFICIENCY

Definition/overview
Cobalt deficiency (pine) occurs in many countries worldwide where there are low soil concentrations. This may be further complicated by dietary factors and parasitic gastroenteritis, which may interfere with absorption of vitamin B12.

Aetiology
Cobalt has its only biological role as a constituent of vitamin B12 manufactured by rumen microflora.

Clinical presentation
Clinical signs of cobalt deficiency are most commonly observed in grazing lambs after weaning. Signs include lethargy, poor appetite, poor wool

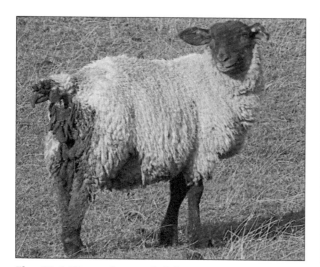

Fig. 14.1 Trace element deficiency states are often insidious in onset and present as poorly-grown lambs during late summer/early autumn with few specific clinical features.

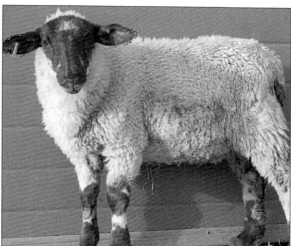

Fig. 14.2 There is considerable interplay between chronic parasitism, poor nutrition, and trace element deficiencies.

quality with an open fleece, small size and very poor body condition despite adequate nutrition (**Figs 14.3, 14.4**) and epiphora with staining of the cheeks. Pale mucous membranes, especially of the conjunctivae, develop late in the deficiency state.

Ovine white liver syndrome (**Fig. 14.5**) has been described in grazing lambs in many countries and is attributed to cobalt deficiency. In severe cases a secondary hepatic encephalopathy develops with a variety of neurological signs including depression (**Fig. 14.6**) extending to stupor and aimless wandering (**Fig. 14.7**).

It is reported that cobalt-deficient sheep suffer from non-specific immunosuppression and are more susceptible to infectious diseases, including clostridial diseases and pasteurellosis.

Cobalt deficiency is less common in adults but is reported to cause reduced fertility and poor mothering ability but these signs may be related to more generalized poor body condition.

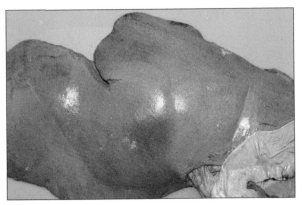

Fig. 14.3 Clinical signs of cobalt deficiency are most commonly observed in grazing lambs after weaning.

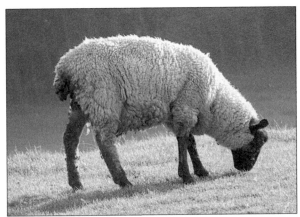

Fig. 14.4 Clinical signs of cobalt deficiency include lethargy, poor appetite, a poor fleece and very poor body condition despite adequate nutrition.

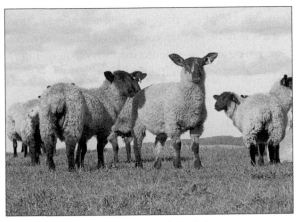

Fig. 14.5 Ovine white liver syndrome is attributed to cobalt deficiency.

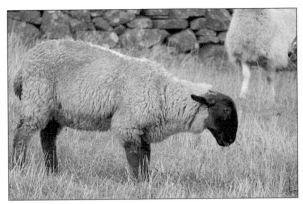

Fig. 14.6 In severe cobalt deficiency secondary hepatic encephalopathy develops, with signs including altered behaviour and stupor.

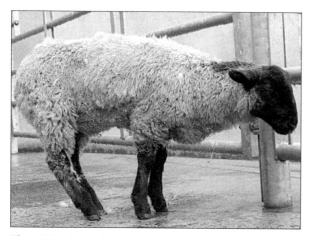

Fig. 14.7 Secondary hepatic encephalopathy may extend to stupor and aimless wandering.

Differential diagnoses

There is considerable interaction between chronic parasitism, malnutrition and trace element deficiency states, such that it may prove difficult to determine which is the most important problem. Diagnosis is often compounded by the fact that lambs may have been recently treated with an anthelmintic and moved onto better pasture immediately before veterinary examination.

The main differential diagnoses for cobalt pine are conditions that affect a large proportion of the lamb crop and include:

- Poor ewe nutrition or overstocked pasture mean that lambs do not have a good start to life.
- Poor grazing or overstocked pasture after weaning.
- Coccidiosis and nematodirosis can cause a serious growth check in 4–12-week-old lambs with protracted convalescence.
- Parasitic gastroenteritis is a very common cause of poor lamb growth. There is an increasing number of reports of multiple resistant nematode species in many countries worldwide.

Cases of ovine white liver disease showing neurological signs should be distinguished from coenurosis, polioencephalomalacia, sulphur toxicity and focal symmetrical encephalomalacia.

Diagnosis

Diagnosis is based upon clinical signs in areas with known cobalt-deficient soils supported by low plasma and/or liver vitamin B12 concentrations. As a general guide, a growth response is expected when the mean plasma vitamin B12 concentration falls below 500 pg/ml, and is likely to be significant below 250 pg/ml. A minimum of 10 blood samples is recommended to determine the mean plasma vitamin B12 concentration but this number is likely to be limited by cost considerations. These blood samples must be collected as soon as possible after the sheep have been gathered as values increase significantly during confinement. Liver vitamin B12 concentration can be determined following collection by biopsy which, while recommended by certain authors, is not regularly undertaken in general practice. A dose-response is expected in sheep with a mean liver cobalt concentration below 110 nmol/l; concentrations of 110–220 nmol/l are considered marginal.

Perhaps the best, and most cost effective, method for determining any growth retardation resulting from cobalt deficiency is to undertake a supplementation trial over 4–6 weeks and compare supplemented and control lambs' performance. 10 to 12 lambs could be left untreated until such time as a demonstrable difference can be appreciated, thereby reducing the impact of leaving more lambs non-supplemented. Typically, a 2–4 kg improvement in growth rate over controls would be expected over this time period.

Methylmalonic acid (MMA) accumulates in plasma and has been used to determine cobalt deficiency with concentrations higher than 5 μmol/l considered abnormal.

Packed cell volume (PCV) can readily be determined in the practice laboratory by microhaematocrit but anaemia may also result from infestations such as haemonchosis and chronic fasciolosis, and in association with many chronic bacterial infections.

Gross postmortem examination is non-specific revealing an emaciated carcase with serous atrophy of fat. There is bone marrow hypoplasia (**Fig. 14.8**). In severe cases of cobalt deficiency, the liver is enlarged, pale and friable.

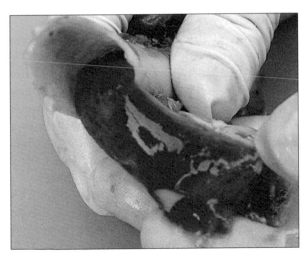

Fig. 14.8 There is bone marrow hypoplasia in severe cobalt deficiency.

Treatment

Treatment is more quickly effected by a combination of intramuscular injection of vitamin B12 and drenching with up to 1 mg/kg bodyweight of cobalt sulphate than by oral supplementation alone. Thereafter, monthly drenching with cobalt sulphate should ensure normal weight gain.

Management/prevention/control measures

Oral cobalt supplementation is very cheap and certain anthelmintics belonging to Group 1-BZ and Group 2-LM may already contain a cobalt supplement. Monthly dosing from around 3 months old should supply sufficient cobalt to growing lambs in most situations.

Cobalt oxide boluses, which lodge in the reticulum to provide a continuous supply of cobalt, are expensive in those lambs which require supplementation for only 2–3 months.

Soluble glass boluses containing cobalt, selenium and copper are available in some countries but are a very expensive means of supplying cobalt and are only indicated in situations where all three deficiency conditions are considered to exert a negative influence on health.

Economics

Oral cobalt supplementation costs less than 1 penny per 25 kg lamb with labour the major cost factor in drenching sheep. Conversely, soluble glass boluses containing cobalt, selenium and copper cost £1 per lamb with care required for administration. The high cost of cobalt-containing fertilizers has curtailed their use as a means of increasing soil and herbage cobalt content.

COPPER DEFICIENCY

Definition/overview

Copper deficiency is common when sheep graze pasture in certain geographic areas, often as a consequence of antagonists present in the soil such as iron, molybdenum and sulphur, and management practices such as lime application which increases soil pH. The clinical manifestation of copper deficiency varies worldwide with swayback more common in the UK, poor wool quality and anaemia in Australia and osteoporosis in New Zealand.

As well as being susceptible to copper deficiency, certain sheep breeds are prone to copper accumulation and toxicity. There is considerable breed variation with respect to copper absorption and therefore to copper deficiency and toxicity.

Aetiology

Copper forms an integral part of numerous enzyme systems in the body.

Clinical presentation

Copper deficiency during mid-gestation may lead to swayback (**Figs 14.9, 14.10**) which is described in Chapter 8, Neurological Diseases.

In growing lambs copper deficiency may result in a poor fleece without its natural 'crimp' which has been described as 'steely wool'. Other reports describe poor weight gain, anaemia and increased susceptibility to bacterial infections.

Osteoporosis leading to long bone fractures, often during handling procedures, has been reported in New Zealand as a consequence of copper deficiency.

Differential diagnoses

The differential diagnoses of swayback are described in Chapter 8, Neurological Diseases. Long bone fractures occur sporadically in growing lambs during handling procedures in poorly designed facilities.

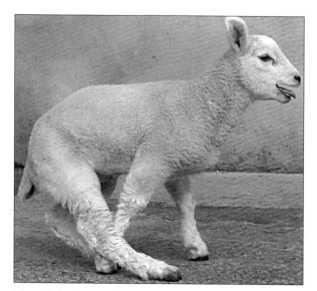

Fig. 14.9 Copper deficiency during mid-gestation may lead to delayed swayback in lambs.

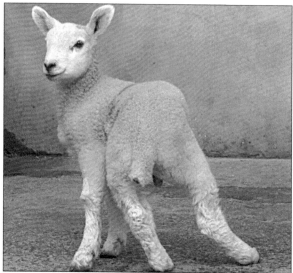

Fig. 14.10 Progressive hindlimb weakness appears from 2–4 months old in delayed swayback.

Diagnosis

Swayback is provisionally diagnosed on clinical examination and confirmed following histopathological examination of the spinal cord.

Copper deficiency is most reliably diagnosed in growing lambs based upon a dose/response study but this is rarely practicable under most farm conditions and farmers are generally reluctant to leave some sheep non-supplemented.

In situations where copper absorption is inadequate there is depletion of liver reserves followed by depletion at non-essential sites; clinical disease follows depletion at essential sites. In a deficiency situation, copper stores are mobilized from the liver to maintain plasma concentrations; low plasma concentrations therefore indicate depletion of liver reserves.

Plasma samples are most commonly submitted for analysis; concentrations below 9.4 μmol/l are considered to indicate depletion of liver reserves, but may not yet have exerted an adverse effect on growth. It is reported that hypocuprosis does not limit lamb performance until plasma concentrations fall below 3 μmol/l. The copper-dependent enzyme superoxide dismutase declines more slowly in a copper deficit situation; therefore, low concentrations are considered more likely to reflect negative influences on health and growth (normal concentrations above 0.4 and 0.3 IU/mg haemoglobin for lambs and adult sheep, respectively).

Liver copper concentrations below 157 μmol/kg dry matter (DM) are considered to indicate exhaustion of liver reserves, although biopsy is rarely undertaken in the UK. The liver can be readily imaged using transabdominal ultrasonography which may assist biopsy.

Treatment

Treatment of delayed swayback is described in Chapter 8, Neurological Diseases.

Management/prevention/control measures

Prevention of copper deficiency in growing lambs is much more important than treatment because irreversible changes have often taken place in the fleece, and full compensatory growth may not result after supplementation. Furthermore, treatment of swayback is hopeless and emphasis must be placed upon preventive measures.

While copper deficiency is often a perennial problem on certain farms, farmers must always be made aware of the risks of copper toxicity. Therefore timing and type of copper supplementation should be specified in the veterinary flock plan, with specific notes made regarding no other source of extra copper. Sheep must not be given a copper supplement prior to, or during, housing. Toxicity could result from a number of sources including using more than one method of copper supplementation and use of feeds with high copper content; such feeds are often distillery by-products. Change of sheep breed may result in an incident of copper poisoning because certain breeds are particularly susceptible to copper toxicity, e.g. if the same supplementation method is used, but Texel lambs are purchased rather than the usual Suffolk or Scottish Blackface lambs.

Copper is usually given by injection as copper heptonate; copper salts such as calcium copper edetate and cuproxiline are rapidly absorbed from the site of injection and may be toxic to sheep. Certain copper injections are irritant and may cause large local reactions. Care must be exercised that the injection is given correctly because abscessation, and in some cases tracking of infection to the cervical spinal canal, have been observed after incorrect injection technique.

Supplementation can be effected with copper oxide needles administered orally in a gelatin capsule at a dose rate of 0.1 g copper oxide per kg liveweight. Sheep should not be re-treated for 12 months unless signs of copper deficiency recur.

Appropriate supplementation of the ewe during mid-gestation will prevent the development of swayback in her progeny. Weather conditions, in particular snow cover, determine a low-risk year in the UK because of reduced intake of inhibitor substances from soil. Solutions containing copper administered twice during late gestation to prevent swayback have been largely replaced by other forms of supplementation due to reducing handling requirements during late gestation.

The contribution of copper-containing fertilizers is dependent upon soil type and is too variable in most practical situations.

Economics
Copper supplementation costs 30–50 pence for injectable preparations and gelatin capsules containing copper oxide needles.

SELENIUM AND VITAMIN E DEFICIENCY

(syn. white muscle disease, nutritional muscular dystrophy, stiff lamb disease)

White muscle disease occurs in the UK with recognized risk factors such as feeding home grown cereals and root crops, and incorrectly mineralized rations; however, disease prevalence is generally low. It is reported that 20–30% of the flock can be affected with white muscle disease in certain areas of New Zealand where low selenium concentration in soil results in low plant concentrations.

Resistance to bacterial pathogens is reported to be lower in selenium-deficient animals, which show increased disease levels.

Definition/overview
Selenium deficiency occurs in soils of certain geographic areas worldwide leading to pasture/crop deficiency. Vitamin E concentrations are high in green crops but fall rapidly under drought conditions. Certain root crops are known to be low in both selenium and vitamin E. Feeding grain treated with propionic acid may increase the risk of white muscle disease.

Aetiology
Selenium and vitamin E act as cellular antioxidants protecting cells against free radicals and lipid peroxides. These, if unchecked, cause membrane damage and tissue necrosis. Skeletal, cardiac and respiratory muscle cells and blood cells are especially susceptible to oxidative stress, and selenium and vitamin E deficiency may lead to disease of these body systems.

Clinical presentation
Congenital white muscle disease has been reported in lambs that are stillborn or die soon after birth, often from starvation.

In the UK, white muscle disease typically affects rapidly growing 2–6-week-old lambs, often ram lambs of meat breeds such as the Suffolk and Texel. There is sudden-onset stiffness with lambs reluctant to move such that they are easily caught. Affected lambs are bright, alert and suck well but have a painful expression with the head held lowered. After 1–2 days, affected lambs are unable to rise and remain in sternal recumbency (**Fig. 14.11**) with the ewe searching out the lamb at feeding times rather than *vice versa*. During the early stages the major skeletal muscle groups may be swollen and are painful under digital pressure. Stress factors such as recent handling or turnout to pasture may precipitate white muscle disease. It is reported that older lambs may suffer respiratory distress, which is often accompanied by secondary pneumonia.

Selenium-responsive poor growth in lambs has been reported in certain geographic areas of Australia and New Zealand, where dramatic improvements result after supplementation.

Early embryonic loss/failure to implant has been attributed to selenium deficiency. In ewes an increased lamb crop with fewer barren ewes has been reported after selenium supplementation before the mating period but these responses were highly variable.

Differential diagnoses

- In the UK, the main differential diagnosis for stiffness leading to recumbency is bacterial polyarthritis, particularly *S. dysgalactiae* affecting the atlanto-occipital joint.
- Erysipelas polyarthritis is common in this age group of lambs but presents with obvious lameness.
- Vertebral empyema of a cervical vertebra will cause recumbency but is uncommon in lambs less than 4 weeks old.
- Chronic debilitating infections may result in weakness and eventual recumbency but these signs contrast with the previous rapid growth and excellent condition of lambs before they show signs of white muscle disease.
- There are many causes of poor growth in growing lambs including cobalt deficiency, poor pasture management, and parasitic gastroenteritis.
- Likewise there are many causes of returns to service including infertile rams (ewes returning at 17 day intervals), toxoplasmosis and Border disease (ewes returning at intervals greater than 17 days).

Diagnosis

Histopathological examination of myocardium is often necessary to detect the congenital form of white muscle disease.

A provisional diagnosis of white muscle disease in young lambs is based upon clinical signs in rapidly growing healthy lambs, with the presence of some of the risk factors listed above. The serum creatine kinase concentration is massively increased during the acute phase of disease, typically to 10,000–20,000 IU/l but it can be as high as 100,000 IU/l (normal concentration = <500 IU/l). White striations may be visible in the gluteal and psoas muscles during gross postmortem examination (**Fig. 14.12**).

Most laboratories determine glutathione peroxidase as the indicator of selenium status with concentrations below 20 IU/l packed red blood cells at 30°C deemed to be at increased risk, although reference ranges may vary between laboratories.

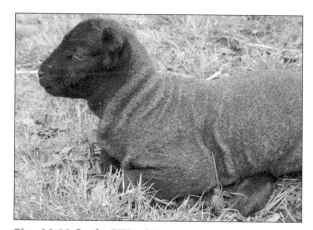

Fig. 14.11 In the UK, white muscle disease typically affects rapidly growing 2–6-week-old lambs.

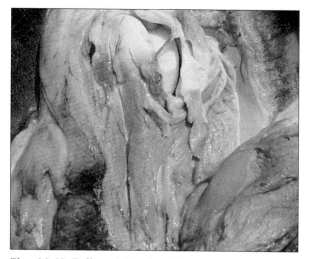

Fig. 14.12 Pallor of the gluteal muscles revealed during gross postmortem examination of this lamb with nutritional muscular dystrophy.

With respect to vitamin E, plasma α-tocopherol concentrations below 1 μmol/l are regarded as carrying increased risk of disease even if the selenium status is normal (as determined by glutathione peroxidase concentration).

Soil analysis can be undertaken but it is more usual to determine selenium concentration in tissues such as liver or kidney with liver tissue samples collected by biopsy. There is little between animal variation, and three to five samples afford an accurate assessment of selenium status.

Treatment

Intramuscular or subcutaneous injection with 0.75–1.5 mg selenium as potassium selenate and 34–68 mg vitamin E (dl α-tocopherol acetate) results in return to full mobility within 2–3 days.

Management/prevention/control measures

Several methods can be used to supply selenium and/or vitamin E including in-feed medication, targeted drenching, depot injection and intraruminal glass bolus or pellet. It is generally accepted that free-access licks/minerals are unreliable because of highly variable intakes.

As white muscle disease is seen most commonly in young lambs, prevention can be achieved by either correct supplementation of the dam's ration during late gestation or injection of all newborn lambs with a selenium and vitamin E preparation. The presence of feeds which increase the likelihood of white muscle disease, such as root crops, weathered hay and propionic acid-treated grain, necessitates higher levels of dietary supplementation.

Supplementation of growing lambs is best achieved by drenching and provides adequate selenium for 1–3 months. The standard selenium inclusion rate in an anthelmintic preparation is 0.4 mg/ml of elemental selenium with the anthelmintic combination product given at 1 ml per 5 kg bodyweight. Great care must be exercised when formulating a supplementation programme because toxicity can occur following over-dosage, especially in young lambs. The preparation must be shaken vigorously prior to use to ensure thorough mixing. In breeding sheep, selenium supplementation via drenching is given 1–2 months before the start of the breeding season.

Economics

Selenium supply via regular drenching is a cheap and reliable means of supplementation for growing lambs. Intraruminal glass boluses are a very expensive means of supplementing with selenium but are a useful method where other trace element deficiency states occur concurrently.

In the absence of a split flock trial, it is very difficult to calculate the cost benefit of selenium supplementation with respect to reproductive wastage. If doubts exist regarding poor reproductive performance, ewes should be drenched at regular intervals prior to mating. The low cost of selenium supplementation may result in more flocks receiving selenium preparations than is necessary rather than the converse situation.

IODINE DEFICIENCY

Definition/overview

Iodine is used in the synthesis of the thyroid hormones thyroxine (T4) and tri-iodothyronine (T3). Iodine deficiency can arise from a primary lack in the soil or, more commonly, secondarily to the action of goitrogens in leguminous crops which interfere with iodine metabolism. Feeding brassicas for long periods during pregnancy in New Zealand is related to iodine deficiency and manifests as poor survival of newborn lambs, especially during unfavourable weather conditions. The prevalence and severity of iodine deficiency may vary between years because of differing grazing and management conditions. Clinical signs are more severe in the Merino than in other breeds.

Clinical presentation

It is reported that iodine deficiency may be related to poor embryo survival. Iodine deficiency during pregnancy typically results in late abortion or the birth of weakly lambs with markedly swollen thyroid glands (goitre). It is reported that in severe cases lambs are born with little fleece, rendering them highly susceptible to hypothermia. Goitre is also recognized in adult sheep associated with goitrogen intake from fodder.

Differential diagnoses

There are many causes of perinatal lamb mortality in extensively managed sheep. Determination of thyroid gland to liveweight ratio would be only part of the lamb necropsy investigation.

Diagnosis

Diagnosis of iodine deficiency during pregnancy can be determined by the thyroid gland weight of a minimum of 15 lambs, with deficiency indicated by thyroid gland weights >0.4 g/kg liveweight. Histopathology can also be performed on thyroid glands. Plasma thyroid hormone concentrations, prior to and during pregnancy, are unreliable guides to reproductive performance and the appearance of goitre in lambs.

Treatment

Clinical goitre has been successfully treated with oral potassium iodide (20 mg per lamb).

Management/prevention/control measures

Ewes can be supplemented prior to mating with an intramuscular injection of iodized oil which is claimed to last for 2 years. Alternatively, ewes can be drenched twice during pregnancy with potassium iodide.

Economics

It may prove difficult to determine the true cost of iodine deficiency in commercial flocks because losses vary from one year to another, depending upon nutrition during gestation. A split flock supplementation study offers the most accurate and practical means of determining real costs of iodine deficiency.

Welfare implications

Increased perinatal mortality has an obvious welfare cost.

COPPER TOXICITY

Definition/overview

Chronic copper toxicity is a common occurrence in intensively-managed sheep. It results once the liver's capacity for lysosomal copper storage has been exceeded, causing lipid peroxidation and intravascular haemolysis with the appearance of jaundice (**Fig. 14.13**). The prognosis is grave once signs of jaundice appear in sheep.

Aetiology

Acute poisoning may occur after accidental overdose with excessive quantities of soluble copper salts when treating suspected deficiency states with drenches or certain injectable preparations.

Chronic copper toxicity is much more common in sheep and results from ingestion of relatively high levels of copper over a prolonged period; the term 'relatively high levels' is very important because dietary molybdenum and sulphur exert considerable influences on copper availability. During periods of high copper intake liver copper storage increases

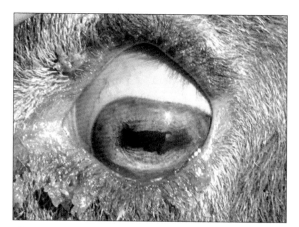

Fig. 14.13 Chronic copper toxicity presents with obvious jaundice of mucous membranes, most noticeably affecting the conjunctivae.

until critical levels are exceeded. This results in a sudden massive release of copper into the circulation, causing lipid peroxidation and intravascular haemolysis. The haemolytic crisis may be precipitated by stressors including such factors as advanced pregnancy, adverse weather, transportation, housing and sudden reduction in feeding, which may occur during winter storms. The precipitation of chronic copper toxicity may occur some days to weeks after removal of the copper source from the ration.

Concentrations of aspartate transaminase (AST) are markedly raised for several days to weeks before the haemolytic crisis with values commonly above 400 IU/l (normal range = 20–60 IU/l).

There is a wide variation in susceptibility to copper toxicity; UK native breeds such as the North Ronaldsay, Soay and Texel are especially prone whilst Scottish Blackface sheep are much less so when fed equivalent rations.

Hepatogenous copper toxicity, which occurs after the liver has been damaged by toxins, causing an increased avidity for copper, is uncommon in sheep.

Clinical presentation

Acute copper toxicity causes severe gastroenteritis with colic signs, diarrhoea and rapid dehydration. The affected sheep are very depressed and anorexic and death usually ensues within 3 days. If the sheep survive this per-acute phase, haemolysis and haemoglobinuria may be seen.

In cases of chronic copper toxicity the appearance of clinical signs is associated with the haemolytic crisis, which may be precipitated by the variety of stressors listed above. Affected sheep are weak, very dull and depressed (**Fig. 14.14**) and separate from others in the group. The rectal temperature is normal or slightly elevated (<40.2°C). They have a poor appetite and foetid diarrhoea with considerable mucus present. There is evidence of dehydration and obvious jaundice of mucous membranes, most noticeably affecting the conjunctivae. The heart and respiratory rates are increased, and an increased abdominal effort may be noted. There is no ruminal activity. The urine is dark red due to the presence of haemoglobin. Affected animals have a grave prognosis despite specific treatment with ammonium tetrathiomolybdate (where available)

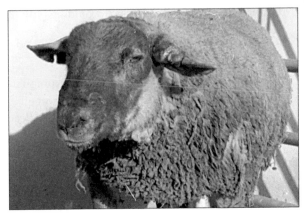

Fig. 14.14 Sheep with chronic copper toxicity are weak, very dull and depressed.

and supportive therapy; careful consideration must be given to humane destruction of sheep with these clinical signs.

Differential diagnoses

The diagnosis is relatively simple once jaundice becomes apparent. Differential diagnoses of sudden onset depression, weakness and anorexia may include pneumonic pasteurellosis, acute fasciolosis, clostridial diseases such as blackleg and bighead, urolithiasis in rams and ovine pregnancy toxaemia in ewes.

Diagnosis

Diagnosis is based on history, with a source of excess copper, and clinical findings of jaundice in chronic toxicity. The diagnosis is supported by laboratory findings of a massively increased serum AST concentration commonly above 1000 IU/l (normal range = 20–60 IU/l) and a serum gamma glutamyl transferase concentration more than 10 times normal (normal range = 27–31 IU/l). The serum total bilirubin concentration is greatly increased (more than 10 times normal). There is evidence of anaemia that worsens during the haemolytic crisis, with PCV falling as low as 0.10 l/l. Red blood cells typically show anisocytosis and large numbers of normoblasts are observed in blood smears. Surprisingly, serum copper concentrations measured during the haemolytic crisis are frequently only marginally increased and prove of little diagnostic significance.

Necropsy findings: Acute copper poisoning produces severe gastroenteritis with erosion of the abomasal mucosa. In chronic copper toxicity there is jaundice of the carcase, most noticeable in the omentum. The kidneys are swollen and dark grey with dark red urine in the bladder. The liver is enlarged and friable (**Fig. 14.15**). The spleen is enlarged and appears dark brown/black on cut section.

Kidney copper concentrations are massively elevated often in excess of 3000 μmol/kg DM (normal = <314 μmol/kg DM). Liver copper concentrations are usually also elevated but such determinations are not as reliable as kidney copper determination.

Treatment

The suspected copper source must be removed immediately but this has often already taken place before clinical signs of illness are first noted. Treatment of severely affected sheep is rarely successful and euthanasia for welfare reasons should be carefully considered. The best results are achieved by selecting those sheep most at risk by determining serum AST concentrations and treating these animals with ammonium tetrathiomolybdate by intravenous or subcutaneous injection (where available). Alternatively, all at-risk sheep can be treated using this regimen but this can prove expensive.

The dose rate of ammonium tetrathiomolybdate is either 1.7 mg/kg administered intravenously or 3.4 mg/kg injected subcutaneously on two to three occasions 2 days apart. There is no ammonium tetrathiomolybdate preparation licensed for use in food-producing animals and its use in suspected cases of chronic copper toxicity is poorly defined from a regulatory standpoint. A meat withdrawal period of at least 6 months has been recommended, thus preventing its use in fattening lambs. Treatment of sick individuals should be carefully monitored and failure to observe improvements by the second ammonium tetrathiomolybdate treatment indicates a grave prognosis.

Renal failure often develops in those animals that survive the initial acute haemolytic crisis and monitoring blood urea nitrogen and creatinine concentrations is strongly recommended. Blood urea nitrogen and creatinine concentrations more than five times normal indicate a hopeless prognosis and euthanasia is indicated. Concentrations of blood urea nitrogen and creatinine more than 10–20 times normal are not uncommon during the agonal stages.

Management/prevention/control measures

Copper supplementation must be carefully considered and the reader is directed to the section detailing management and prevention of copper deficiency.

Copper toxicity may arise after feeding cattle feed to sheep (**Fig. 14.16**). This situation occurs more commonly on hobby farms with small numbers

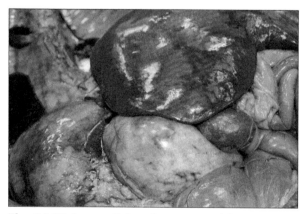

Fig. 14.15 A case of chronic copper toxicity at necropsy presents with findings of an enlarged friable liver; the kidneys are swollen and dark grey/black.

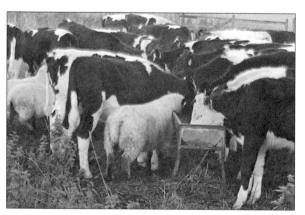

Fig. 14.16 Copper toxicity may arise following feeding cattle feed to sheep, albeit unintentionally.

of sheep. Incorrect mineral supplementation of proprietary concentrates may occur. However, copper concentrations are strictly regulated in the UK to levels below 15 mg/kg as fed in complete feeds. The interactions of copper antagonists such as molybdenum and sulphur are also of critical importance, and toxicity may result in certain breeds/situations where the copper concentration is within permitted legal levels but these antagonists are not included in the proprietary feed.

Economics

An outbreak of copper toxicity rarely results in the death of more than 5% of sheep at risk provided the source of copper is removed immediately. The longer-term consequences of copper toxicity, defined as those sheep with elevated serum AST concentrations that are not treated with ammonium tetrathiomolybdate, are much more difficult to quantify. It is claimed that nursing ewes do not lactate well with resultant poor lamb growth rates, although there are no specific data.

Welfare implications

The welfare of sheep showing severe depression and jaundice is of particular concern. Euthanasia is indicated if there is no improvement after injection with ammonium tetrathiomolybdate.

OVINE PREGNANCY TOXAEMIA

(syn. twin lamb disease)

Definition/overview

Ovine pregnancy toxaemia (OPT) occurs in all countries worldwide. In the UK the incidence of ovine pregnancy toxaemia is about 0.5% and most commonly encountered in lowground flocks affecting multiparous ewes carrying three or more lambs during the last 2 weeks of gestation. Where production relies almost exclusively upon pasture-based feeding with little supplementary concentrates, ovine pregnancy toxaemia is seen in severely underfed twin-bearing ewes. Several factors, such as severe lameness, may precipitate disease in individual ewes; however, the appearance of OPT generally indicates an energy underfeeding problem in the flock and the likely occurrence in other at-risk ewes.

Aetiology

Flock factors: OPT follows a period of severe energy shortage, whether the result of poor roughage quality, inadequate concentrate allowance or high foetal demand, but clinical signs can be precipitated by a sudden stressful event such as adverse weather conditions, handling, vaccination or housing. Parasitism, in particular liver fluke infestation, causing depletion of body reserves may be an important factor leading to OPT, although such chronic conditions more commonly result in chronic intrauterine growth retardation with consequent reduced energy demands of small foetus(es).

Individual ewe factors: Individual ewe factors such as obesity, severe lameness, vaginal prolapse or other disturbance such as acidosis or hypocalcaemia causing temporary inappetance, may also predispose to OPT.

Pathophysiology

Severe energy deficiency, whether primary due to management errors or secondary due to reduced appetite, results in excess fat mobilization and fatty infiltration of the parenchymatous organs.

Clinical presentation

The early clinical signs of OPT include disorientation leading to isolation from the remainder of the flock (**Fig. 14.17**). Occasional bleating may be heard from ewes during these early stages associated with blindness and separation from the remainder of the group. Over the next 24–48 hours affected ewes wander aimlessly because of blindness and may become caught in fences. While the sheep appear dull and depressed they are often difficult to restrain to administer treatments because they are hyperaesthetic to tactile stimuli.

There is a lack of menace response (**Fig. 14.18**) but pupillary light reflexes are normal. Abnormal behaviour including head pressing, dorsiflexion of the neck ('star gazing'), and frequent teeth grinding (bruxism) usually develops. Continuous fine muscle fasciculations causing movement of the overlying skin may be observed around the muzzle and affecting the ears.

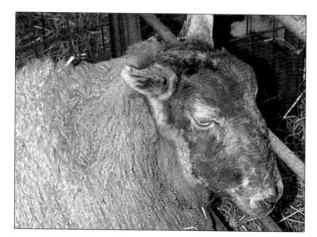

Fig. 14.17 The early clinical signs of ovine pregnancy toxaemia include disorientation leading to isolation from the remainder of the flock.

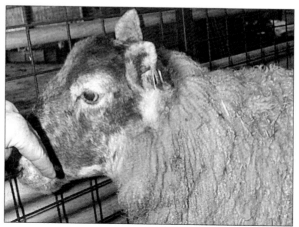

Fig. 14.18 There is a lack of menace response in ovine pregnancy toxaemia but the pupillary light reflexes are normal.

Unresponsive ewes may become recumbent with the hips extended caudally and the hindlimbs held out behind the ewe. There is a loss of abdominal wall musculature and the abdomen appears flattened dorsoventrally and 'spread out'. The foetuses can be balloted easily through both sides of the caudal abdomen. Inability to stand leads to urine scalding. Abortion as a consequence of OPT is uncommon. Death can occur 7–10 days after first appearance of clinical signs.

Differential diagnoses

Common differential diagnoses of OPT (often affecting more than one ewe in the flock at the same time) include:

- Several ewes affected:
  - Hypocalcaemia.
  - Listeriosis.
  - Acidosis resulting from carbohydrate overfeed.
  - Impending abortion.
  - Polioencephalomalacia.
  - Copper poisoning.
- Individual ewes:
  - Sarcocystosis.
  - Peripheral vestibular lesion (middle ear infection).
  - Space-occupying brain lesion such as coenurosis or abscess.

Diagnosis

Each of the conditions listed above can lead to isolation, reduced appetite and/or recumbency during late gestation. The diagnosis of pregnancy toxaemia is based upon history and clinical findings in a multigravid, multiparous ewe. While serum 3-OH butyrate concentrations above 3.0 mmol/l are suggestive of OPT, such values are not pathognomonic because concentrations can rise in sheep when there is high foetal demand for glucose and insufficient energy intake resulting from inappetance of relatively short duration.

Treatment

The response of OPT to treatment is generally poor even with early detection of clinical signs. Housed ewes should be penned separately and offered palatable feeds to promote appetite. If ewes are housed, turnout to good pasture may promote appetite although such grazing is seldom available. Treatment with oral propylene glycol and glucocorticoid injection is successful in approximately 30% of OPT cases that are still ambulatory when treatments commence.

Some authors recommend 60–100 ml of 40% dextrose injected intravenously twice daily, but this is seldom practical. Ten to 15 litres of fluids containing rumen stimulants can be easily administered by orogastric tube twice daily. Transfaunation can be undertaken in valuable ewes. Abortion/premature lambing can be induced after day 136 of pregnancy by injection of 16 mg dexamethasone, which may improve prognosis but the ewe must be very closely monitored for first stage labour and metritis is common following delivery of the lambs. The administration of a long-acting glucocorticoid injection is claimed to have similar glucogenic effects to dexamethasone but does not result in abortion.

Some practitioners routinely administer subcutaneous 40% calcium borogluconate to recumbent ewes suffering from OPT because serum analysis often reveals marginal hypocalcaemia. However, there is no convincing field evidence that calcium administration improves the recovery rate. Hypocalcaemia can readily be differentiated from OPT during clinical examination.

Ewes with OPT must be checked at least twice daily for signs of abortion/lambing because they may be too weak to expel the foetuses/lambs. Failure to expel dead foetuses leads to autolysis, with rapid development of toxaemia causing death of the ewe.

The decision to perform a caesarean operation must be made during the early clinical stages of disease to achieve best results from this salvage procedure. However, caesarean operations performed to save the life of the ewe have a poor success rate due to the emaciated state of the ewe and fatty infiltration of the liver, kidneys and heart. In addition, retention of the foetal membranes commonly leads to septic metritis (**Fig. 14.19**).

Ewes that do recover from OPT are rarely able to nurse a single lamb and are generally culled once they have regained body condition, although wool slip commonly occurs.

Postmortem findings: Postmortem findings include fatty infiltration of the parenchymatous organs, especially the liver (**Fig. 14.20**). The presence of two or more well-developed foetuses *in utero* is suggestive of, but not pathognomonic for, OPT. The necropsy findings can be supported by an aqueous humor 3-OH butyrate concentration >2.5 mmol/l or a cerebrospinal fluid (CSF) value >0.6 mmol/l, which correspond to ante-mortem serum concentrations >3.0 mmol/l, and absence of other significant lesions.

Management/prevention/control measures

Multigravid ewes must be fed appropriate levels of high-quality roughages and supplementary concentrate feeding during the last 6 weeks of pregnancy (**Fig. 14.21**). Foetal number can be determined by ultrasonography at 45–90 days post mating, allowing grouping based upon energy demands. Dietary energy sufficiency can be accurately determined by measuring ewes' serum concentrations of 3-OH butyrate four to six weeks prior to lambing.

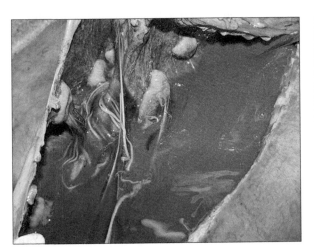

Fig. 14.19 Retention of the foetal membranes after an elective caesarean operation commonly leads to septic metritis.

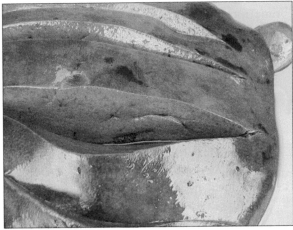

Fig. 14.20 Postmortem findings of ovine pregnancy toxaemia include fatty infiltration of the parenchymatous organs, especially the liver.

HYPOCALCAEMIA

Definition/overview

Hypocalcaemia is reported in all countries worldwide when sheep are managed intensively. A UK survey reported 0.4% prevalence of hypocalcaemia, more commonly in three-crop or older ewes maintained at pasture during late gestation, but also occurring sporadically during early lactation. Hypocalcaemia is often observed when ewes are brought down off hill grazing onto improved pastures prior to lambing. 'Outbreaks' of hypocalcaemia can result from errors in formulating home-mix rations, incorrect mineral supplementation, stress related events such as dog-worrying, movement onto good pastures prior to lambing or following housing.

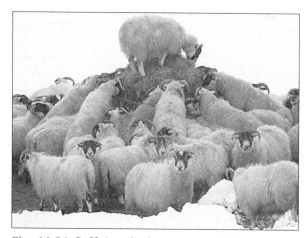

Fig. 14.21 **Sufficient feeders are essential to ensure adequate roughage intake as well as concentrate allowance.**

Aetiology

The highest demand for calcium in non-milk sheep occurs 3–4 weeks prior to parturition due to calcification of foetal bones. Mobilization of calcium from bone stores takes more than 24 hours; therefore, periods of transient hypocalcaemia may result.

Clinical presentation

During the early stages of hypocalcaemia affected ewes become isolated from the flock (**Fig. 14.22**). A small percentage of sheep appear disorientated and hyperaesthetic and may have a rapid respiratory rate ('panting'). Over 2–6 hours the ewe becomes dull, weak and unable to stand even when supported (**Fig. 14.23**). The head is held on the ground. There is a menace response and no cranial nerve deficit. There is rumen stasis with the development of bloat. The rectum is flaccid and may contain pellets of dried faeces that are not voided (**Fig. 14.24**). Passive reflux of rumen contents may occur with green fluid present at the external nares and around the lower jaw. These findings, together with the presence of stridor, result in the shepherd treating the ewe for respiratory disease, with a consequent delay in the request for veterinary assistance. There may be partial prolapse of the vagina. Unlike cattle, sheep do not assume lateral recumbency in the advanced stages of hypocalcaemia. Without appropriate therapy, the condition develops to coma, and death follows 24–48 hours after onset of recumbency.

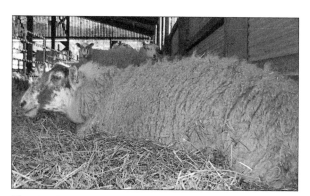

Fig. 14.22 **Ewes with hypocalcaemia are weak and become isolated from the group.**

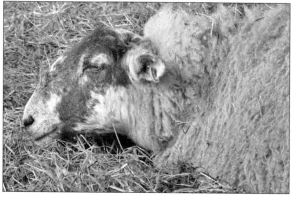

Fig. 14.23 **Ewes with hypocalcaemia become dull, weak and unable to stand even when supported.**

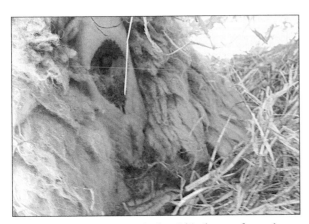

Fig. 14.24 The rectum is flaccid in hypocalcaemic sheep and may contain pellets of dried faeces which are not voided.

Differential diagnoses
- OPT.
- Listeriosis.
- Acidosis resulting from carbohydrate overfeed.
- Copper poisoning.
- Rhododendron poisoning.
- Polioencephalomalacia.

Diagnosis
In sheep recumbent due to hypocalcaemia, serum calcium concentrations are <1.0 mmol/l. Serum 3-OH butyrate concentrations can be elevated, especially if the ewe has been inappetent for more than 12 hours. The immediate response to intravenous calcium infusion confirms the diagnosis.

Treatment
There is an immediate response to slow intravenous administration of 20–40 ml of a 40% calcium borogluconate solution given over 30–60 seconds (45–80 kg ewes). Eructation is observed 1–2 minutes after intravenous calcium administration. Characteristically, ewes will stand within 5 minutes of intravenous injection (**Figs 14.25–14.27**; see **Fig. 14.23**), urinate, defaecate and wander off to rejoin the rest of the flock. There is no requirement to give any subcutaneous calcium; relapses do not occur. The diagnosis should be questioned if there is no immediate response to intravenous calcium injection.

The response to subcutaneous administration of 60–80 ml of 40% calcium borogluconate solution injected over the thoracic wall behind the shoulder may take up to 4 hours, especially if the solution has not been warmed to body temperature and injected at one site.

Management/prevention/control measures
Addition of appropriate minerals to the ration during pregnancy and thorough mixing are essential. Outbreaks of hypocalcaemia occurring over 2–3 days may still result after stressful events such as movement or housing, but these sheep respond promptly to appropriate therapy. At present, sheep rations are not formulated on the basis of cation–anion balance because hypocalcaemia has a sporadic occurrence with excellent treatment response, providing affected sheep are treated by a veterinarian.

Economics
The cost of calcium borogluconate is approximately £2 per 400 ml sufficient to treat 5–10 ewes. Incorrect diagnosis will result in death of the ewe(s), which may total up to 5% of the flock in situations where the condition results from incorrect feed mineralization/mixing and where veterinary attention is not sought immediately.

Welfare implications
Incorrect diagnosis and/or inappropriate treatment will result in unnecessary loss from a disease which has a 100% treatment response rate. Subcutaneous calcium injection is painful and much less effective than intravenous administration.

HYPOMAGNESAEMIA

Definition/overview
Hypomagnesaemia is reported as a very occasional cause of sudden death in lactating ewes but there are few detailed clinical reports of hypomagnesaemia in sheep. Shepherds' reports of hypomagnesaemia or 'staggers' in the UK usually refer to hypocalcaemia. Findings of sudden death in ewes nursing twins on recently-fertilized lush pasture are not sufficient for a diagnosis of hypomagnesaemia, unless

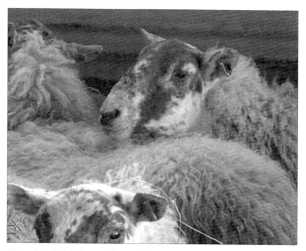

Fig. 14.25 Hypocalcaemic ewes will stand within 5 minutes of intravenous calcium injection (see Fig. 14.23).

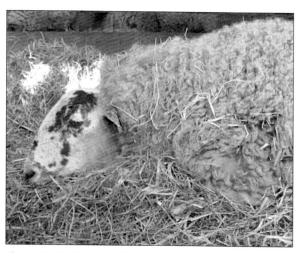

Figs 14.26 Ewe with hypocalcaemia shown before treatment (see Fig. 14.27).

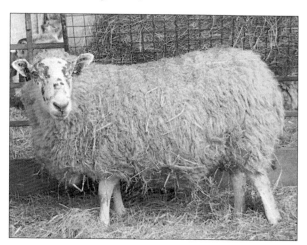

Fig. 14.27 Hypocalcaemic ewes will stand within 5 minutes of intravenous calcium injection.

the postmortem is supported by the absence of significant findings of other potential causes of death and an aqueous humor or CSF magnesium concentration below 0.2 mmol/l.

Aetiology

Hypomagnesaemia has been reported in ewes nursing twin lambs, 4–8 weeks after parturition, managed on lush pastures which have received large applications of artificial fertilizers containing high levels of nitrogen and potassium.

Clinical presentation

Sudden death of ewes grazing lush pasture during early lactation is often attributed to hypomagnesaemia without justification because such deaths are rarely investigated in detail. It is reported that recumbency can occur in ewes nursing twin lambs 4–8 weeks after parturition, managed on lush pastures; these ewes have low serum magnesium and calcium concentrations that do not respond to intravenous calcium alone, but recover following injection of subcutaneous magnesium sulphate.

Other reports detail initial depression but muscle tremors, seizure activity and opisthotonus occur once these sheep are disturbed. Spontaneous horizontal nystagmus, tachycardia and tachypnoea are also reported. Death ensues within 4–6 hours.

Differential diagnoses

Common differential diagnoses for recumbency/ seizure activity include:

- Polioencephalomalacia.
- Listeriosis.
- Vestibular disease.

Common differential diagnoses for sudden death in lactating ewes grazing lush pasture include:

- Bloat following lateral or dorsal recumbency.
- Focal symmetrical encephalomalacia (FSE) in unvaccinated stock.
- Pasteurellosis (*Mannheimia haemolytica*).
- Clostridial enterotoxaemia.
- Per-acute gangrenous mastitis (*Pasteurella* spp. and *Staphylococcus aureus*).

Diagnosis

Careful clinical examination must exclude the common diseases listed under differential diagnoses. A diagnosis of hypomagnesaemia is based upon finding an hyperaesthetic, frequently laterally recumbent, ewe 4–8 weeks post lambing, grazing lush pasture with a serum magnesium concentration below 0.2 mmol/l.

Treatment

Because making an accurate diagnosis of hypomagnesaemia is difficult, the assessment of treatment protocols is problematic. Twenty to 40 ml of 25% magnesium sulphate should be injected subcutaneously in addition to 40 ml of 40% calcium borogluconate injected intravenously. Unlike cattle, there are no reports of sedation as part of the treatment protocol for hypomagnesaemia in sheep. There are no published reports of slow intravenous injection of magnesium/calcium combination products in sheep, unlike the situation in cattle.

Management/prevention/control measures

Unlike beef and dairy cattle, losses from hypomagnesaemia in sheep are uncommon in the UK and no special control measures are undertaken. It is recommended that early season fertilizer applications do not contain potash, thereby reducing potassium interference with magnesium absorption.

Economics

Hypomagnesaemia is not an important economic factor in sheep production in the UK.

PARASITIC DISEASES

GASTROINTESTINAL NEMATODE INFESTATIONS

Gastrointestinal nematode infestations comprise the most important group of conditions limiting intensive sheep production worldwide. Infestations range from acute disease with profuse diarrhoea and possible death (**Fig. 15.1**) to chronic disease with reduced performance (**Fig. 15.2**), extending to weight loss and emaciation. Nematode infestations raise concerns because of their prevalence, effects on production, very considerable control costs with reliance upon chemical control and animal welfare consequences. In many developed countries the growth of the organic food sector has highlighted the need for more integrated approaches to parasite control.

The major gastrointestinal nematode parasites in the UK are:

- *Teladorsagia circumcincta* and *Haemonchus contortus* in the abomasum.
- *Trichostrongylus vitrinus* in proximal small intestine.
- *Nematodirus battus* in the small intestine.

Gastrointestinal nematode infestations are a major problem in many sheep-producing countries but especially in Australia and other southern hemisphere countries, where widespread resistance to the three 'older' anthelmintic groups (Groups 1–3) poses serious challenges. Monepantel (Group 4-AD) and derquantel plus abamectin (Group 5-SI) anthelmintics have been introduced in the past 5 years with some disease modelling studies suggesting drug efficacy for the next 20 years.

In the UK, Groups 4 and 5 anthelmintics are classified POM-V, meaning that they can only be prescribed by a veterinary surgeon. Expert veterinary advice as part of the flock health plan is regarded as

critically important if these products are to retain their efficacy. However, such regulatory control over these products is regarded as too restrictive by the UK sheep industry and does not operate worldwide. Previous expert advice to rotate Group 1-3 anthelmintics annually to delay the development of anthelmintic resistance, widely promoted by the veterinary profession, is now regarded as having been wholly ineffective and possibly counter-productive.

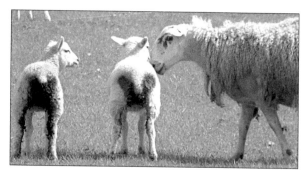

Fig. 15.1 Gastrointestinal nematode infestations, in this case nematodirosis, can cause acute disease with profuse diarrhoea and possible death.

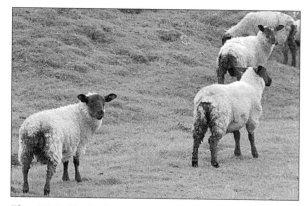

Fig. 15.2 Typically, parasitic gastroenteritis causes chronic disease with reduced performance and even weight loss.

There are nematode control programmes in operation in many countries, and within particular regions of those countries. In the UK the sustainable control of ovine parasites forum (SCOPS; www.scops.org.uk) disseminates expert advice to farmers and veterinary practitioners but studies have revealed a very poor uptake of these recommendations and there is concern that the refugia concept is far too complex for most farmers to understand fully and adopt.

In the UK (the example country in this particular section) the important parasitic infestations are:

- Nematodirosis affecting young lambs during late spring.
- Parasitic gastroenteritis (PGE) affecting growing lambs from mid-summer onwards.
- Liver fluke in sheep of all ages.

Nematodirosis in young lambs
Definition/overview
Nematodirosis is an important disease affecting young lambs, particularly during late spring when losses can be high before remedial action is taken.

Aetiology
Outbreaks of diarrhoea and sudden death occur in young lambs grazing pastures contaminated with large numbers of infective larvae that have synchronously hatched from eggs deposited by lambs during the previous grazing season. *Nematodirus battus* is much more pathogenic than *Nematodirus fillicolis* because of this synchronous hatching and massive larval challenge. As few as 2000 parasites cause clinical disease.

Clinical presentation
Only lambs are affected (**Fig. 15.3**); ewes do not show disease (**Fig. 15.4**). There is acute onset of profuse watery diarrhoea in 4–10-week-old lambs with faecal staining of the wool of the tail and perineum (**Fig. 15.5**). The lambs are dull and rapidly develop a gaunt appearance with obvious dehydration and condition loss. It is not unusual with severe larval challenge for 5% of lambs to die within a few days. Convalescence following anthelmintic treatment is protracted with affected lambs having a greatly extended period to market.

Differential diagnoses
The initial clinical presentation of severe larval challenge may be sudden death of young lambs without diarrhoea. In this situation the important differential diagnoses include pasteurellosis and pulpy kidney disease. More characteristically, the appearance of large numbers of lambs with profuse diarrhoea would suggest coccidiosis.

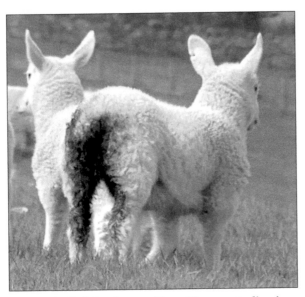

Fig. 15.3 Only lambs are affected by nematodirosis with acute onset of profuse watery diarrhoea.

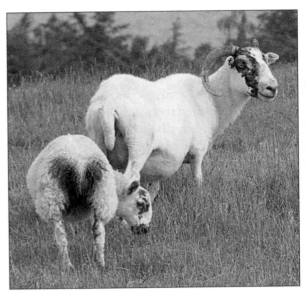

Fig. 15.4 Ewes are not affected by nematodirosis.

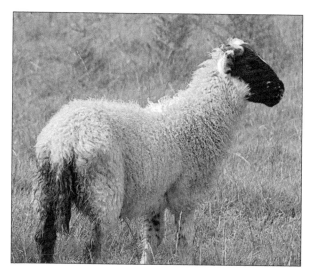

Fig. 15.5 Nematodirosis causes profuse watery diarrhoea in lambs with resultant faecal staining of the wool of the tail and perineum.

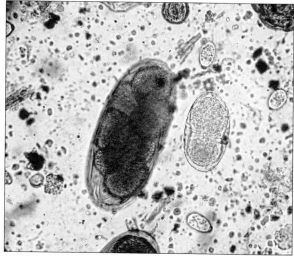

Fig. 15.6 Characteristic microscopic appearance of *Nematodirus battus* egg; brown colour and approximately three times larger than the strongyle egg present on the right-hand side of image.

Diagnosis

Faecal egg count monitoring (**Fig. 15.6**) to time *Nematodirus* treatments is too risky because acute disease is caused by developing larvae and adults before egg laying (prepatent infestation).

Postmortem examination may reveal very large numbers of developing larvae and adults within the lumen of the small intestine but often they have been expelled during the diarrhoeic phase. Confirmation of disease may necessitate microscopic examination of the small intestine.

Treatment

Sheep should be moved from infested pastures whenever possible. Anthelmintic resistance is not a problem with *N. battus* and a Group 1 anthelmintic (benzimidazoles; white drench) is commonly recommended because this group is of little use for other nematode parasites (**Fig. 15.7**). An alternative anthelmintic group should be administered if the faecal examination reveals other strongyle eggs such as *Teladorsagia* spp.

Administration of oral fluid therapy is possible but time-consuming for large numbers of lambs; intravenous fluid is not an option for logistical/cost reasons.

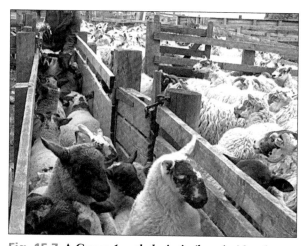

Fig. 15.7 A Group 1 anthelmintic (benzimidazole; white drench) is commonly recommended to treat nematodirosis.

Management/prevention/control measures

Prevention is based upon avoidance of pastures grazed by lambs during the previous grazing season because adult sheep are highly resistant to infection and only lambs produce significant numbers of eggs (**Fig. 15.8**).

The infective third stage larva (L3) is very resistant to desiccation and low temperatures and overwinters readily on pasture, still within the egg. After

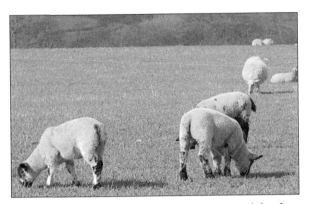

Fig. 15.8 To avoid nematodirosis do not stock lambs on pastures grazed by lambs during the previous season.

a period of cold exposure the L3 hatches once the maximum environmental temperature exceeds 10°C for several days. While this simultaneous hatch occurs every year on permanent pasture, nematodirosis only results when the mass hatch coincides with grazing activity of young susceptible lambs. Warm spring weather results in L3 larvae hatching en masse before lambs start grazing. While it has been demonstrated experimentally that young dairy calves can also act as hosts to *N. battus*, this epidemiology is very uncommon in practice.

Reducing patent *N. battus* infestations in lambs during the previous grazing season by regular anthelmintic treatments can limit the build-up of larval infection on pasture. This programme will not eliminate all egg deposition on pasture and anthelmintic prophylaxis remains necessary to avoid overt disease. The timing of anthelmintic prophylaxis is guided by environmental temperature during the spring. Typically, for lambs born from mid-March onwards (UK) in 'normal risk' years on contaminated pasture, anthelmintic treatments are given 3 weeks apart during May. In 'high-risk' years, three anthelmintic treatments are often given, extending the drenching period into June.

Economics
Chemical prophylaxis is relatively inexpensive (0.1–0.5% of the sale value of a lamb depending on the class of anthelmintic chosen) but drenching is time-consuming, especially when attempting

to gather large numbers of sheep from a semi-extensive grazing system. Reliance on chemical control raises environment and sustainability issues.

Welfare implications
Profuse diarrhoea in severe infestations may cause death and severe condition loss. While blowflies are not normally active in May in the UK, fleece contamination can persist and attract flies later in the grazing season.

Parasitic gastroenteritis of growing lambs
Definition/overview
Gastrointestinal nematode infestations are a major problem in many sheep-producing countries but especially in Australia and other southern hemisphere countries, where resistance to the three older anthelmintic groups (Group1 BZ, benzimidazoles; Group 2 LV, levamisole; Group 3 ML, macrocyclic lactones) poses serious challenges. Monepantel (Group 4-AD, amino-acetonitrile derivative) and derquantel (Group 5-SI spiroindoles) anthelmintics have been introduced in the past 5 years. Derquantel and abamectin are marketed together as a dual active product.

Diarrhoea with faecal contamination of the fleece attracts blowflies, which leads to cutaneous myiasis. Many countries have developed integrated nematode control programmes that are specific to their grazing and climatic conditions and such specialist advice should be consulted first and foremost. In most situations, the farmer's own veterinary surgeon is best placed to advise their client after consulting regional forecasts. This section deals in general terms with parasite control in the UK and may not be applicable to other situations where different host/parasite/climate relationships exist.

Aetiology
In the UK the important genera causing PGE are *Teladorsagia* (formerly *Ostertagia*) and *Trichostrongylus* (nematodirosis has been described above). In many countries *Haemonchus contortus* is a serious threat to intensive sheep production.

Clinical presentation

Infestations usually cause profuse diarrhoea, leading to dehydration and reduced performance and extending to considerable weight loss and emaciation. In haemonchosis the most important clinical sign is anaemia. The severity of clinical signs of parasitism depends on the age of the host, the current nutritional status (especially protein intake), the immune status of the animal, the trace element status and genotype. The classical signs of PGE are observed in growing lambs exposed to large numbers of infective larvae on contaminated pasture during warm wet summer months.

Teladorsagiosis: Disease (type I) is typically seen in growing lambs, with diarrhoea, dehydration and reduced weight gain/condition loss (**Figs 15.9, 15.10**). Weight loss results from a number of factors including reduced appetite, changes in the abomasal wall with loss of mature functional cells and protein loss across the compromised mucosa.

Another form of the disease has been described (type II) but its importance has not been fully investigated on commercial sheep farms. Type II disease occurs during late winter when large numbers of hypobiotic larvae emerge simultaneously from the gastric glands.

Haemonchosis: As a consequence of *H. contortus* feeding on blood, haemonchosis presents with anaemia (**Fig. 15.11**), submandibular oedema (**Fig. 15.12**), and increased heart and respiratory rates; diarrhoea is not a feature of this nematode infestation (**Fig. 15.13**).

Ingestion of large numbers of larvae over a short period of time causes acute disease with lethargy, weakness and rapid loss of condition. This form of the disease is more commonly seen in growing lambs. Ingestion of smaller numbers of infective stages over several weeks to months causes a more general loss of condition, which progresses to emaciation.

Trichostrongylosis: Trichostrongylosis is normally seen during early winter and affects 8–10-month-old lambs (**Figs 15.14, 15.15**) but also yearlings and adult sheep. The most prominent clinical feature

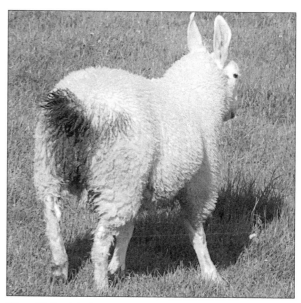

Fig. 15.9 Teladorsagiosis is typically seen in growing lambs with diarrhoea, dehydration and reduced weight gain.

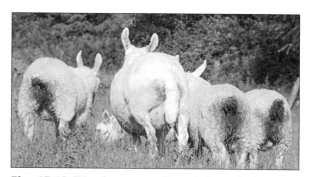

Fig. 15.10 Diarrhoea caused by teladorsagiosis affecting lambs grazing permanent pasture.

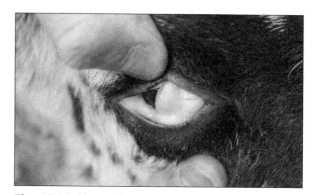

Fig. 15.11 Sheep affected by haemonchosis present with anaemia.

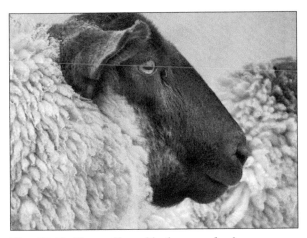

Fig. 15.12 Sheep affected by haemonchosis may present with submandibular oedema.

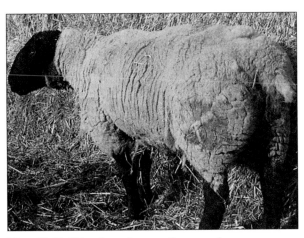

Fig. 15.13 Diarrhoea is not a feature of haemonchosis.

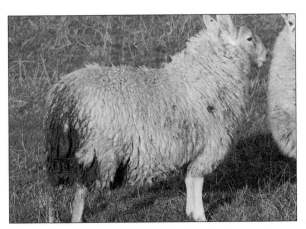

Fig. 15.14 Trichostrongylosis is seen during early winter and typically affects 8–10-month-old lambs.

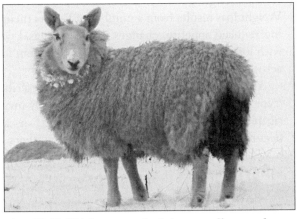

Fig. 15.15 Trichostrongylosis is normally seen during early winter when many farmers are not thinking about parasitism.

is profuse dark-coloured, foul-smelling diarrhoea with copious mucus present in the worst affected sheep. Other sheep in the group are less severely affected but have lost weight and present in poor condition.

Differential diagnoses

Teladorsagiosis and trichostrongylosis

- On a group/flock basis the common causes of poor growth/weight loss include poor grazing conditions and overgrazing, especially during adverse weather.
- Trace elements act synergistically with chronic parasitism to cause poor growth and it

may prove difficult to determine the primary cause.

- Cobalt (vitamin B12) status should be monitored in the group.
- Selenium status should be investigated in geographically deficient areas.
- Salmonellosis and yersiniosis should be considered in the differential diagnosis of trichostrongylosis.

Haemonchosis

- On a group/flock basis the common presenting features of peripheral oedema, anaemia and chronic weight loss must be differentiated from chronic fasciolosis, although the seasonal occurrence of these infestations differs markedly (summer versus winter, respectively).

- Other chronic nematode infestations can also cause weight loss but with diarrhoea.
- On an individual basis, adult sheep with paratuberculosis typically present with chronic weight loss, mild anaemia, absence of diarrhoea and submandibular oedema in some advanced cases.
- Numerous chronic bacterial infections result in weight loss extending to emaciation.

Diagnosis

Teladorsagiosis and trichostrongylosis: Faecal egg counts are routinely used to aid diagnosis of nematode infestations but they have inherent limitations. Due to numerous factors the faecal egg count may not accurately indicate the adult nematode population present within the gastrointestinal tract at that time. Pathology is most often caused by developing larval stages before infestations become patent, and also by hypobiotic stages.

It is not easy to differentiate members of the trichostrongyle genera *Teladorsagia*, *Trichostrongylus*, *Haemonchus* and *Cooperia* on examination of their eggs in a McMaster preparation. Differentiation necessitates specialized coproculture and identification of L3 larvae on the appearance of the tail. By identifying the eggs only as trichostrongyles, it is possible for less pathogenic species to make a disproportionate contribution to the total egg count. As a general rule, a trichostrongyle egg count of 400 epg is considered moderate while 700–1000 epg is considered high and worthy of anthelmintic treatment.

Gross postmortem examination of the abomasal surface can be undertaken for *Teladorsagia* and *Haemonchus* worms.

Haemonchosis: Identification of anaemia is a reliable indicator of haemonchosis in countries with endemic disease (FAMACHA system), whereby sheep are selected for anthelmintic treatment on the basis of ocular mucous membrane colour assessed against a colour guided chart (scale 1–5; normal pink mucous membranes to white). This highly practical assessment guides treatment and reduces the number of sheep treated with an anthelmintic,

thereby selecting for more resilient animals; sheep requiring regular treatments should be considered for culling. Such targeted anthelmintic treatment has been adopted against other nematode species based upon growth rate rather than anaemia, and has many advantages with respect to reducing the risk of selecting nematode species resistant to anthelmintics.

Faecal worm egg counts are often very high in patent *Haemonchus* spp. infestations, with counts >10,000 epg not uncommon. At necropsy very large numbers of adults are visible on the surface of the abomasum of untreated sheep.

Treatment

Treatment involves the use of an effective anthelmintic (see also Anthelmintic resistance). All drugs within a class have a similar mode of action. The five major anthelmintic classes, defined by the active chemical, comprise:

- Group 1-BZ benzimidazoles, probenzimidazoles (white wormers). Benzimidazoles such as albendazole and fenbendazole have a similar mode of action. Febantel, netobimin and thiophanate are probenzimidazoles, which are converted to benzimidazoles in the body.
- Group 2-LM imidazothiazoles, tetrahydropyrimidines (yellow wormers). Levamisole and tetramisole are imidazothiazoles. Morantel and pyrantel are tetrahydropyrimidines.
- Group 3-AV avermectins, milbemycins (clear wormers). Preparations that contain avermectins include doramectin and ivermectin, and milbemycins such as moxidectin.
- Group 4-AD monepantel (orange wormers).
- Group 5-SI derquantel and abamectin (dual active) (purple wormers).

Closantel and nitroxynil can be used in situations where *H. contortus* is the major parasite.

Drenching practice: It is essential that a representative number of sheep are weighed before treatment and treatment is based on the heaviest sheep in the group. If there is a large range of weights, consider subdividing the group, for example when there are

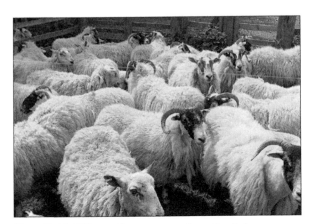

Fig. 15.16 Where there are two breeds of sheep present with different weights the farm should consider subdividing the group to ensure accurate dosing.

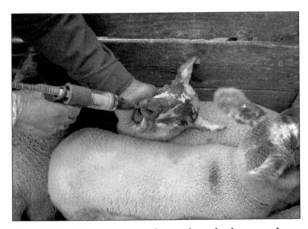

Fig. 15.17 Sheep are not always drenched correctly; there is the risk that this lamb will jump forward causing pharyngeal injury.

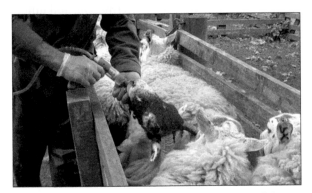

Fig. 15.18 The ewe's head should be restrained from behind with the nozzle of the drenching gun carefully placed over the back of the tongue (not as shown).

two breeds of sheep present with different weights (**Fig. 15.16**).

- Calibrate drenching guns using a syringe.
- Maintain drenching guns in good working order.
- Restrain sheep in a raceway and carefully place the nozzle of the drenching gun over the back of the tongue and discharge the contents slowly. Sheep are not always drenched correctly (**Figs 15.17, 15.18**).

Management/prevention/control measures

Experts emphasize the need for sustainable parasite control programmes written by veterinary surgeons for individual farms based upon their unique circumstances and management. It is accepted that once pastures have become heavily contaminated with infective nematode larvae it is almost impossible to achieve good lamb growth rates. Repeated anthelmintic treatments, even at short intervals, do not prevent such poor performance because it is the continuous larval challenge from pasture that causes much of the poor performance and not simply the adults within the gastrointestinal tract. It is therefore essential to reduce larval challenge to susceptible sheep as much as possible whilst at the same time enabling the establishment of a protective immunity. With traditional management of sheep on permanent pasture in the UK, PGE in growing lambs results from ingestion of very large numbers of infective larvae from the pasture during mid-summer. *Teladorsagia circumcincta*, and in warmer areas *H. contortus*, larvae appear first in the summer months with *Trichostrongylus* spp. appearing during the autumn.

Pasture larvae arise from two sources:

- Periparturient rise in ewe faecal egg output.
- Over-wintered L3 on pasture.

Periparturient rise in ewe faecal egg output: The periparturient relaxation of host immunity permits a significant increase in nematode egg production during the last few weeks of gestation that may persist until 8 weeks post lambing (**Fig. 15.19**). This reduction in host immunity is influenced by numerous factors including ewe body condition, nutritional status and litter size. Reduction in host immunity can be

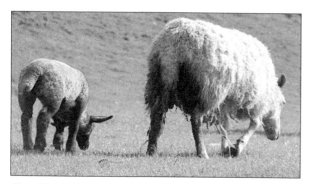

Fig. 15.19 Periparturient relaxation of host immunity causing diarrhoea may persist until 8 weeks post lambing.

largely overcome by dietary undegradable digestible protein supplementation but this is costly. Under suitable environmental conditions eggs develop to infective larvae within 3 weeks but maximum levels may not be present on the pasture for up to 6 weeks. These infective larvae are the major source of infestation for young lambs.

Over-wintered L3 on pasture: Young lambs may also ingest over-wintered infective larvae from pasture and these develop to adult nematodes. The large numbers of eggs produced by adult nematodes resident in the gastrointestinal tract of young lambs results in the appearance of significant numbers of infective larvae on pasture during mid-summer ('mid-summer rise'). Clinical parasitism results unless appropriate action is taken.

Use of prophylactic anthelmintics

Periparturient rise in faecal egg output: Anthelmintic treatment to prevent the periparturient rise in egg output by ewes can be given at various times depending on the farm management system (e.g. when housing ewes during mid-gestation, at the same time as vaccination against the clostridial diseases 4–6 weeks prior to lambing, or immediately prior to turnout to pasture when lambs are 1–2 days old). The aim of anthelmintic treatment of ewes around lambing time is to reduce pasture contamination with eggs and subsequent larval challenge to lambs.

It is important that the anthelmintic chosen to counter the periparturient rise is effective against hypobiotic larval stages. To gain maximum benefit

from the residual activity of drugs such as moxidectin, ewes should be drenched/injected at turnout to pasture with their lambs rather than at housing; this affords up to 7–11 weeks' residual action. The importance of good ewe nutrition during early lactation should not be underestimated with respect to parasitic gastroenteritis. In addition, ewes that are well fed also produce more milk, so the lambs reach market weight before the peak of the mid-summer pasture larval challenge.

Ewes grazing contaminated pastures: Ewes grazing contaminated pastures may need a persistent anthelmintic treatment to prevent immediate re-infection from the pasture. All adult sheep should be treated in these circumstances.

Ewes turned out onto clean pasture: Ewes turned out onto clean pasture after lambing only require a short acting anthelmintic treatment. Consider leaving ewes in good body condition nursing single lambs untreated; these ewes probably have the lowest parasite burdens and shed fewest parasite eggs but this practice should reduce the selection pressure for anthelmintic resistance by allowing some contamination of pasture by susceptible strains.

Nematodirosis: The timing of early season prophylactic anthelmintic administration to control nematodirosis in lambs has been discussed earlier but essentially it comprises a strategic anthelmintic drench depending on weather data. While these disease forecasts are reasonably accurate, local factors may operate with the result that two drenches are often given to lambs grazing contaminated pasture 2–3 weeks apart from early May (UK).

Other gastrointestinal parasites: Control from mid-summer onwards is based on susceptible lambs not grazing potentially heavily infested pastures (**Fig. 15.20**). Avoidance of infested pastures from July onwards can be integrated into most farm management systems by moving weaned lambs on to hay or silage aftermaths from mid-June onwards (**Fig. 15.21**) or to re-seeded pasture (**Fig. 15.22**). On some mixed farms it may be possible to rotate pastures annually between cattle and sheep (**Fig. 15.23**) and operate a 'modified' 2-year safe grazing system.

Where there are no alternatives and lambs graze heavily infested pastures throughout the summer months, anthelmintics have been administered at approximately monthly intervals to reduce pasture contamination; however, lamb performance will still be adversely affected by developing larvae. This approach is unsustainable and a more responsible and sustainable use of anthelmintics must be

developed as part of the farmer's veterinary flock health plan.

Where lambs graze permanent grassland, anthelmintic treatments can be based upon growth rate (**Fig. 15.24**) and the adoption of strategic targeted treatments when lambs fail to record target gains. While such a policy of targeted anthelmintic treatments is time-consuming it results in far fewer treatments (around 40% in some studies) and slows the rate of selection for anthelmintic resistance

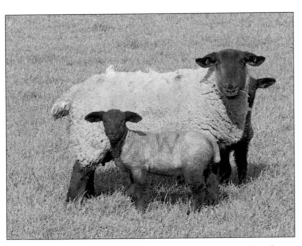

Fig. 15.20 Lambs grazing clean pastures – prior farm planning is essential.

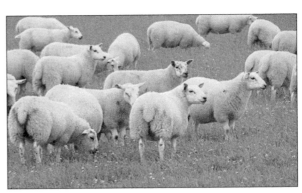

Fig. 15.21 Avoidance of infested pastures from July onwards can be achieved by moving weaned lambs on to hay or silage aftermaths.

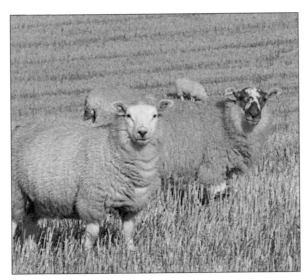

Fig. 15.22 Farm planning must ensure full use of re-seeded pasture in parasite control programmes.

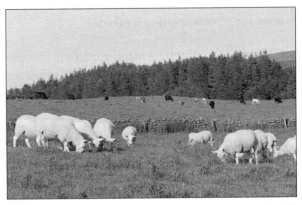

Fig. 15.23 On mixed livestock farms pastures should be rotated annually between cattle and sheep where possible.

by ensuring susceptible parasite strains in refugia. Treating only those lambs with evidence of diarrhoea (**Fig. 15.25**) and/or poor performance as selection criteria could be considered where regular weight recording is not possible. Electronic identification tags and automatic weighing greatly facilitate recording and selection of lambs for anthelmintic treatment. Such automation will become increasingly common over the next decade.

Grazing heavily contaminated pasture with reliance on repeated chemical prophylaxis/treatment is unsustainable, and lambs fail to grow to their potential under such management. A more integrated pasture management policy is much more preferable, cheaper, and yields better growth rates.

Economics

The major cost of nematode infestations is lost production in terms of lower fleece weight and poorer quality wool, and poorer live weight gain with an extended interval to marketing.

Nematode control is expensive in terms of drugs and labour (**Fig. 15.26**). The appearance of resistance to certain anthelmintics in many countries has placed almost total reliance on newer, more expensive anthelmintics.

Welfare implications

Nematode infestations can lead to severe loss of body condition and emaciation with obvious welfare concerns. Diarrhoea with faecal contamination of the

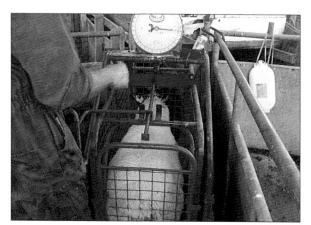

Fig. 15.24 Targeted anthelmintic treatment can be based upon growth rate; this lamb is growing well and there is no evidence of significant parasitism; therefore, anthelmintic treatment is not needed.

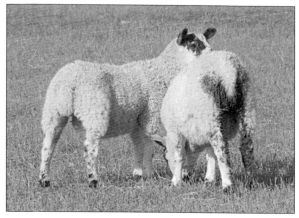

Fig. 15.25 Anthelmintic treatment of only those lambs with evidence of diarrhoea could be considered where regular weighing is not possible.

Fig. 15.26 Nematode control is expensive in terms of drugs and labour and a more integrated approach is necessary on many farms.

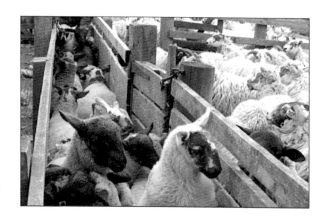

fleece surrounding the perineum is a major risk factor for cutaneous myiasis.

Anthelmintic resistance

Anthelmintic resistance has been defined as the heritable ability of a parasite to tolerate a normally effective dose of anthelmintic. Gene(s) conferring resistance to an anthelmintic may be present at a very low frequency within a nematode population. Utilization of that anthelmintic alone leaves only resistant nematodes, with the appearance of clinical disease once the resistant adult nematode population exceeds a threshold. It is imperative that these resistant alleles are not afforded any survival advantage as a consequence of unnecessary anthelmintic treatments and poor farm management.

Once resistance to a member of an anthelmintic group has emerged, that group of drugs can no longer be used to control PGE in that flock. Anthelmintic resistance may first manifest simply as poor growth in lambs before diarrhoea, and possibly death, occur in the flock. However, gastrointestinal nematodes can still be adequately controlled by integration of strategic anthelmintic treatments into an evasive farm management policy.

Since the mid 1980s, anthelmintic resistance has become a very important issue in many intensive sheep production systems, particularly in southern hemisphere countries such as Australia, many South American countries and South Africa. This demographic emergence of anthelmintic resistance is related to intensive management practices, often using irrigated pastures, and climatic conditions that permit a greater number of nematode generations per annum compared with western European countries. Resistance to benzimidazoles has been recognized as widespread in the UK and resistance to all members of the anthelmintic Groups 1–3 ('triple' or 'multiple resistance') has been identified since 2001.

Various strategies have been recommended to delay the progress of anthelmintic resistance; some strategies, such as annual rotation between Groups 1–3 anthelmintics adopted in the 1990s, appear to have been much less successful than predicted.

Detection: The emergence of anthelmintic resistance in a nematode population on a particular sheep enterprise can easily be overlooked because clinical signs may be limited to reduced performance and diarrhoea rather than mortality. The most common technique to detect anthelmintic resistance on a sheep farm is the faecal egg count reduction test. Individual faecal egg counts are undertaken on 10–15 animals, which are then weighed and drenched with the recommended volume of anthelmintic. The individual faecal egg counts are repeated 10 days later. Failure to effect a reduction in geometric faecal count greater than 95% strongly suggests the presence of resistance to that anthelmintic group although production losses may not be evident until efficacy falls below 80%.

In-vitro egg hatch assays can be used to identify benzimidazole resistance.

Control strategies

Effective treatment

- All drenching/injection equipment must be regularly calibrated.
- Sheep must be weighed and the dose rate calculated for the heaviest group members, not the average.
- Withholding feed has been recommended when using Group 1-BZ and 3-AV drenches because reduced rumen fill delays passage of the drug. This fasted state often exists in sheep transported to market, purchased then transported to their destination; therefore, drenching on arrival is strongly recommended rather than after a few days' delay when pasture contamination could have resulted. Administration of low volume formulations may also increase the likelihood of anthelmintic drench deposition into the rumen.

Management practices to delay the onset of anthelmintic resistance in UK flocks are not clearly defined. Most recommendations are based on theoretical principles, or on practical experience of anthelmintic resistance in Australia, New Zealand and South Africa, where sheep management and the epidemiology of PGE may not reflect the situation in the UK.

The selection pressure for anthelmintic resistance is influenced by:

- The frequency and timing of anthelmintic treatment.
- The anthelmintic dose rate.
- Drug efficacy.
- The life expectancy and fecundity of the adult nematodes.
- The proportion of the susceptible population exposed to the anthelmintic compared with that on pasture (in refugia).
- The parasite generation time.

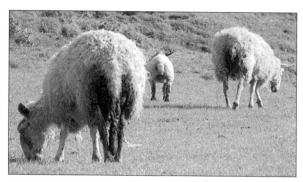

Fig. 15.27 Ewe treatments should be targeted at eliminating the periparturient rise in egg output.

Reduction in treatment frequency: Fewer treatments necessitate a more structured approach than presently operated by many farmers and adoption of more fully integrated grazing programmes. For example, in many UK sheep flocks, ewe treatments should be targeted at eliminating the periparturient rise in egg output (**Fig. 15.27**); prebreeding treatments are largely unnecessary.

In growing lambs, movement on to clean grazing can avoid the mid-summer challenge from large numbers of infective larvae on permanent pasture. Anthelmintic treatment at the time of movement is causing concern because of the risk posed by only resistant worms remaining after anthelmintic treatment and contaminating the 'safe' or 'clean' grazing. By removing all susceptible strains, only resistant nematode strains remain. It has been recommended that 5–10% of the strongest lambs should be left untreated (**Fig. 15.28**) to dilute the effects of potentially emerging resistant strains on clean grazing where there may be few, if any, susceptible parasites in refugia.

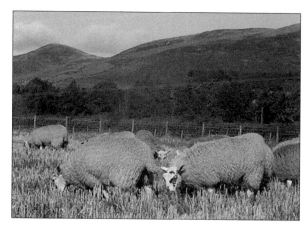

Fig. 15.28 Approximately 5–10% of the strongest lambs could be left untreated when moved on to clean grazing.

Many farmers routinely treat ewes with an anthelmintic prior to the mating season but this is unnecessary in most flocks (**Fig. 15.29**). It would suffice to treat only those ewes with diarrhoea and in poorer body condition than other sheep in the group (see **Figs 15.30–15.33**).

On the contrary, rams are often neglected in parasite control programmes (**Fig. 15.34**) but are highly susceptible to PGE and regular monitoring of faecal worm egg count (FWEC) is recommended as part of the whole flock parasite control strategy.

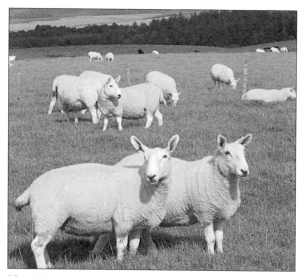

Fig. 15.29 It is not necessary to treat all ewes with an anthelmintic prior to the mating season.

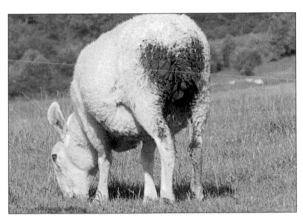
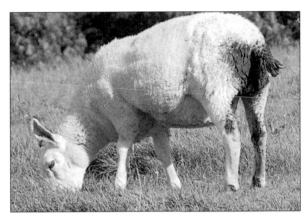

Figs 15.30, 15.31 Anthelmintic treatments should be targeted at those ewes with diarrhoea and in poorer body condition.

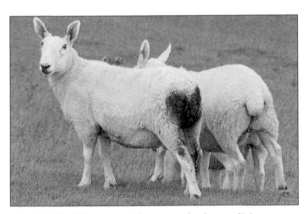

Fig. 15.32 The ewe with poorer body condition and diarrhoea (on the left) should be treated with an anthelmintic; the ewe on the right should remain untreated.

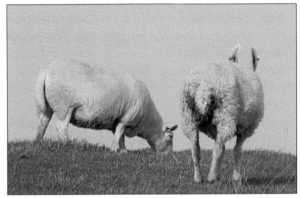

Fig. 15.33 The ewe with poorer body condition and diarrhoea (on the right) should be treated with an anthelmintic; the ewe on the left should remain untreated.

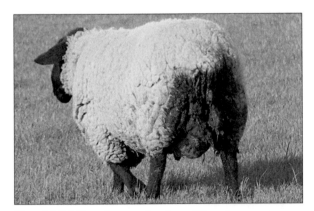

Fig. 15.34 Regular monitoring of faecal worm egg counts of the ram stud is often overlooked on sheep farms.

Testing for anthelmintic resistance: The faecal egg count reduction test (FECRT) is a reliable test for resistance to each of the anthelmintic groups. Approximately 10 sheep are randomly allocated to each of control or treatment groups (one group for each class of anthelmintics to be tested). A FWEC is then undertaken for all sheep and repeated 10 days later for Group 2-LV sheep and 14 days later for control sheep and Groups 1-BZ and 3-ML (there is no known resistance for 4-AD and 5-SI groups in the UK at present); these specific timings are not essential and it may be impractical to handle sheep twice in quick succession. Anthelmintic resistance is suspected where the mean FWEC is less than 95% of the percentage reduction in the control group.

Bioassays for anthelmintics belonging to Groups 1 and 2 are available but not yet commonly used in practice.

Anthelmintic treatment of introduced sheep – quarantine treatments: All introduced sheep should be assumed to be potential sources of multiple anthelmintic resistance and be treated with an effective anthelmintic or combination of products upon arrival. These animals should then be yarded for 48 hours to ensure that any viable nematode parasite eggs have been voided before they are turned onto pastures which might be grazed by sheep within the next 6 months. After quarantine treatment, sheep should be turned out onto pasture that has been grazed by sheep this season so that any parasites left after treatment make up a very small percentage of an otherwise (assumed) susceptible population.

The current SCOPS recommendations are to use a combination of anthelmintic drugs with different mechanisms of action. Quarantine arrangements are essential to reduce the risk of introducing anthelmintic-resistance worms of species such as *H. contortus* and *T. circumcincta.* Current best practice involves sequential full dose treatments with either 4-AD monepantel (Zolvix) or 5-SI derquantel and abamectin (Startec) and moxidectin. All introduced sheep should be grazed separately from the main flock for at least 1 month. This quarantine period allows inspection for a range of diseases that can be introduced onto the farm but are not visible at sale such as sheep scab, lice, and footrot.

Goats are a serious risk for nematodes with multiple anthelmintic resistance and must never be grazed with sheep.

Misuse of liver fluke and anthelmintic combination products: There are several flukicide and anthelmintic combination products marketed for both liver fluke and PGE treatment. Use of these combination products at the wrong time of year for nematode control simply introduces an extra unnecessary treatment which will accelerate selection for anthelmintic resistance nematode species.

TAPEWORM (CESTODE) INFESTATIONS

Sheep as the final host
Definition/overview
Tapeworms with their adult stage in sheep occur in all major sheep-producing areas but they are of no clinical concern. Segments of tapeworms are often seen in the faeces of young growing lambs in the UK (**Fig. 15.35**) but they exert no adverse effects on growth rate.

Aetiology
Only the genus *Monezia* occurs in the UK. Free-living oribatid mites act as the intermediate stage.

Clinical presentation
Tapeworm segments are readily recognized in faeces of young lambs as white ribbon-like structures up to 10 mm wide.

Diagnosis
Diagnosis is based on the finding of tapeworm segments in the faeces.

Treatment
Treatment is not considered necessary because tapeworms are non-pathogenic. Only members of the benzimadazole group (1-BZ) are effective against adult tapeworms.

Management/prevention/control measures
No control measures are necessary for tapeworms.

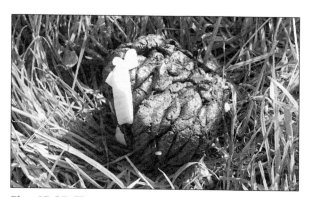

Fig. 15.35 Tapeworm segments are often seen in the faeces of growing lambs but are of no clinical significance.

Sheep as the intermediate host

Definition/overview

Sheep also act as the intermediate host for cestode parasites that have dogs as their definitive host. Cestode infestation causes no disease in the dog but these infestations are important because of their space-occupying nature in the case of the intermediate (metacestode) stage of *Taenia multiceps*. Ovine cysticercosis caused by the intermediate stages of *T. ovis* and *T. hydatigea* may result in carcase condemnation in very heavy infestations.

Aetiology

The intermediate stage of *T. multiceps* infection is *Coenurus cerebralis* with cyst(s) developing in the brain. *Cysticercus tenuicollis* is the intermediate stage of *T. hydatigea* infection, while *C. ovis* is the intermediate stage of *T. ovis*.

Clinical presentation

The clinical signs of coenurosis (gid) are presented in Chapter 8, Neurological Diseases. Ovine cysticercosis causes no clinical signs but may be a common cause of rejection of the heart and liver, and perhaps the whole carcase, at meat inspection. *C. tenuicollis* appears as cysts attached to the omentum, liver and serosal surfaces (**Figs 15.36, 15.37**). Excessive scarring of the liver capsule (hepatitis cysticercosa) can result in liver condemnation. *C. ovis* is reported to be a common cause of rejection of ovine hearts during meat inspection although severe infestations can result in whole carcase rejection.

Diagnosis

Diagnosis is based upon the finding of tapeworm cysts at meat inspection.

Treatment

There is no treatment of the intermediate (metacestode) stages.

Management/prevention/control measures

Control measures are based upon regular cestode treatment of dogs, prevention of faecal contamination of sheep feed stores and immediate proper disposal of all sheep carcases.

FASCIOLOSIS

(syn. liver fluke)

Definition/overview

Fasciolosis is a major parasitic disease of sheep in many countries worldwide. This section relates to disease caused by *Fasciola hepatica* as it presents in the UK. Acute and subacute fasciolosis have become major problems in areas of the country where such infestations had not been seen for decades, caused by sheep movements,

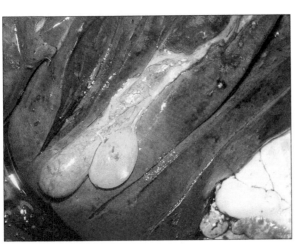

Fig. 15.36 *Cysticercus tenuicollis* attached to the liver capsule.

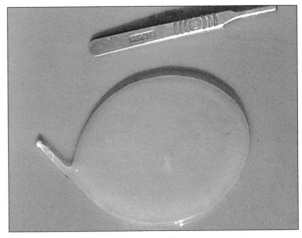

Fig. 15.37 *Cysticercus tenuicollis* may extend to 8–10 cm in diameter.

poor biosecurity measures and changing weather patterns with consecutive wet summers. In certain countries of the world, *F. gigantica* and *Dicrocoelium dentriticum* are important.

Aetiology

F. hepatica has the liver as its site of infection in both cattle (**Fig. 15.38**) and sheep (**Fig. 15.39**). The intermediate stages involve snails of the genus Lymnaea, mostly *Galba truncatula*. The important stages of the life cycle of *F. hepatica* require moisture and an environmental temperature above 10°C. Essentially, late spring/early summer infestation of snails by miracidia results in an autumn metacercariae challenge to sheep, with immediate acute disease, subacute disease over the following weeks (**Figs 15.40, 15.41**) or chronic disease apparent several months later (**Figs 15.42, 15.43**), depending on the level of challenge.

Clinical presentation

Acute fasciolosis: During a wet summer grazing sheep can ingest very large numbers of metacercariae over several days with invasion of the liver parenchyma causing acute disease. Affected sheep die suddenly from haemorrhage and liver damage, with the first evidence of a problem being sudden deaths in previously healthy sheep from August to December. Inspection of others in the group reveals lethargy and reduced grazing activity. Gathering

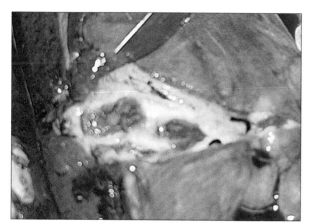

Fig. 15.38 The liver fluke *Fasciola hepatica* infests cattle as well as sheep.

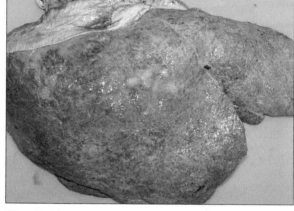

Fig. 15.39 Necropsy finding of severe subacute fasciolosis in a sheep.

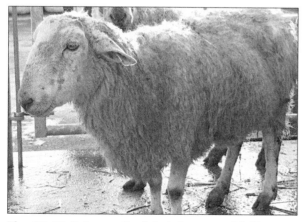

Fig. 15.40 Subacute fasciolosis has caused dullness, inappetance with reduced rumen fill and marked weight loss over 7–10 days.

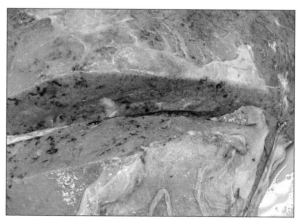

Fig. 15.41 Necropsy findings of subacute fasciolosis (see Fig. 15.40).

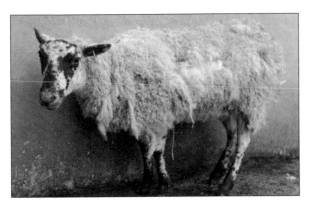

Fig. 15.42 Emaciation, reduced rumen fill and very poor fleece quality caused by chronic fasciolosis.

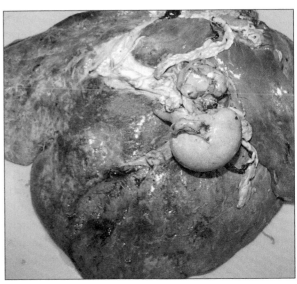

Fig. 15.43 Necropsy findings of chronic fasciolosis with enlarged hepatic lymph nodes (see Fig. 15.42).

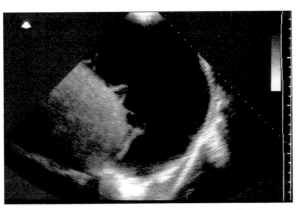

Fig. 15.44 Sonogram of the right anterior abdomen; there is marked accumulation of inflammatory exudates with fibrin deposits on the liver capsule caused by migrating immature flukes (see Fig. 15.45).

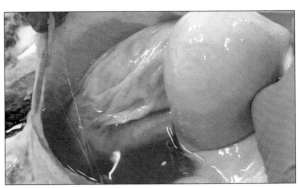

Fig. 15.45 Necropsy confirms a large volume of inflammatory exudate and fibrin tags in the abdomen.

may prove difficult because the sheep are reluctant to run. Closer examination reveals pale mucous membranes. Liver enlargement and ascites/peritoneal exudate have been described (**Fig. 15.44, 15.45**).

Subacute fasciolosis: Subacute fasciolosis results from ingestion of metacercariae over several weeks/months. The major presenting clinical findings are rapid weight loss causing very poor body condition score and poor fleece quality despite adequate flock nutrition. Losses typically occur from December onwards but may be much earlier (October) with

severe challenge. Affected sheep show marked anaemia, most noticeably affecting the conjunctivae. Liver enlargement is reported but is not easy to appreciate during clinical examination. Ascites cannot usually be appreciated clinically without recourse to ultrasonographic examination, except in extreme cases.

Typically, some sheep in the group present with severe depression, inappetence and weakness and may be unable to stand (**Fig. 15.46**). Body condition is very poor but contrasts with abdominal distension due to fluid accumulation. The sheep have a painful expression and gentle palpation of the anterior

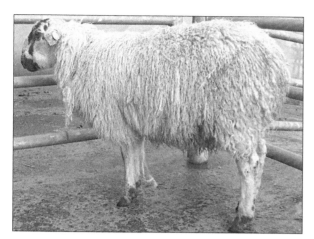

Fig. 15.46 Subacute fasciolosis; this sheep presents with severe depression, inappetence and weakness.

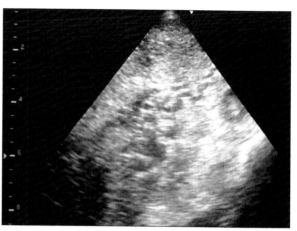

Fig. 15.47 Sonogram of sheep with subacute fasciolosis reveals complete loss of the normal ultrasonographic appearance of the liver.

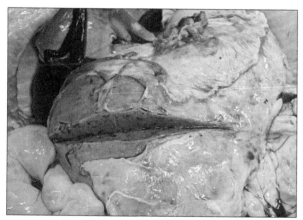

Fig. 15.48 Extensive fibrin deposits on the liver capsule of a sheep with subacute fasciolosis.

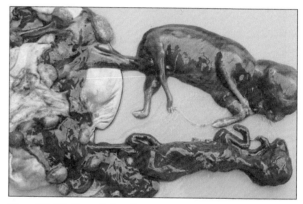

Fig. 15.49 Foetal death/resorption is seen after severe liver fluke infestation, which causes high barren rates and a much lower scanning percentage.

abdomen reveals obvious pain, which is markedly unusual in sheep where their naturally stoic nature reveals little.

Ultrasonographic examination has revealed dramatic reaction to migrating flukes in some sheep, with considerable peritoneal exudate and fibrinous adhesions between the liver and the body wall (**Fig. 15.45**). There is also loss of normal liver architecture (**Fig. 15.47**). The liver capsule has a hyperechoic appearance due to fibrin deposition. Necropsy fully reveals the extent of the peritoneal exudate and fibrinous reaction (**Fig. 15.48**).

Foetal death/resorption (**Fig. 15.49**) causing high barren rates and much lower litter size is reported after severe liver fluke infestation. Indeed, where disease has not been seen before, very poor scanning results may be the first indication that there is a serious liver fluke problem on the farm; this may be limited to only one group of sheep depending upon their autumn/winter grazing.

Chronic fasciolosis: The major clinical findings are low body condition score and poor fleece quality despite an appropriate ration (**Fig. 15.50**). There is submandibular oedema in many sheep (**Figs 15.51, 15.52**). Affected sheep show marked anaemia (**Fig. 15.53**) with packed cell volume (PCV) values as low as 0.06 l/l. Affected sheep may die in

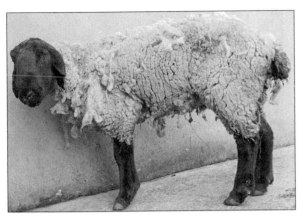

Fig. 15.50 The major clinical findings of chronic fasciolosis are emaciation and very poor fleece quality.

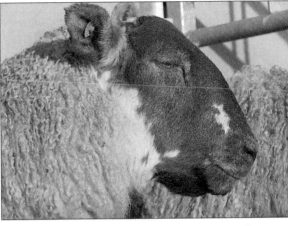

Fig. 15.51 Submandibular oedema is present in many sheep with chronic fasciolosis.

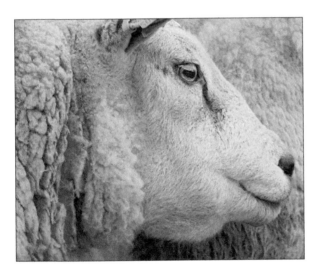

Fig. 15.52 Submandibular oedema is present in a Texel ram with chronic fasciolosis.

an emaciated state, especially when infestation is compounded by the metabolic demands of advanced gestation/early lactation.

Differential diagnoses

Differential diagnoses of sudden death caused by acute fasciolosis and, less commonly, subacute fasciolosis are:

- Clostridial disease: pulpy kidney disease, black-leg, black disease, braxy.
- Pasteurellosis or other septicaemic disease secondary to tick-borne fever.
- Louping-ill.
- Abdominal catastrophe, e.g. volvulus of the abomasum or small intestine.

- Poisoning (e.g. nitrate or ammonia).
- Acidosis if fed grain.

Differential diagnoses of emaciation resulting from subacute and chronic fasciolosis include:

- Group problem:
  - Poor flock nutrition.
  - Chronic parasitism including anthelmintic-resistant strains.
  - Footrot.
  - Cobalt deficiency (lambs).
- Individual problem:
  - Paratuberculosis.
  - Chronic suppurative pneumonia or other septic focus.

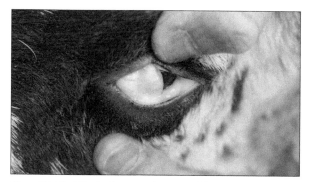

Fig. 15.53 Marked anaemia caused by chronic fasciolosis.

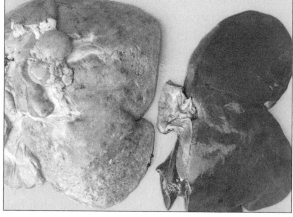

Fig. 15.54 The liver is grossly enlarged in subacute fasciolosis (normal liver on right).

- Poor dentition, especially cheek teeth.
- Chronic severe lameness.
- Ovine pulmonary adenocarcinoma.
- Visceral form of caseous lymphadenitis.
- Intestinal adenocarcinoma.
- Visna.

Diagnosis

Acute fasciolosis: Diagnosis of acute fasciolosis is based on the epidemiological data (high-risk year) and massively raised liver enzymes (e.g. aspartate transaminase, AST), indicating acute liver insult, and is confirmed at necropsy of sudden deaths.

Subacute fasciolosis: Subacute fasciolosis can be diagnosed by raised serum AST and glutamate dehydrogenase (GLDH) concentrations. Increased serum gamma glutamyl transferase (GGT) concentrations, which indicate bile duct damage, are also commonly used to establish the diagnosis. These three liver enzymes are typically increased 5–30-fold but, in the case of AST, fall to near normal concentrations within 10–14 days of flukicide treatment. Serum GGT and GLDH remain elevated for at least 1 month after flukicide treatment and are therefore the biochemical determinations of choice for subacute fasciolosis.

The serum albumin concentration is reduced within a range of 12–20 g/l and the serum globulin concentration is massively increased to >65 g/l and

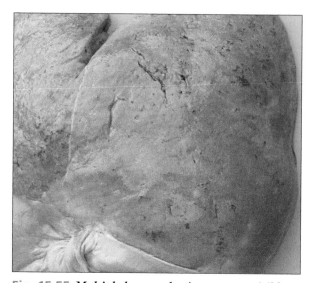

Fig. 15.55 Multiple haemorrhagic tracts are visible beneath the liver capsule in subacute fasciolosis.

often >75 g/l. There are few bacterial infections that give such a dramatic serum protein profile, and certainly none on a group basis; therefore, serum protein analysis should be included with liver enzymes in the biochemistry profile. At necropsy, the liver is grossly enlarged (**Fig. 15.54**) with multiple haemorrhagic tracts visible under the liver capsule (**Fig. 15.55**) and throughout its substance (**Fig. 15.56**). Immature flukes can be demonstrated within the bile ducts and gall bladder.

Chronic fasciolosis: Chronic fasciolosis is diagnosed by demonstration of fluke eggs in faecal samples (**Fig. 15.57**) and by raised serum GGT concentrations; however, these values may only be increased 2–3-fold in some cases. Many sheep show profound anaemia, hypoalbuminaemia and hyper-gamma-globulinaemia. Mature flukes are demonstrated within the bile ducts and gall bladder at necropsy. Nodular hyperplasia of the liver is commonly seen (**Fig. 15.58**).

The coproantigen enzyme-linked immunosorbent assay (ELISA) detects digestive enzymes produced by migrating (late immature) and adult flukes which are released into the bile and detected in faeces, thereby confirming active infestation. Fluke infestation can be detected after 3–4 weeks but more reliably after 6–9 weeks, 2–3 weeks before eggs can be detected in faeces. The test can identify as few as five adult flukes. The coproantigen reduction test has been promoted as a suitable screen for triclabendazole resistance with negative results 1–2 weeks after successful treatment.

Treatment

Triclabendazole is effective at killing all fluke stages. Drenched sheep should be moved to clean pasture. Re-treatment should be based upon risk and may be necessary 3 and 6 weeks after the first treatment in high-risk years where there is no alternative pasture or housing. Thereafter, treatment with closantel should be considered to avoid selecting for triclabendazole resistant strains of liver fluke but noting that closantel is effective only against developing flukes from 6–8 weeks old. Nitroxynil and oxyclosanide should be used for the treatment of adult flukes during late winter/spring.

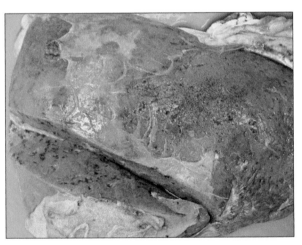

Fig. 15.56 Multiple haemorrhagic tracts are present throughout the liver parenchyma in subacute fasciolosis.

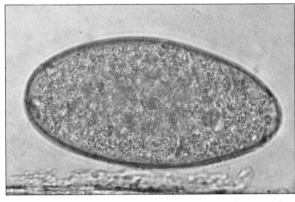

Fig. 15.57 Chronic (patent) fasciolosis is diagnosed by microscopic demonstration of fluke eggs in faecal samples.

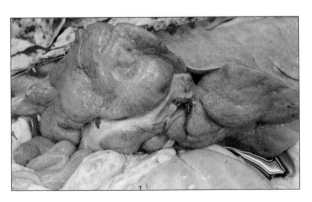

Fig. 15.58 Nodular hyperplasia of the liver is commonly seen in chronic fasciolosis.

Management/prevention/control measures

While most emphasis has been placed on the use of triclabendazole against immature flukes, a major component of liver fluke control is to reduce as far as possible future egg output by mature flukes that will comprise next year's challenge. This protocol will reduce metacercarial challenge the following autumn; however, it is not possible to remove all challenge, especially during high-risk years.

In areas with endemic fasciolosis, control is founded on strategic flukacide drenches. During low-risk years, triclabendazole is given to sheep in October and December (may also use closantel in January depending upon local veterinary advice), and either nitroxynil or oxyclosanide is administered in May. In years when epidemiological data indicate a high risk of fasciolosis, an additional triclabendazole treatment should be given in November. Feedback from slaughter plants may provide useful data regarding fluke prevalence and severity in some situations (**Fig. 15.59**).

While it may be possible to eliminate fluke from the flock on a farm by strategic drenching, there are risks from wildlife species and cattle that harbour flukes. Drenching based on the appearance of clinical disease in a few sheep represents a considerable risk because serious losses could result in the flock before treatment can be effected. Therefore, it is strongly recommended that strategic drenching is undertaken every year with additional treatments in high-risk years, the latter based upon forecast data. Advice from the farmer's veterinary surgeon is essential to qualify more generic control principles.

Fencing off snail habitats (**Fig. 15.60**) is rarely practicable and in most situations is cost prohibitive, as these are often extensive sheep enterprises; many farms are also subject to environmental controls.

Economics

Fasciolosis can have a very serious financial impact on a sheep farm but can be largely controlled by strategic drenching with appropriate flukicides as outlined in the flock health plan. Losses can result when infested sheep are brought onto a farm and contaminate pasture and infest snails, with subsequent challenge to the home flock during the following autumn, causing disease. Problems may also arise after a succession of wet summers that allow

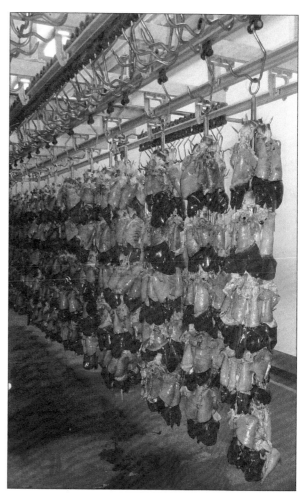

Fig. 15.59 Feedback from slaughter plants may provide useful data regarding fluke prevalence and severity in some situations.

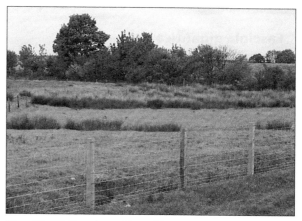

Fig. 15.60 Fencing off snail habitats is rarely practicable and in most situations is cost prohibitive.

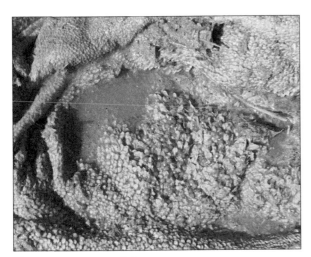

Fig. 15.61 Rumen flukes.

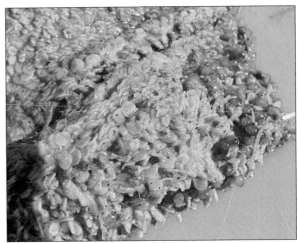

Fig. 15.62 Rumen flukes.

snail numbers to increase dramatically, providing an abundance of intermediate hosts for the developing fluke stages.

Welfare implications

There are obvious welfare concerns arising from sheep that die of acute and subacute fasciolosis but the greater concern is the welfare of large numbers of emaciated sheep as they approach late pregnancy. These ewes are more prone to ovine pregnancy tox-aemia, have poor colostrum stores and give birth to low birthweight lambs. The latter two factors result in an unacceptably high perinatal lamb mortality rate from starvation and increased susceptibility to environmental pathogens.

Fasciola gigantica

The life cycle of *F. gigantica* is broadly similar to that of *F. hepatica*. The intermediate stages involve the snail *Lymnaea auricula*. Both acute and chronic forms of the disease occur in sheep. Control measures are similar to those for *F. hepatica*.

Paramphistomes (rumen flukes)
Definition/overview

Paramphistome infestations are now considered common in sheep in the UK but adult flukes present in the rumen may not cause clinical disease.

Aetiology

Calicophoron daubneyi affects cattle and sheep and was probably introduced into the UK with cattle imported from Europe. *C. daubneyi* has a similar two host life cycle to *F. hepatica* but uses a different intermediate snail host.

Clinical presentation

Adult flukes reside in the ventral walls of the rumen (**Figs 15.61, 15.62**) and may not cause clinical signs although large numbers of migrating immature rumen flukes cause transient diarrhoea.

Diagnosis

Mature rumen flukes are readily identified at necropsy. Eggs of *C. daubneyi* can be detected by the same sedimentation technique as for *F. hepatica*.

Treatment

Treatment is not considered necessary because rumen flukes are thought to cause little clinical disease.

Management/prevention/control measures

Prevention and control measures are not usually necessary because rumen flukes cause little clinical disease.

TICK-BORNE DISEASES

Diseases transmitted by ticks include tick-borne fever, heartwater, louping-ill, tick pyaemia and Lyme disease; however, these diseases are not present in all tick-infested areas.

Tick-borne fever

Definition/overview

Tick-borne fever can be a sporadic but serious cause of abortion in sheep not previously exposed to the rickettsial infection. It is important in endemically infected flocks because impairment of the immune status predisposes to other infections such as tick pyaemia. Infection is encountered in northern Europe on grazing land that provides suitable habitat for ticks.

Aetiology

Tick-borne fever is caused by the rickettsial microorganism *Ehrlichia phagocytophila*. The vector is the nymph and adult stages of the tick *Ixodes ricinus*. A carrier state develops with recurrence of parasitaemia during stressful periods. Deer may act as a reservoir for tick-borne fever which may explain the occasional appearance of disease in sheep flocks.

Clinical presentation

Exposure of non-pregnant sheep to infected ticks results in a brief period of malaise with pyrexia, depression and reduced appetite. The resultant leucopenia renders sheep prone to infections such as tick pyaemia in lambs and louping-ill in unvaccinated yearlings. Re-exposure may result in mild transient illness but abortion does not result.

In most situations, lambs and yearlings exposed to tick-borne fever do not encounter infection for the first time when they are pregnant. Exposure of susceptible (purchased) pregnant ewes to tick-borne fever can produce disastrous consequences with abortion rates >90% reported and high mortality in ewes after abortion. Tick-borne fever may also exacerbate existing respiratory tract infections.

Differential diagnoses

The common causes of abortion:

- *Chlamydophila abortus* infection.
- Toxoplasmosis.
- *Salmonella* serotypes.
- *Campylobacter fetus intestinalis*.
- *Listeria monocytogenes*, *Pasteurella* spp.

Diagnosis

Diagnosis is based on the clinical signs and history of recent exposure of susceptible sheep to a tick-infested area. There may be evidence of all three stages of the tick life cycle feeding on the sheep; particular attention should be paid to the groin and axillae. Initially, there is a profound lympho-paenia followed by a neutropaenia, which slowly return to normal values after 2–3 weeks in uncomplicated cases. Focal bacterial infection will affect these values over time with a developing mature neutrophilia.

During the first week parasites can be observed microscopically in granulocytes of Giemsa-stained blood films. Seroconversion indicates recent infection and is perhaps of most use in establishing the potential role of tick-borne fever in abortion cases.

Treatment

While uncomplicated cases of tick-borne fever can be successfully treated with oxytetracycline, clinical signs would not be noted unless secondary or associated diseases occurred.

Metaphylactic antibiotic injection with long-acting oxytetracycline could be attempted in the face of an abortion problem, in addition to removing sheep from infested pasture and treatment for ticks.

Management/prevention/control measures

In some countries with extensive management systems it is not possible to avoid tick-infested pastures. Tick activity in spring coincides with the return of ewes and their lambs to hill/mountainous areas such that young lambs are especially susceptible to tick-borne fever and tick pyaemia. Lambs are protected from louping-ill by passively-derived antibody.

Control measures involve the use of synthetic pyrethroid pour-on acaricides such as deltamethrin or flumethrin before turnout to infested areas; these provide control for up to 6 weeks after topical application. The use of pour-on preparations has numerous advantages over plunge dipping. In some situations the injection of all lambs with long-acting oxytetracycline is used in addition to a topical acaricide.

Economics

Application of a synthetic pyrethroid pour-on acaricide costs approximately 0.5% of the value of the ewe. A single injection of long-acting oxytetracycline for a 10 kg lamb costs approximately 1% of the value of the lamb.

Welfare implications

Tick-borne fever has no specific welfare concerns *per se* but the associated condition of tick pyaemia raises serious welfare concerns because of the crippling affects of polyarthritis and vertebral empyema.

Tick pyaemia

Definition/overview

Tick pyaemia is typically seen in lambs 10–14 days after exposure to tick-infested pastures where tick-borne fever (*Ehrlichia phagocytophila*) is present; however, not all lambs with tick-borne fever develop tick pyaemia.

Aetiology

Infection of lambs with tick-borne fever causes a leucopenia and this may be followed by bacterial infection of the feeding sites.

Clinical presentation

Lambs are generally turned away to hill (tick-infested) pastures when approximately 1–2 weeks old and infection is observed in lambs 3–4 weeks old. Infection of skin bite wounds with bacteria, commonly *Staphylococcus aureus*, results in large subcutaneous abscesses. Bacteraemia with localization in joints and the vertebral column causes septic joints and eventual paralysis caudal to the affected vertebra, respectively. Severely affected lambs on extensive grazing systems fall prey to opportunist predators with the extent of these losses not known until first gathering or weaning. Lambs with polyarthritis are severely lame when only one limb is affected and unable to stand/move if two or more limbs are affected. Unlike most other cases of polyarthritis in young lambs, affected joints become markedly distended with viscous green pus. In many cases the skin overlying aspects of the joint capsule is much thinner than normal, with hair loss typical of an underlying abscess, although the joint contents rarely discharge. The clinical manifestation of infection of the vertebral column is described in detail in Chapter 8, Neurological Diseases.

Differential diagnoses

- Other causes of polyarthritis include *Streptococcus dysgalactiae*, typically seen in lambs less than 2 weeks old, and *Erysipelas rhusiopathiae* in older lambs, which can be differentiated on clinical examination and bacteriology of joint fluid or synovial membrane.
- Vertebral empyema should be differentiated from delayed swayback and, possibly, white muscle disease.

Diagnosis

Diagnosis of tick pyaemia is based on clinical findings and history of tick exposure. It is unlikely that there will be evidence of *E. phagocytophila* in blood films from lambs with chronic bacterial infections.

Treatment

Subcutaneous abscesses can be lanced but lambs with vertebral empyema and polyarthritis must be euthanased for welfare reasons.

Management/prevention/control measures

There are no specific control measures for tick pyaemia. Tick control is described in the section on tick-borne fever.

Economics

Considerable losses can result from mortality associated with tick pyaemia. Preventive measures are relatively inexpensive and topical application of synthetic pyrethroid can be repeated where necessary.

Welfare implications

Crippled lambs with septic joints or vertebral empyema present a serious welfare concern. Many lambs succumb to starvation and/or predation in extensive management systems. When found alive, these lambs must be humanely destroyed for welfare reasons.

Louping-ill

Definition/overview

Louping-ill is an acute, tick-transmitted viral infection of the central nervous system of sheep and, much less commonly, a range of other species including man. The disease is confined to certain tick-infested areas in certain countries of northern Europe, in particular Scotland, with a seasonal occurrence reflecting tick activity.

Aetiology

Louping-ill is caused by a flavivirus and is transmitted by the tick *Ixodes ricinus*. The severity of clinical signs is exacerbated following concurrent infection with tick-borne fever. The majority of cases occur during the spring but a distinct autumn feeding population of ticks gives rise to disease much later in the year.

Clinical presentation

All ages of sheep appear susceptible to infection but in endemically-infected areas clinical signs are most common following waning of passive protection; thus disease is seen in weaned lambs associated with an autumn tick quest, and during the following spring as yearlings.

The clinical signs are variable and range from mild ataxia to sudden death. The neurological signs reported include ataxia and seizure activity progressing to opisthotonus. The severity of clinical signs and mortality are increased with concurrent infection with *E. phagocytophila*. It is reported that recovered sheep exhibit posterior paralysis for weeks to months after infection.

Differential diagnoses

- Posterior paresis in weaned lambs could result from delayed swayback and sarcocystosis. Numerous sheep may present with sarcocystosis

over a period of 7–10 days after movement on to pastures contaminated by dog faeces, but no acute deaths result.
- Vertebral empyema of the thoracolumbar vertebral column may cause posterior paresis for a few days but this rapidly progresses to paralysis. Such cases occur sporadically and not as an outbreak.
- Oubreaks of acute coenurosis have been reported but would probably differ from louping-ill with respect to epidemiology.
- Acute cases of listerial encephalitis may present with many of the neurological signs of louping-ill although fewer losses would occur and the epidemiology would almost certainly differ.
- Seizure activity and opisthotonus are common presenting signs of polioencephalomalacia.
- Focal symmetrical encephalomalacia should be considered in unvaccinated lambs.
- Sudden death in sheep grazing extensive pasture may result from acute fasciolosis or clostridial disease, in particular black disease. Losses could also result from systemic pasteurellosis and other acute bacterial infections.

Diagnosis

Diagnosis is based on clinical signs affecting a number of susceptible sheep within weeks of moving on to tick-infested pasture. The provisional diagnosis is supported by histopathological examination of brain tissue from carcases and virus isolation. For safety reasons, the sheep's head should be submitted for laboratory examination rather than removing the brain under field conditions. Blood smears may reveal the presence of *E. phagocytophila*. Seroconversion would be evident in recovered sheep; the presence of IgM antibody provides evidence of infection within the preceding 10 days.

Treatment

There is no treatment and efforts are directed at prevention by vaccination (where available) and tick control.

Management/prevention/control measures

While tick control programmes using pour-on acaricides may limit all tick-transmitted diseases, these regimens are not completely effective at eliminating tick populations; therefore, control of louping-ill must incorporate a vaccination policy. In endemic areas all replacement breeding stock, including rams, are vaccinated at least 28 days before exposure to tick-infested pastures. Thereafter, vaccination every 2 years is recommended, which should be given prior to lambing to ensure passive antibody protection of lambs during their first spring.

Economics
Vaccination (where available) is relatively expensive (5% of the value of the ewe) but is essential on all endemically affected farms.

Welfare implications
Vaccination is indicated on affected farms for both economic and welfare reasons.

Heartwater
(syn. cowdriosis)

Definition/overview
Heartwater is an important production-limiting disease of sheep in sub-Saharan African countries.

Aetiology
Heartwater is caused by infection with *Cowdria ruminantium* and is transmitted by ticks of the genus *Amblyomma*. The natural tick life cycle may involve non-domesticated ruminants.

Clinical presentation
After an incubation of approximately 2 weeks, sheep show marked pyrexia. In mild infections sheep are dull and inappetent. Respiratory distress, with tachynpoea and an abdominal component to breathing, is present in many cases, resulting from pulmonary oedema and effusion within the chest and pericardium. This state rapidly progresses to death. Vague neurological signs may also be observed including hyperaesthesia and seizure activity. In peracute situations sheep may simply be found dead. Losses are higher in introduced breeds and may exceed 50%.

Diagnosis
Diagnosis is based on clinical findings and history of exposure to tick-infested pasture, particularly with non-indigenous breeds. Typical necropsy findings include marked pericardial and pleural effusions and widespread carcase petechiae. Brain smears should be examined carefully for the presence of intracytoplasmic rickettsiae in endothelial cells.

Treatment
Treatment with oxytetracycline is unsuccessful in most cases because of the advanced changes present when sick sheep are identified.

Management/prevention/control measures
Indigenous breeds have a higher level of resistance to heartwater than introduced breeds. Cross-breeding programmes offer the best compromise to acquiring desired genetic traits whilst still maintaining some degree of resistance to local disease conditions.

A vaccine is reported to be available in South Africa and Zimbabwe but this presents many practical difficulties. Controlled exposure, with oxytetracycline treatment once pyrexia or clinical signs are noted, is one method of acquiring some degree of natural immunization but this is time-consuming and not without risk of severe disease from overwhelming challenge.

Control of tick infestation in sheep also involves a programme of intensive acaricide application to cattle, but infestations involving non-domesticated hosts limit the efficacy of this approach.

Economics
Losses accrue not only from deaths involving indigenous breeds but also from limitations to the importation of desirable genetics in other sheep breeds.

Welfare implications
Respiratory distress associated with the more severe presentation of the disease raises obvious welfare concerns; however, these issues are tempered by problems arising from famine and other natural disasters in these areas of the world.

Lyme disease

Definition/overview

Lyme disease is a rare tick-transmitted infection of large mammals including sheep, cattle, horses, deer and man. Lyme disease is only of concern because of the remote zoonotic risk.

Aetiology

Lyme disease is caused by the spirochaete *Borrelia burgdorferi* and transmitted by *Ixodes* species ticks.

Clinical presentation

Few, if any, clinical signs have been attributed to Lyme disease in sheep; seroconversion has been reported without any ill health. It has been suggested that Lyme disease can give rise to arthritis in lambs. Infection of tick feeding sites with bacteria, commonly *S. aureus*, results in large subcutaneous abscesses and, often, bacteraemia with localization within joints leading to septic joints.

Differential diagnoses

The more common causes of outbreaks of polyarthritis include *S. dysgalactiae* and *E. rhusiopathia*e,
which can be differentiated on clinical examination and bacteriology of synovial fluid or joint capsule.

Diagnosis

Clinical signs are rarely recognized; seroconversion typically occurs without overt disease.

Treatment

Treatment is not necessary.

Management/prevention/control measures

Tick control is operated on most farms for the much more important tick-transmitted diseases tick-borne fever and tick pyaemia.

Economics

Lyme disease presents no economic concerns.

Welfare implications

The disease is largely asymptomatic and presents no welfare concerns as recognized to date.

SCHMALLENBERG VIRUS

Definition/overview

Between August and October 2011, outbreaks of disease in adult cattle causing mild to moderate fever, reduced milk yield, loss of appetite, loss of body condition and diarrhoea were reported in both the Netherlands and Germany. Testing for common causes proved negative. From December 2011, abortions and stillbirths associated with foetal abnormalities, affecting mainly sheep but also cattle and goats, were identified in the Netherlands, Germany and Belgium. A new virus was identified in November 2011 as the cause of both conditions. This was named 'Schmallenberg virus' (SBV) after the German town where the virus was first identified.

Aetiology

SBV is in the Simbu serogroup of the Orthobunyavirus group. SBV is similar to some other animal disease pathogens including Akabane and Shamonda viruses, which are transmitted by vectors such as midges, mosquitoes and ticks. SBV can infect and cause disease in sheep, cattle and goats.

SBV transmission has not yet been confirmed. The potential for direct transmission from one animal to another is therefore unknown. If biting insect vectors are the major route of transmission, significant spread is believed unlikely during the winter period when biting insects are usually inactive. However, this premise has been questioned by the birth of congenitally infected animals, infected during 'non-transmission' periods. It is believed SBV was circulating widely in sheep and cattle in the Netherlands and in a part of western Germany between August and October 2011. It is likely that initial introduction of the virus to the UK resulted from wind-blown insect vectors.

On January 23rd 2012, SBV was reported on four sheep farms in Norfolk, Suffolk and East Sussex. In these initial cases, the disease was diagnosed following the testing of deformed lambs. By March 5th 2012, SBV infection had been identified on 121 farms in England. Eight positive cases were diagnosed in cattle and 113 in sheep. Cattle and sheep in the south, south-west and east of England were at the highest risk of showing signs of the disease.

In the Netherlands and Germany outbreaks of SBV disease in cattle have caused clinical signs including fever, reduced milk yield, inappetence, loss of body condition and diarrhoea. Outbreaks of disease have lasted 2–3 weeks, with individual affected animals recovering over several days. These clinical signs are broadly similar to bluetongue, another midge-borne viral disease familiar to UK livestock farmers.

Clinical presentation

Clinical signs have not been reported in adult or growing sheep, although there is anecdotal evidence of milk drop in milking sheep in Netherlands. Seroconversion to SBV has occurred without observed clinical signs. In most flocks the impact of SBV has been low, but a small percentage of flocks have experienced considerable losses.

Malformations in newborn animals and foetuses include brain deformities and marked damage to the spinal cord. Arthrogryposis is reported to be a common birth defect. Some animals are born with a normal appearance but have nervous signs such as a 'dummy' presentation or blindness, ataxia, recumbency, an inability to suck and sometimes seizures. The foetal deformities vary depending on when infection occurred during pregnancy.

Differential diagnoses

Arthrogryposis can also be inherited as an autosomal recessive condition, therefore veterinary investigation is essential. Genetic causes of birth defects will generally be traced to the introduction of a particular ram into the flock.

Diagnosis

SBV is suspected after a high prevalence of congenital abnormalities, particularly arthrogryposis, and confirmed after demonstration of viral sequences using real time polymerase chain reaction (PCR) on tissues. Paired serology confirms recent SBV infection. A positive enzyme-linked immunosorbent assay (ELISA) will confirm previous exposure or vaccination.

Treatment

Malformations affecting lambs exposed to the virus *in utero* may lead to lambing difficulties. Excessive force must not be used during lambing as this may risk injury to both the ewe and lamb. Farmers should contact their veterinary surgeon because safe delivery may necessitate a caesarean operation. Lambs delivered alive with severe deformities must be euthanased for welfare reasons.

Management/prevention/control measures

An inactivated vaccine is currently available which is injected at least 1 month before the mating period.

Public health

SBV is not a notifiable disease but UK farmers and veterinarians should remain vigilant and report any suspicious cases to AHVLA for testing, as part of enhanced surveillance. The European Centre for Disease Prevention and Control suggests that there is a low likelihood of any risk to public health. However, as this is a new virus, work is ongoing to identify whether it could cause any health problems in humans. Farmers and veterinary surgeons are advised to take sensible hygiene precautions when working with livestock and abortion material. Although several members of the group of related viruses can affect humans, the ability to do so is thought to be due to a gene sequence which is not present in SBV. Pregnant women should not have contact with sheep and goats at lambing/kidding time due to risk of exposure to other disease-causing organisms.

BLUETONGUE

Definition/overview

Bluetongue is a viral disease affecting sheep, cattle, deer, goats and camelids (camels, llamas, alpacas, guanaco and vicuña). Although sheep are most severely affected, cattle are the main mammalian reservoir of the virus and are very important in the epidemiology of the disease. Bluetongue is a notifiable disease in the UK. The UK was declared free of bluetongue in 2011 after the last case in 2008.

The geographic distribution of bluetongue is dependent upon the *Culicoides* (midge) host which was until recently restricted to the African continent. Since 1999 there have been widespread outbreaks of bluetongue in Greece, Italy, Corsica (France) and the Balearic Islands (Spain). Cases also occurred in Bulgaria, Croatia, Macedonia and Kosovo. Bluetongue serotypes 2, 4, 9 and 16 have been involved. It appears that the bluetongue virus spread from both Turkey and North Africa. Bluetongue serotype 8 (BTV-8) was first found in the Netherlands, Belgium, Luxembourg, Western Germany, and in parts of north-eastern France in the summer of 2006.

In 2007, northern Europe experienced a dramatic increase of new BTV cases in all existing infected areas, and cases numbered into the many tens of thousands as disease steadily spread across Europe. Affected countries witnessed increased mortality rates in animals and production losses. Bluetongue is also widespread within the USA, and has also been identified in Australia but is not associated with overt disease in sheep.

Aetiology

Bluetongue is caused by an arthropod-borne reovirus. There are currently 24 distinct serotypes. The virus is transmitted by biting midges of the *Culicoides* genus; bluetongue cannot be transmitted directly between animals.

Clinical presentation

The clinical signs, which vary depending on viral strain and sheep breed, follow an incubation period of 4–12 days. Only a small percentage of viraemic sheep may develop clinical signs. Affected sheep are pyrexic (up to 42.0°C) and appear stiff and very reluctant to move. They often adopt a roached back stance with the neck extended and the head held lowered. There is oedema of the face (**Fig. 16.1**) and ears, and also pulmonary oedema, which may cause dyspnoea. Erosions may appear on the lips and progress to ulcers. There is often profuse salivation and a serous to mucopurulent nasal discharge. There may be hyperaemia of the coronary band (**Fig. 16.2**) and around the muzzle and mouth. The tongue may become swollen, oedematous and appear cyanotic.

Bluetongue infection during the breeding season may result in a large percentage of early embryonic losses, with sheep returning to oestrus at irregular intervals. Viral infection during early gestation may result in central nervous system defects such as hydranencephaly.

Differential diagnoses

The most important differential diagnosis is foot and mouth disease, but in foot and mouth a larger percentage of the flock may be affected with high temperatures, and erosions within the mouth and on the coronary band and interdigital skin.

Differential diagnoses include:

- Foot and mouth disease.
- Contagious pustular dermatitis.
- Photosensitization including outbreaks of facial eczema.
- Peste des petits ruminants.
- Schmallenberg virus infection causing congenital abnormalities.

Diagnosis

Diagnosis is based on clinical signs, virus isolation and/or seroconversion to bluetongue virus.

Treatment

There is no specific treatment. Antibiotics could be used to treat secondary bacterial infections.

Management/prevention/control measures

Control of bluetongue is very difficult because of the large number of potential hosts and virus serotypes. While control is aimed at keeping susceptible animals away from the vector, this is not always practical. Control of the *Culicoides* species vector can be attempted with pour-on insecticides but this is expensive and does not achieve total freedom from the midge. Co-grazing sheep with cattle affords some protection, as midges feed preferentially on cattle.

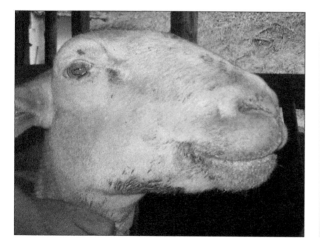

Fig. 16.1 There is oedema of the face in bluetongue infection.

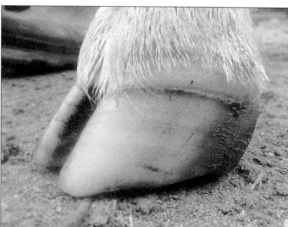

Fig. 16.2 Hyperaemia of the coronary band occurs in bluetongue infection.

Vaccines are used extensively worldwide. Inactivated vaccines were used successfully in the UK in 2007 to control BTV-8. Most modified live vaccines produce a viraemia in the vaccinated animal, which affords the opportunity for further spread. Problems may arise with viral reassortment if viraemic animals are vaccinated with a modified live vaccine. The timing of vaccination will depend on local factors, in particular the occurrence of high-risk periods. In certain areas, lambing time may be changed so that waning of passively derived antibody does not coincide with *Culicoides* species activity.

As the UK is officially free of bluetongue, vaccination is no longer permitted under EU law although this situation may change.

Economics

Bluetongue virus infection has an enormous impact on sheep production in many countries on the African continent and elsewhere. Losses result primarily from mortality, reduced production during protracted convalescence, including poor wool growth, and reduced reproductive performance, including temporary ram infertility.

Welfare implications

Mortality and protracted convalescence with susceptibility to secondary bacterial infections do raise welfare concerns but these may need to be tempered with respect to the impact of bluetongue disease on the agriculture-based community in developing countries.

FOOT AND MOUTH DISEASE

Definition/overview

Foot and mouth disease (FMD) does not occur in Australia, New Zealand or North America because of the very strict quarantine regulations for livestock and strict meat import restrictions. FMD is endemic in many parts of Africa and occurs sporadically in Asia. FMD was reported throughout the UK in 2001 with more than 2000 cases of disease; more than 10 million sheep and cattle were killed (**Figs 16.3–16.7**) in an attempt to control the disease, estimated to cost the UK government more than £8 billion. In 2007 escape of FMD virus from a laboratory facility in England caused a small outbreak involving cattle on four premises.

Aetiology

FMD is caused by a picornavirus that is highly contagious to cattle, sheep and pigs. Disease is readily spread by aerosol and by mechanical vectors such as vehicles and people. In the UK the widespread dispersal of sheep through markets resulted in rapid distribution of the virus in the 2001 epidemic.

Clinical presentation

This author witnessed FMD in sheep during the 2001 epidemic in the UK. The clinical findings observed are described below.

A shepherd suspected FMD when four out of 120 ewes became acutely lame and were unwilling

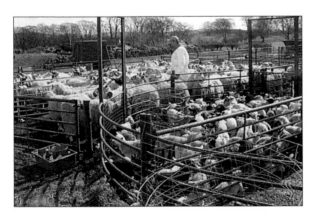

Fig. 16.3 More than 10 million sheep and cattle were killed in the UK in 2001 to control foot and mouth disease (FMD).

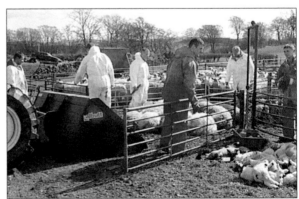

Fig. 16.4 On-farm slaughter of ewes and lambs employing army personnel.

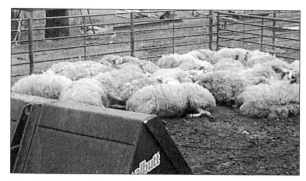

Fig. 16.5 Slaughter of large numbers of ruminants on-farm presents enormous logistical problems.

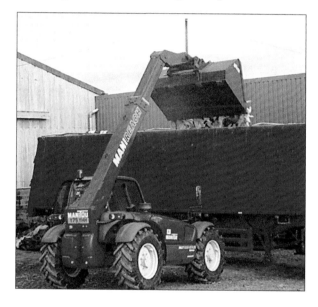

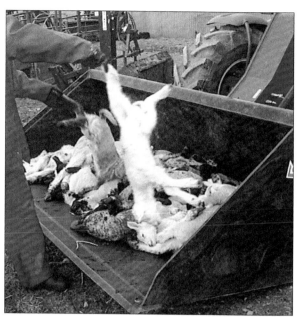

Fig. 16.6 Disposal of dead lambs for burial was undertaken as part of the contiguous cull undertaken in the UK in 2001.

Fig. 16.7 Transport of dead stock for burial was undertaken as part of the contiguous cull undertaken in the UK in 2001.

to stand and walk to the troughs at feeding time. The remaining ewes ate less than one-half of their concentrate ration that morning. The flock had just started lambing and 10 ewes had lambed in the previous 4 days. Examination of the four ewes revealed severe lameness on all four feet. The ewes were reluctant to stand such that two of the ewes were easily caught where they lay in sternal recumbency. The other two ewes were easily shepherded into a corner of the field. All four ewes showed pyrexia of 41.5°C and had not been stressed before being caught. All the ewes had an increased respiratory rate. Examination revealed hyperaemia of the interdigital skin and slight swelling around the coronary band. Two ewes had large vesicles measuring up to 15 mm diameter at the coronary band. There were some

small punctate erosions (2–3 mm in diameter) on the dental pad in all four ewes but no lesions on the tongue. Samples were collected from the coronary band vesicles for virus isolation; these subsequently proved positive for FMD.

Four out of 12 lambs were found dead in the lambing field that morning. The lambs were aged from 1–4 days old and were well-fleshed. Postmortem examination failed to reveal an obvious cause of death; death was not the result of starvation/exposure or of any of the infectious bacterial diseases common in neonatal lambs.

Advanced lesions of approximately 7–10 days' duration are shown in **Figs 16.8–16.11**. It is highly unlikely that such chronic lesions would be encountered in the investigation of an outbreak of FMD because these

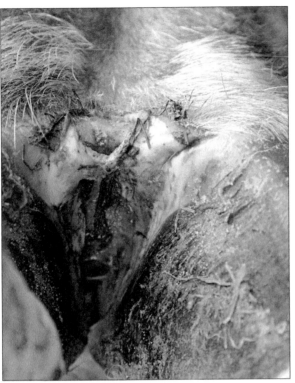

Fig. 16.8 Advanced FMD lesion affects the interdigital skin after vesicle rupture, with exposure of the subcutis.

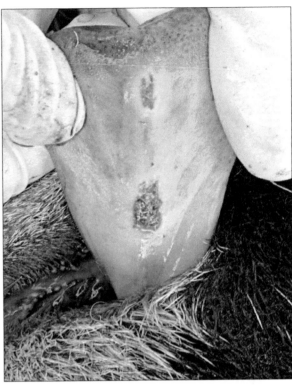

Fig. 16.9 Advanced FMD lesions are present under the tongue after vesicle rupture.

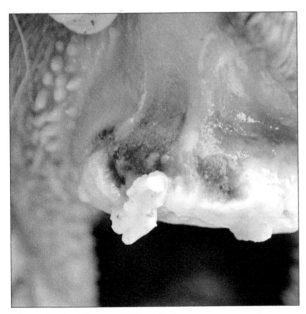

Fig. 16.10 Advanced FMD lesions appear on the dental pad after vesicle rupture.

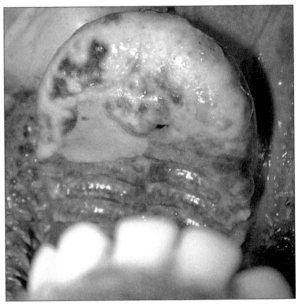

Fig. 16.11 Advanced lesions of FMD represented by healing erosions on the hard palate.

animals would have shown clinical signs for up to 1 week. These lesions were advanced because of a serious logistical delay in the interval to slaughter in 2001.

Differential diagnoses

- A combination of pyrexia and sudden onset of severe lameness with vesicle formation should eliminate other common causes of lameness such as footrot.
- Postdipping lameness can be ruled out by the clinical examination and the history of the sheep not being recently plunge dipped.
- Pyrexia is not uncommon in sheep when gathering takes more than 30 minutes. During the 2001 epidemic in the UK some flocks were falsely diagnosed as having FMD on the basis of pyrexia alone. Chronic lesions present in the mouths of some sheep can readily be differentiated from FMD by their deep-fissured appearance, paucity and distribution on the dental pad only.
- Sudden death in lambs could be caused by lamb dysentery or septicaemic pasteurellosis and during adverse weather conditions. White muscle disease affecting the myocardium causes only sporadic losses.

Diagnosis

Diagnosis is based on clinical signs and confirmed by virus isolation. Retrospective confirmation can be obtained following seroconversion in acute and convalescent samples.

Treatment

Compulsory slaughter of suspected outbreaks of FMD operates in many countries including the UK.

Management/prevention/control measures

Prevention on a national basis involves strict quarantine of imported livestock. On a farm basis, greatly improved biosecurity is necessary on all farms.

National control schemes

Strict regulations regarding importation of animals, meat and meat products operate in many countries. In the UK, for example, a compulsory slaughter and compensation policy operated during the 2001 epidemic. Other countries have operated a ring vaccination policy to control spread of infection, with subsequent slaughter of all vaccinated cattle.

Economics

Outbreaks of FMD can have serious economic consequences. For example, the 2001 epidemic in the UK cost the Treasury in excess of £8 billion.

Welfare implications

There are no special welfare implications from the disease itself and cattle and sheep do recover from infection, albeit with a protracted convalescence. However, movement restrictions, such as those enforced in the UK in 2001, can cause welfare problems because, for example, cattle and sheep cannot be moved across roads or transported home.

PESTE DES PETITS RUMINANTS AND RINDERPEST

Definition/overview

Peste des petits ruminants (PPR) occurs in equatorial Africa, extending into Egypt and, more recently, India and Pakistan. It is not possible to differentiate clinical signs of acute PPR from acute rinderpest. Rinderpest/PPR is not present in the main sheep-producing countries, including Europe, North America, Australia and New Zealand, where strict import controls prevent their introduction.

Aetiology

PPR and rinderpest are caused by a paramyxovirus (genus Morbillivirus). PPR is much more important than rinderpest in sheep and goats. Infection is spread via aerosol.

Clinical presentation

The clinical signs are highly variable, with Indian isolates of PPR causing severe disease in sheep. Susceptible sheep show severe clinical disease with pyrexia (41°C), depression, profuse salivation and serous ocular and nasal discharges that rapidly become purulent. The mucous membranes are congested. There are erosions in the nasal passages and buccal cavity, which coalesce and may ulcerate.

There is profuse foetid diarrhoea with occasional colic signs. Affected sheep develop pneumonia with associated dyspnoea. Inability to eat or drink gives a gaunt, pitiful appearance and rapid dehydration. Severely affected sheep die within 7–10 days; those that survive have an extended convalescence but remain immune for life. Pregnant sheep frequently abort.

Clinical signs of PPR are uncommon in areas where the virus is considered to be endemic and are often restricted to mild oral lesions, diarrhoea and mild respiratory signs.

Differential diagnoses

Differential diagnoses include:

- Foot and mouth disease.
- Sheep pox.
- Bluetongue.

Diagnosis

Diagnosis is based on the clinical signs. Severe disease in susceptible sheep populations causes significant losses, with typical histopathological changes in the lungs. Erosions and ulcers are identified in the buccal cavity and there is a viral-type bronchopneumonia with anteroventral consolidation. Virus can be isolated from lymphoid tissue at necropsy, including lymph nodes, Peyer's patches and spleen.

Disease occurring in endemic areas can be confirmed by seroconversion.

Treatment

In many countries affected sheep are slaughtered as part of a control/eradication programme. There is no specific treatment for PPR or rinderpest; efforts are directed to supportive therapy, including antibiotics and oral fluids.

Management/prevention/control measures

Disease is prevented in many countries by strict quarantine controls. Introduced disease has been eradicated from countries by compulsory slaughter of affected flocks/herds. While live attenuated rinderpest virus has been used successfully in the past, rinderpest control programmes prevent the use of this vaccine in sheep in many endemic countries.

Economics

PPR and rinderpest would have devastating effects on the livestock industry if introduced into disease-free countries; therefore, strict import controls operate.

Welfare implications

Compulsory slaughter would limit any welfare concerns should disease be introduced into many countries.

POISONINGS

Plant poisoning

Plant poisoning is uncommon when sheep are grazing enclosed pastures but it can occur when there is accidental access (rhododendron), poor grazing (bracken) or the sheep are fed exclusively on brassicas. Prevention is based on maintaining sound perimeter fences and practising good husbandry (e.g. giving sheep ready access to good quality forages when folded on brassica crops).

Rhododendron

Rhododendron poisoning occurs sporadically following accidental access to ornamental gardens during periods of temporary starvation, typically during winter storms with deep snow. Affected sheep are weak, often unable to stand, and present with abdominal pain (bruxism and vocalization) and passive regurgitation of rumen contents. Recumbency, ruminal atony and bloat with rumen fluid around the muzzle lead to confusion with hypocalcaemia. Death can occur within hours (more typically in affected goats). Less severely affected animals recover with symptomatic treatment including pethidine (3 mg/kg q12 h where available) and non-steroidal anti-inflammatory drugs.

Bracken

Bracken poisoning causing progressive retinal atrophy (bright blindness) has been described in textbooks in sheep grazed on moorland for many years, but is very uncommon.

Brassicas

Toxicity problems may arise when rape, kale, stubble turnips and roots are introduced too quickly, are fed in too high proportion or are fed for too long. The common presenting feature is poor weight gain but acute deaths can occur with sudden and exclusive exposure.

The potentially toxic substances in brassicas include S-methyl-cysteine sulphoxide (precursor of the haemolytic factor), glucosinolates (goitre), nitrate (when reduced to nitrite causes methaemoglobinaemia) and oxalates.

The anaemia, which varies from mild to severe, relates directly to the amount of S-methyl-cysteine sulphoxide, which itself is dependent on variety and stage of growth. Confirmation of the diagnosis is based on demonstration of anaemia with Heinz–Ehrlich bodies. In acute toxicity there is anaemia and jaundice.

Nitrate ingestion in plants (particularly in roots) is converted into nitrite by the rumen microflora. Following absorption, nitrites combine with haemoglobin to form methaemoglobin. Clinical signs include brown mucous membranes, tachypnoea with an abdominal component, and weakness progressing to recumbency and death, which may be precipitated by forced exercise when gathered. Treatment with 10 mg/kg methylene blue injected intravenously has been described but it would present numerous logistical problems if many sheep were involved.

Poisoning from ingestion of nitrogenous fertilizers is theoretically possible.

Excessive ingestion of oxalates (particularly in the leaves of beets) can induce acute oxalate poisoning with clinical signs of hypocalcaemia. Long-term ingestion of oxalates can result in deposition of insoluble calcium oxalate in the kidneys, causing chronic renal failure. Sheep should be removed from the crop and acute cases treated as for hypocalcaemia with 20–40 ml of 40% calcium borogluconate.

Inorganic poisons

Inorganic poisons tend to result from industrial pollution and often have a distinct geographical distribution (e.g. chronic lead poisoning from mine workings).

Lead poisoning

Typical features of chronic lead poisoning include chronic lameness affecting growing lambs, with brittle bones leading to multiple fractures and bone abnormalities. Diagnosis is based on lead concentrations in faeces, blood and kidney. Acute lead poisoning following ingestion of lead-based paint is possible but is rare.

Control of chronic disease is based on avoidance of mine workings and other sources of pollution. Treatment of acute cases, where recognized, involves intravenous administration of sodium calcium edetate, repeated 2 days later.

CHAPTER 17

ANAESTHESIA

INTRODUCTION

The most common ovine surgical procedures such as caesarean operation, vasectomy and digit amputation are generally undertaken using paravertebral anaesthesia, spinal analgesia and intravenous regional anaesthesia (IVRA), respectively. There are presently few clinical data reporting the positive effects of preoperative non-steroidal anti-inflammatory drug (NSAID) administration in sheep, but extrapolation from other species warrants their use, even when practice situations result in intravenous administration only 5–10 minutes prior to surgery.

Lignocaine is not licensed for food producing animals in EU countries, and procaine is used instead. However, procaine is contraindicated by the extradural and intravenous injection routes; therefore, lignocaine should be used for high and low extradural blocks and IVRA.

GENERAL ANAESTHESIA

There are occasions when general anaesthesia is necessary (e.g. abdominal surgery and eye enucleation), but few products are licensed for use in sheep in the UK. In such situations a standard withdrawal period is observed; in some countries the animal must never enter the food chain.

There are some inherent risks with general anaesthesia in sheep; for example, regurgitation of rumen content with inhalation giving rise to aspiration pneumonia, and bloat compromising respiratory function and venous return to the heart.

It is advisable to remove concentrate feeding for 24 hours prior to any elective procedure to reduce the likelihood of excess gas production by the rumen microflora. Whenever possible the sheep should be positioned in sternal recumbency with the head held lowered to allow drainage of saliva from the buccal cavity.

Xylazine/ketamine

Xylazine is unpredictable as a sedative in sheep. Poor sedative effects often result if the sheep has been stressed prior to sedation and isolated after injection. Whenever possible, the sheep to be anaesthetised should be sedated in a pen next to other sheep, with direct vision, if not direct contact, to reduce the stress of isolation.

Xylazine is given intramuscularly at a dose rate of 0.05–0.07 mg/kg. Sedation should result within 10 minutes but can be very variable; note that xylazine is not licensed for use in sheep in many countries. Medetomidine injected intravenously at 10 μg/kg provides much more predictable sedation but is not licensed for use in sheep.

Induction of anaesthesia is then achieved by intravenous injection of 3 mg/kg ketamine which affords 10–15 minutes surgical anaesthesia. Anaesthesia can be extended following incremental doses of 2–3 mg/kg ketamine injected intravenously, which give a further 10 minutes of surgical anaesthesia.

Alphaxalone

Alphaxalone at 2.2–4.4 mg/kg injected intravenously is very safe in sheep but its short duration of only a few minutes restricts its use to an induction agent when employed in adult sheep. Surgical anaesthesia can then be maintained using halothane or isofluorane, and nitrous oxide and oxygen after intubation.

The duration of surgical anaesthesia is longer in neonatal lambs (up to 10 minutes after single intravenous injection at 4.4 mg/kg) where it is the anaesthetic drug of choice for forelimb fracture reduction, and short surgical procedures (e.g. replacement of intestinal herniation through the umbilicus). Alphaxalone is not licensed for use in sheep.

Propofol

Propofol (6.5 mg/kg in non-premedicated animals) can be used to induce general anaesthesia in adult sheep, but more commonly is used for short duration procedures in neonatal lambs (see above).

SEDATION WITH XYLAZINE AND LOCAL INFILTRATION WITH PROCAINE/LIGNOCAINE

Sedation with xylazine and local infiltration with procaine/lignocaine is used by some practitioners for some surgical procedures in sheep (e.g. vasectomy), but in this situation lumbosacral extradural lignocaine injection is the much better option.

Sedation can be effected in sheep with xylazine at 0.05 mg/kg injected intramuscularly; care must be undertaken when measuring such small volumes. During preparation for vasectomy, infiltration of the spermatic cord with procaine/lignocaine solution may accidentally result in injection into the pampiniform plexus. Furthermore, it proves difficult to block the noxious stimuli generated when traction is applied to each vas deferens.

CAUDAL ANALGESIA

Effective caudal analgesia is essential before replacement of vaginal, uterine and rectal prolapses (**Fig. 17.1**).

Sacrococcygeal extradural injection (low extradural block)

Sacrococcygeal extradural injection (**Fig. 17.2**) is given more easily in standing sheep than in sheep in sternal recumbency. The area over the tailhead is clipped and swabbed with surgical spirit. The first intercoccygeal space can be identified by digital palpation during slight vertical movement of the tail, and a 25 mm 20 gauge needle directed at 10–20° to the tail, which can either be held horizontally, or in such a position that the needle point is introduced parallel to the vertebral canal (i.e. in the standing ewe the needle is introduced horizontally).

Correct position of the needle can be determined by failure to strike bone during travel of the needle point, and lack of resistance to injection of the combined lignocaine and xylazine solution. It is not possible to identify when the point of the needle enters the extradural space by the hanging drop technique because of the shallow angle of the needle. A 40 mm needle may be necessary in sheep heavier than 85 kg.

Combined extradural injection of xylazine and lignocaine

Combined extradural injection of xylazine and lignocaine (0.07 mg/kg and 0.5 mg/kg, respectively) at the first intercoccygeal site provides effective analgesia, permitting replacement of rectal, cervical or uterine prolapses after 5–10 minutes. In practical terms, 2 ml of 2% lignocaine and 0.25 ml of

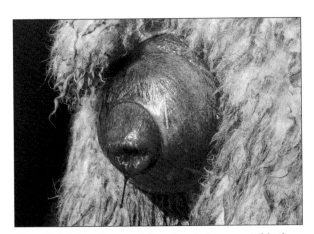

Fig. 17.1 Effective caudal analgesia is essential before replacement of this vaginal prolapse.

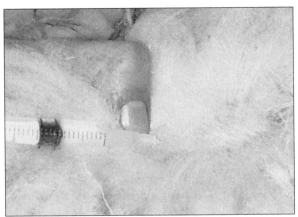

Fig. 17.2 Sacrococcygeal extradural injection is more easily given when the sheep is standing.

2% xylazine are mixed in the same syringe to treat adult ewes weighing 65–80 kg. A correspondingly reduced volume is used in sheep with live weights from 35–60 kg. Xylazine, an alpha-2 adrenergic agonist drug, injected into the sacrococcygeal extradural space, has been used successfully in cattle, horses, llamas and sheep to provide surgical analgesia of the perineal region, with advantages of extended duration of analgesia and less affect on motor innervation compared with lignocaine. In contrast to its effect in cattle, llamas and horses, extradural xylazine does not cause significant sedation in sheep when used at a dose rate of 0.07 mg/kg.

There is loss of tail tone and sensation of the perineum within 2 minutes of successful sacrococcygeal extradural injection, but 10 minutes should elapse before vaginal prolapse replacement is attempted. It may prove difficult to appreciate loss of tail tone in short-docked breeds and in ewes near full-term where there is considerable slackening of the sacrococcygeal ligaments; therefore, sensation of the tail/anus/vulva should be checked before attempting prolapse replacement.

Complications

Inadvertent injection of the combined xylazine and lignocaine solution into fascia and tissues surrounding the sacrococcygeal or first intercoccygeal site causes mild sedation (xylazine) lasting 2–3 hours. In this event, the sacrococcygeal extradural injection should be attempted again but using only lignocaine. This avoids further sedation if the second injection were also to prove unsuccessful. Accidental injection of xylazine at dose rates above 0.07 mg/kg could cause bradycardia and respiratory depression. In some sheep mild hindlimb paresis may persist for up to 48 hours after successful extradural injection.

Caesarean operations

While caesarean operations can be undertaken in ewes under field infiltration with procaine/lignocaine, concerns arise regarding the welfare of the ewe, especially where complicating factors are present, e.g. a foetal malformation caused by Schmallenberg virus infection, which necessitate considerable handling of the uterus during surgery. Possible analgesic options include:

Surgery 40–50 minutes after extradural xylazine (0.07 mg/kg) injection

When tested by needle prick 40–50 minutes after injection, analgesia of the flank was present in 12 of 13 ewes and 8 of 9 ewes following either sacrococcygeal or lumbosacral extradural xylazine injection at 0.07 mg/kg to a volume of 2.5 ml, respectively. The precise interval to onset of surgical analgesia after extradural injection was not determined in the study for welfare reasons. Instead, the interval of 40–50 min between extradural injection and surgery exceeded the interval to onset of flank analgesia in cattle and perineal skin analgesia in llamas at a similar xylazine dose rate. As there is no advantage of lumbosacral over sacrococcygeal administration of xylazine, the sacrococcygeal route is recommended because it is the easier technique.

Surgery 40–50 minutes after sacrococcygeal extradural xylazine (0.4 mg/kg) injection

It is reported that sacrococcygeal injection of 0.4 mg/kg xylazine produces sedation and sufficient analgesia for vasectomy without the disadvantage of hindlimb paralysis associated with extradural lignocaine injection, although individual sheep may exhibit paresis for up to 48 hours after injection. There is deep sedation for up to 1 hour after extradural xylazine injection, with the sheep assuming sternal recumbency and the head rested on the ground.

The use of extradural xylazine injection does not preclude the use of preoperative injection with a NSAID. Indeed, such a multi-modal approach is likely to be additive in terms of analgesia. It is important to remember that neither xylazine nor NSAIDs are licensed for use in sheep in many countries and withdrawal periods before slaughter for human consumption must be strictly observed.

Lumbosacral extradural lignocaine injection

Excellent analgesia for caesarean operation, vasectomy and hindlimb surgery/fracture repair (**Fig. 17.3**) can be achieved after lumbosacral extradural injection of 3 mg/kg of 2% lignocaine solution. This analgesic regimen is recommended for caesarean operations when there is considerable trauma to the posterior reproductive tract, a foetal monster *in utero*

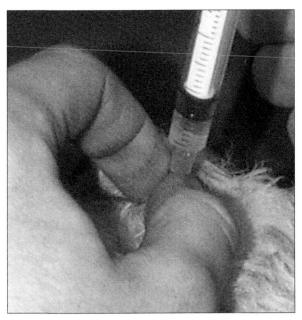

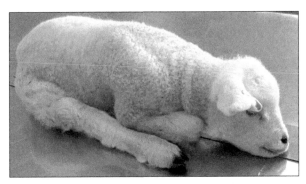

Fig. 17.4 Extradural injection at the lumbar site is facilitated when the sheep is positioned in sternal recumbency with the hips flexed and the hindlimbs extended alongside the abdomen.

Fig. 17.3 Excellent analgesia for hindlimb fracture repair can be achieved after lumbosacral extradural injection of 3 mg/kg of 2% lignocaine solution, even in day-old lambs.

Table 17.1 **Guide to needle length and gauge for extradural injection**

BODYWEIGHT OF SHEEP FOR EXTRADURAL INJECTION	DETAILS OF NEEDLE	
	LENGTH (MM)	GAUGE
Lambs (bodyweight <30 kg)	25	21
Ewes (bodyweight 30–80 kg)	38	20
Rams (bodyweight >80 kg)	50	20

or a concurrent traumatised vaginal prolapse resulting in tenesmus. The ewe can be restrained in sternal recumbency or the sheep can be sedated with 10 µg/kg medetomidine injected intravenously to facilitate positioning for extradural injection.

Extradural injection at the lumbar site is facilitated when the sheep is positioned in sternal recumbency, with the hindlimbs extended alongside the abdomen (**Fig. 17.4**). The site for injection is the midpoint of the lumbosacral space, identified as the mid-line depression between the last palpable dorsal lumbar spine (L6) and the first palpable sacral dorsal spine (S2). This site is approximately 1–3 cm caudal to an imaginary line joining the wings of the ilium. The thumb and middle finger of one hand are placed over the wings of the ilium (**Fig. 17.5**) and the index finger used to palpate the mid-line depression between L6 and S2 (**Fig. 17.6**). The site must be clipped, surgically prepared and between

1–2 ml of local anaesthetic injected subcutaneously. Hypodermic needles are preferred because they can be discarded after single use. Spinal needles with internal stylets are unnecessary. The needle (*Table 17.1*) is slowly advanced over 10 seconds at a right angle to the plane of the vertebral column or with the hub directed 5–10° caudally.

By advancing the needle with only the index finger of the other hand, the changes in tissue resistance as the needle point passes sequentially through the subcutaneous tissue interarcuate ligament and the sudden 'pop' due to loss of resistance as the needle point exits the ligamentum flavum into the extradural space, are easily recognised (**Fig. 17.7**). Should the needle be accidentally advanced into the dorsal subarachnoid space, cerebrospinal fluid (CSF) will well up in the needle hub within 2–3 seconds.

The lignocaine solution is warmed to body temperature prior to injection. The large volume of 2%

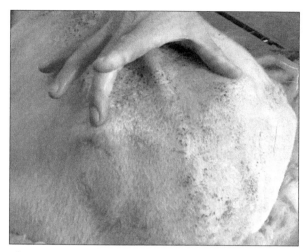

Fig. 17.5 The dorsal view of lumbar extradural injection demonstrated in the sequential images (Figs 17.5–17.8). The thumb and middle finger of one hand palpate the wings of the ilium.

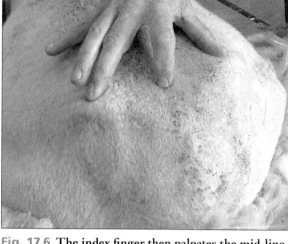

Fig. 17.6 The index finger then palpates the mid-line depression between L6 and S2 which is approximately 1–3 cm caudal to an imaginary line joining the wings of the ilium.

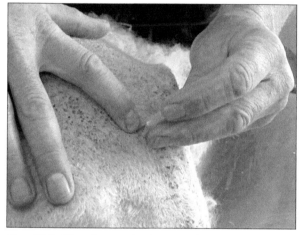

Fig. 17.7 The changes in tissue resistance are easily appreciated by slowly advancing the needle using gentle index finger pressure.

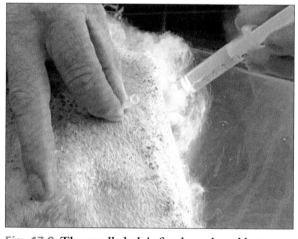

Fig. 17.8 The needle hub is firmly anchored between thumb and index finger before attaching the syringe.

lignocaine solution (12 ml for a 80 kg ewe) should be injected slowly over 30–60 seconds, with the needle hub firmly anchored between thumb and index finger (**Fig. 17.8**). The ewe is held in left lateral recumbency with the head elevated for approximately 10 minutes after injection, during which time there is onset of hindlimb paralysis. During surgery via the left flank approach the ewe's head should remain elevated relative to the vertebral column. To prevent hypothermia and overlying, lambs delivered by caesarean operation must be given colostrum by orogastric tube immediately and placed under a heat lamp or in a warming box until the ewe is ambulatory.

If the point of the needle accidentally punctures the arachnoid mater, CSF will appear within the hub. In this event the needle should be withdrawn into the extradural space and the dose rate reduced to two-thirds that calculated, as a precautionary measure. Further reduction of the dose rate may fail to achieve complete analgesia of the flank. Sheep should be confined to a small well-bedded pen until ambulatory, which is usually 2–4 hours after extradural injection. Unfortunately, the duration of hindlimb paralysis after injection, and requirement for precise injection technique, has resulted in few veterinary practitioners adopting the lumbosacral extradural lignocaine regimen for potentially difficult caesarean operations.

INTRAVENOUS REGIONAL ANAESTHESIA

Digit amputation under intravenous regional anaesthesia gives excellent results. Intravenous NSAID injection is given prior to amputation. Lignocaine (5 ml of 2% or equivalent) is injected into a superficial vein after application of a rubber tourniquet above the hock or carpus. The lateral saphenous vein is readily identified on the dorso-lateral aspect of the mid-metatarsal region for amputation of a hindlimb digit (**Fig. 17.9**). A thumb can be placed alongside the vein to aid stabilisation for intravenous injection (**Fig. 17.10**). Insertion of the 20–21 gauge 25 mm into the distended superficial vein releases 5–10 ml of blood under pressure; blood flow then quickly reduces to the occasional drop if the tourniquet is effective. Some clinicians prefer to use a 21 gauge butterfly needle (**Fig. 17.11**), which allows some latitude if the sheep draws its foot away during the injection. Analgesia should be effective within 2 minutes and is tested by pricking the coronary band. The rapid onset of analgesia allows the digit amputation to be undertaken quickly (**Fig. 17.12**), reducing veterinary time and thereby cost to the client. The low cost of materials and rapid onset of effective analgesia after intravenous regional anaesthesia (IVRA) means that cost is not an issue when dealing with septic pedal arthritis, which is a common very painful lesion.

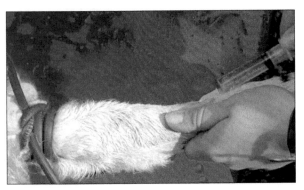

Fig. 17.9 A rubber tourniquet is usually applied above the hock with intravenous injection into the lateral saphenous vein.

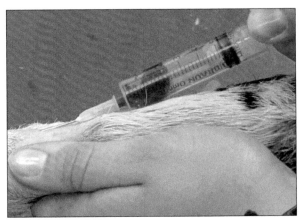

Fig. 17.10 A thumb can be placed alongside the vein to aid stabilization for intravenous injection.

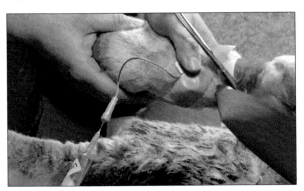

Fig. 17.11 A butterfly needle is inserted into a superficial vein after application of a thick rubber tourniquet.

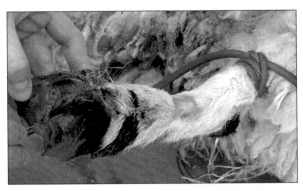

Fig. 17.12 Amputation of the infected digit under intravenous regional anaesthesia.

CHAPTER 18

CLINICAL CASES

CASE QUESTIONS

The answers to the questions can be found on pages 405–420.

CASE 1

Results of serum protein concentrations and faecal samples collected as part of a preliminary investigation of poor condition score in a group of six ewes (**Fig. 18.1**) (study sheep 2–7 sheep; sheep 1 normal control ewe) are presented in *Table 18.1*.

1. How would you interpret these findings?

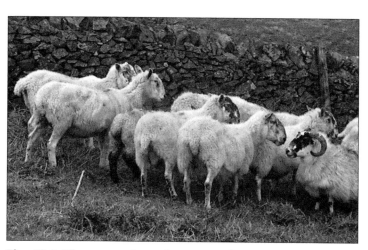

Fig. 18.1 **The group of ewes in poor condition.**

Table 18.1 **Serum protein and faecal egg count in a group of sheep in poor body condition**

	1	2	3	4	5	6	7
Albumin (g/l)	34.1	28.3	12.5	14.1	21.1	24.3	22.5
Globulin (g/l)	44.1	39.1	37.1	40.1	62.7	42.1	64.1
Faecal worm egg count (epg)	100	400	50	6100	100	150	150

CASE 2

A sheep farmer complained of high perinatal lamb mortality in his lowground flock last year. While the overall flock scanning percentage was 207% at 45–90 days of gestation, the weaning percentage was only 160%, with most lamb losses occurring during the first 3 days of life.

This year the flock was housed 3 weeks ago and penned according to litter size. The sheep are fed *ad libitum* clamp silage and 200 g of mineralized barley (twins and triplets). Serum samples collected 5 weeks before the expected lambing date (*Table 18.2*) are ranked according to litter size. Abnormal concentrations are depicted in bold text.

1. Which are the important data in *Table 18.2* (see Russel A, Nutrition of the pregnant ewe. *In Practice* 7:23–29 for excellent review of this subject)?
2. Why not measure plasma glucose and non-esterified fatty acid concentrations?
3. Comment upon the protein status of these sheep.
4. Are mineral (calcium, magnesium, inorganic phosphate) analyses useful in such profiles?

Table 18.2 **Serum samples collected from sheep 5 weeks prior to expected lambing date**										
EWE NUMBER	1	2	3	4	5	6	7	8	9	10
Parity	3	2	2	3	4	3	2	2	5	3
Litter size	1	1	2	2	2	2	3	3	3	3
Body condition score	3	3.5	3.5	3.5	3	3	3	3	2.0	2.5
Butyrate (mmol/l)	0.2	0.4	0.4	0.5	**1.1**	**0.9**	**1.1**	**1.5**	**1.9**	**1.6**
Urea-N (mmol/l)	2.6	2.9	**2.0**	3.5	2.6	4.5	2.6	3.5	2.4	3.4
Albumin (g/l)	34	36	33	**29**	31	34	30	31	**28**	30
Globulin (g/l)	44	46	39	41	45	43	42	42	46	41

CASE 3

A pregnant Blackface ewe was noted 2 days ago to be isolated from the rest of the flock. The ewes are being fed *ad libitum* average quality big-bale silage plus 200g/head/day of a 16% crude protein concentrate. The flock is due to start lambing in approximately 2 weeks. The ewe is in poorer bodily condition (1.5; scale 1–5) compared with other sheep in the group at a similar stage of pregnancy (2.5–3.0). The ewe is dull and depressed. There is lack of menace response (**Fig. 18.3**) but papillary light reflexes are normal. The ewe is hyperaesthetic to tactile and auditory stimuli. The rectal temperature is normal.

1. What conditions would you consider (most likely first)?

2. How could you confirm your diagnosis?
3. What treatment(s) would you give?
4. What control measures could be adopted?

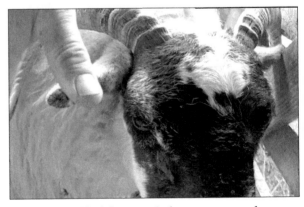

Fig. 18.3 A Blackface ewe in late pregnancy shows a lack of menace response but papillary light and other cranial nerve reflexes are normal.

CASE 4

A sheep client complains that approximately 15 of 200 lambs (ca. 8%) are very lame on one or more limbs. The lameness appears when the lambs are approximately 5–7 days old and have been at pasture for 2–5 days (**Fig. 18.4**). A typical lamb is bright and alert but reluctant to rise and appears very stiff on one or more limbs. The rectal temperature is normal. There is swelling of the joint(s) caused by joint effusion, and enlargement of drainage lymph node(s).

1. What conditions would you consider?
2. What treatment would you administer?
3. What control measures could you introduce?

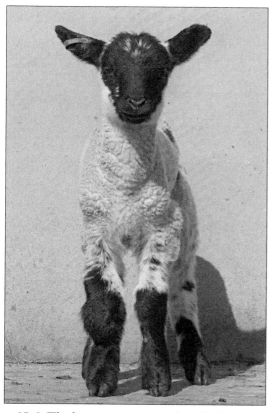

Fig. 18.4 The lameness appears when the lambs are approximately 5–7 days old.

CASE 5

After severe weather conditions of driving wind and snow, a shepherd complains that a number of heavily-pregnant ewes on the hill have suddenly become blind. The ewes are markedly photophobic with blepharospasm and epiphora with tear staining of the cheeks (**Fig. 18.5**). Clinical examination reveals pronounced conjunctivitis and keratitis. In some eyes there is also corneal ulceration, more clearly observed after fluorescein dye strips have been placed in contact with the eye.

1. What conditions would you consider?
2. What treatments would you recommend?
3. What action would you recommend?

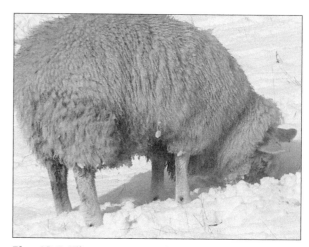

Fig. 18.5 The ewes are markedly photophobic with blepharospasm and epiphora with tear staining of the cheeks.

CASE 6

During early February a pedigree Suffolk ewe is found separated from the remainder of 25 ewes due to lamb in 2 weeks. On clinical examination the ewe is very dull and depressed (**Fig. 18.6**) with an elevated rectal temperature (41.0°C). The mucous membranes are congested. The abdomen is drawn in, which contrasts to the normal distension of late gestation. The ewe's vulva is slightly swollen with evidence of a foetid red/brown fluid discharge. The udder is poorly developed and there is no accumulated colostrum in the glands. The flock is closed with no contiguous sheep flocks.

1. What is your diagnosis?
2. What further tests could be carried out?
3. What treatments would you consider?
4. What control measures could be adopted?

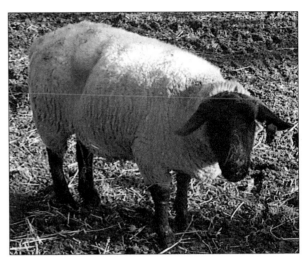

Fig. 18.6 A pedigree Suffolk ewe with a foetid red/brown fluid discharge is found separated from the remaining group of 25 ewes due to lamb in 2 weeks.

CASE 7

Towards the end of the lambing period you are presented with a 6-day-old Texel lamb with sudden weakness affecting all four limbs (**Fig. 18.7**). The rectal temperature is normal. There are no joint swellings and no swollen lymph nodes. There is evidence of cervical pain and gentle manipulation of the neck is resented. The reflex arcs are increased in all four limbs. The umbilical stump is dry and brittle.

1. What is your diagnosis (most likely first)?
2. How could you confirm your diagnosis?
3. What treatments would you administer?
4. What preventive measures could be adopted?

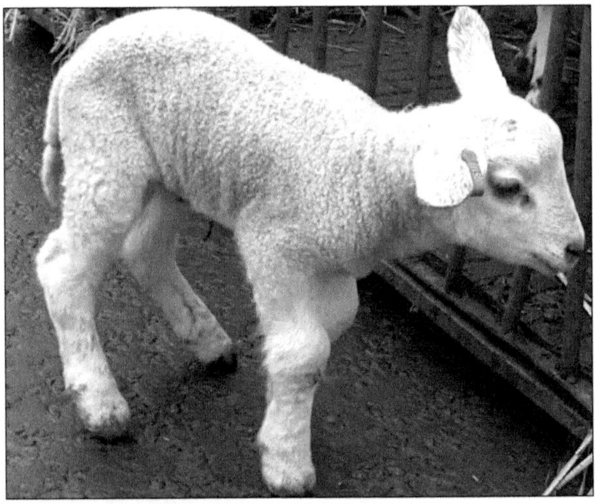

Fig. 18.7 A 6-day-old Texel lamb presents with sudden onset tetraparesis.

CASE 8

In early autumn a farmer reports the loss of two Blackface yearlings 3 weeks after transfer to poor-quality pasture. The farmer had noted no prior signs of illness.

1. What common conditions could cause sudden death in these sheep?
2. What action would you take?

CASE 9

A Suffolk ram presents with an 18 cm diameter area of skin erosion on the brisket covered by granulation tissue (**Fig. 18.9**).

1. What is the likely cause?
2. What treatment would you recommend?
3. What alternative husbandry practices would you recommend?

CASE 10

A farmer complains that approximately 5% of the ewes in his lowground flock have given birth to very small singleton or twin lambs (approximately 2.5–3.0 kg). The lambs are lively and well-fleshed, but 2–4 kg lighter than they should be (**Fig. 18.10**). Examination of the dams of three such litters reveals very low body condition scores of 1.0–1.5 (scale 1–5), while the majority of ewes in the flock are in good body condition (around 3.0).

1. What condition do you suspect?
2. What could be done in future years to prevent this problem?

CASE 11

A lowground farmer in the Scottish Borders reports two lamb deaths and others with diarrhoea in a group of 6-week-old Suffolk cross lambs on permanent pasture with their dams during early May (**Fig. 18.11**).

1. What common conditions would you consider (most likely first)?
2. What tests could be undertaken to support your provisional diagnosis?
3. What control measures would you recommend?

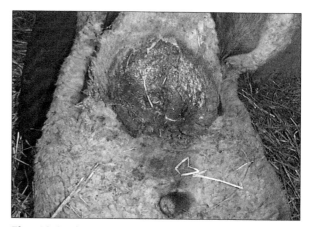

Fig. 18.9 Skin erosion on the brisket covered by granulation tissue in a Suffolk ram.

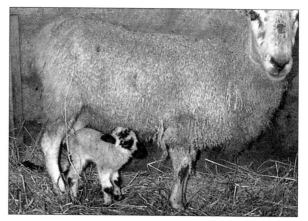

Fig. 18.10 A small percentage of lambs are lively, well-fleshed but very small.

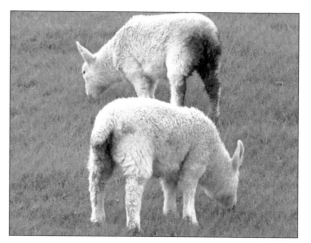

Fig. 18.11 A farmer reports two lamb deaths and others with diarrhoea grazing permanent pasture with their dams during early May.

CASE 12

While selecting ewes in October to retain for the next breeding season, a sheep client finds 10 of 700 1- to 3-crop ewes to be in very poor body condition. You are presented with two emaciated 4-year-old ewes typical of this group (**Fig. 18.12a**). In both ewes, the fleece is open and poor. The rectal temperature is normal. The eyes appear sunken which is thought to be largely due to the absence of intraorbital fat. The mucous membranes appear pale. There is no evidence of diarrhoea.

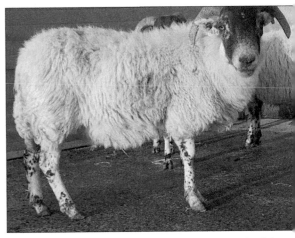

Fig. 18.12a An emaciated 4-year-old ewe, which is one of 10 sheep affected in a flock of 700.

1. What is your provisional diagnosis (most likely first)?
2. What tests would you undertake?
3. What action would you recommend?
4. What control measures could be adopted?

CASE 13

During early April you are presented with a recumbent 6-crop Greyface ewe that lambed 1 week ago and is nursing twin lambs. The ewe was at pasture with 40 other recently lambed sheep, which are being fed 1 kg of 18% crude protein concentrates per head per day plus access to clamp silage. The ewe has been brought indoors for examination. She appears dull and does not respond to your approach. The menace response is present but slow. There are no cranial nerve deficits but the ewe is salivating continuously (**Fig. 18.13a**). The rectal temperature is 39.5°C. The rectum is flaccid and contains a ball of pelleted faeces. The mucous membranes appear normal. The heart rate is 60 bpm. The respiratory rate is 18 breaths per minute. There is reduced ruminal movement with mainly gaseous sounds. There is reduced rumen fill. There is no mastitis. There is no vulval discharge or swelling.

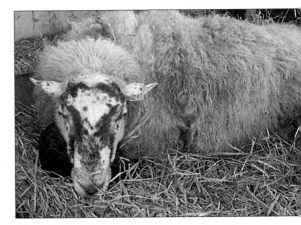

Fig. 18.13a A recumbent six-crop Greyface ewe that lambed 1 week ago and is nursing twin lambs; there is a slow menace response and she is salivating continuously.

1. What conditions would you consider (most likely first)?
2. What treatment would you administer?
3. What control measures would you recommend?

CASE 14

A yearling female sheep presents with a cervico-vaginal prolapse during first stage labour. The sheep is straining vigorously and is in considerable distress. The vaginal mucosa is congested, oedematous, friable and dirty (**Fig. 18.14**). Foetal membranes protrude through the cervix which is dilated to approximately 2 cm.

1. How will you provide proper analgesia in this case?
2. What action will you take?
3. What are the economics of your proposed action plan?

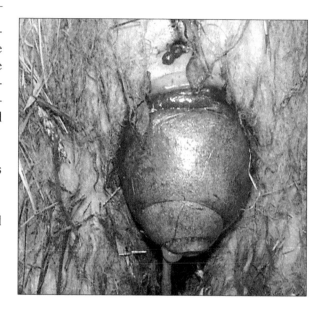

Fig. 18.14 A female sheep presents with a cervico-vaginal prolapse during first stage labour.

CASE 15

During late March you are presented with an obtunded 2-year-old Leicester ram that is weak on the right side of the body and leans against a wall for support (**Fig. 18.15a**). The sheep shows drooping of the right ear, deviated muzzle towards the right side, flaccid right lip and lowered right upper eyelid (ptosis). There is lack of menace response in the right eye and profuse salivation with a flaccid right cheek with impacted food material (**Fig. 18.15b**).

1. What conditions would you consider (most likely first)?
2. What laboratory tests could be undertaken to confirm your provisional diagnosis?
3. What treatments would you administer?
4. What control measures would you recommend?

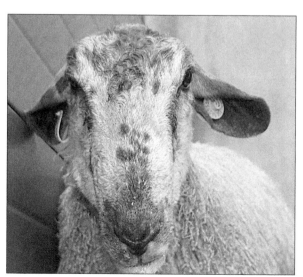

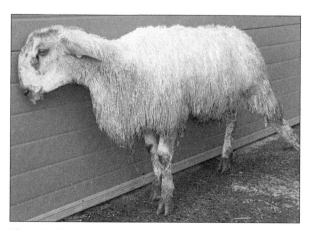

Fig. 18.15a An obtunded 2-year-old Leicester ram presents weak on the right side of the body.

Fig. 18.15b The sheep also shows drooping of the right ear, deviated muzzle towards the right side, flaccid right lip and lowered right upper eyelid.

CASE 16

A yearling pedigree Suffolk ram presents with colic of 6 hours' duration. The ram shows abdominal straining, but only a few drops of urine rather than a continuous flow are voided. The urine is slightly blood-tinged. There are no calculi on the preputial hairs. There is frequent bruxism (teeth grinding). The rectal temperature is normal (39.5°C). The heart rate is increased to 90 bpm. The mucous membranes are normal. Auscultation of the chest fails to reveal any abnormalities. There are reduced rumen sounds.

1. What conditions would you consider (most likely first)?
2. What action would you take?
3. What further investigation could be undertaken?
4. What sequelae could result in neglected cases?
5. What control measures would you recommend?

CASE 17

A white-faced sheep grazing a new grass ley during mid-summer suddenly presents with swollen oedematous head and ears. Clinical examination reveals lachrymation and sensitive erythematous non-pigmented skin with oozing of serum (**Fig. 18.17**). The rectal temperature is normal.

1. What conditions would you consider (most likely first)?
2. What are the possible causes?
3. What treatment would you administer?
4. What control measures would you introduce?

CASE 18

During lambing time a sheep client complains that a large number of neonatal lambs have tear staining of the face, leading to blindness in some cases (**Fig. 18.18a**). Closer examination reveals conjunctivitis, episceral injection and corneal ulceration in some lambs.

1. What is your diagnosis (most likely first)?
2. What treatments would you administer?
3. What are the consequences of no action/treatment?
4. What preventive measures could be adopted?

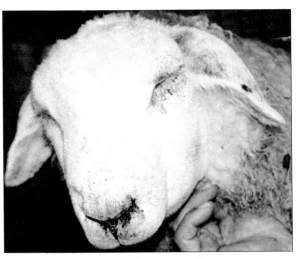

Fig. 18.17 A white-faced sheep grazing a new grass ley during mid-summer suddenly presents with swollen oedematous head and ears.

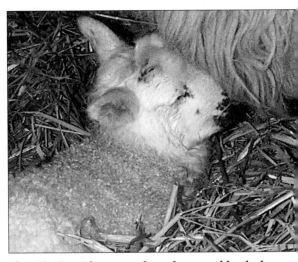

Fig. 18.18a A large number of neonatal lambs have tear staining of the face leading to blindness in some cases.

CASE 19

In mid-winter an 11-month-old Greyface ewe lamb is presented in very poor body condition (BCS 1). The farmer reports that the group of 68 ewe lambs are in poor condition (BCS 1.5) despite being lightly stocked on permanent grass supplemented with hay. The farmer reports that the ewe lambs had been treated with oxfendazole 3 months previously. On clinical examination the hogg is dull, depressed and emaciated. The rectal temperature is normal.

There is obvious pallor of the mucous membranes. Auscultation of the heart and lungs fails to reveal any abnormalities. There is little rumen fill but normal contractions are heard. No other abnormalities are found during clinical examination.

1. What conditions should be considered?
2. What further tests would be appropriate?
3. What treatment would you suggest?

CASE 20

This sonogram (**Fig. 18.20a**) was obtained from a recently purchased ram using a 5.0 MHz linear transducer connected to a real-time, B-mode ultrasound machine.

1. Describe the sonogram (both testicles were similar).
2. What further fertility assessment(s) could be undertaken?
3. What simple selection criterion could farmers adopt at ram sales?
4. What advice would you offer?

CASE 21

You are asked to undertake a postmortem examination on a 2-year-old sheep maintained at pasture with twin lambs during June. The farmer had noted no signs of illness before the sheep was found dead this morning.

1. What conditions causing sudden death would you include in your differential diagnosis list?
2. Comment upon the gross postmortem findings (**Fig. 18.21**).

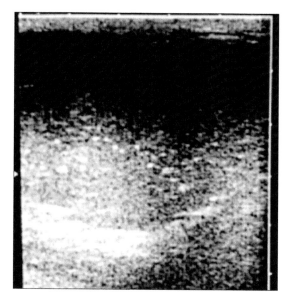

Fig. 18.20a Sonogram obtained from a recently purchased ram using a 5.0 MHz linear transducer.

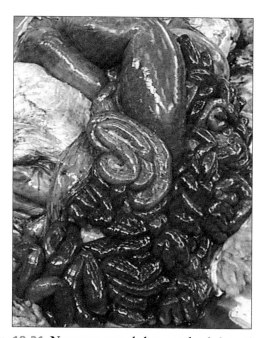

Fig. 18.21 Necropsy reveals haemorrhagic intestines.

CASE 22

Several 4-month-old Texel lambs experience difficulty in raising themselves to their feet and have a stilted gait. Lameness was first noted at 6 weeks old. There was a poor response to long-acting oxytetracycline injection administered after the lambs had been lame for several days to 1 week. Four of the six lambs have bilateral carpal swellings (**Fig. 18.22**) with associated enlargement of the prescapular lymph nodes. There is little joint effusion but marked thickening of the joint capsule, which physically restricts joint excursion.

1. What conditions would you consider?
2. What is the likely cause?
3. How would you confirm the cause?
4. What treatment would you administer?
5. What control measure(s) would you recommend?

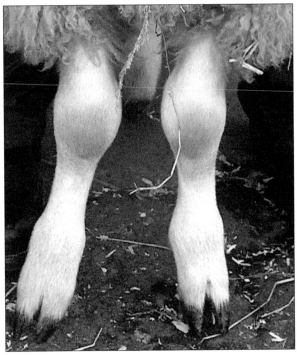

Fig. 18.22 Four of the six lame lambs examined have bilateral carpal swellings with associated enlargement of the prescapular lymph nodes.

CASE 23

You are presented with a pedigree Texel ram which has been dull and inappetent for the past 6 days. The ram has a tucked-up abdomen consistent with a poor appetite. The ram often adopts a wide stance with the hindlimbs placed further back than normal and the head held lowered. There is frequent bruxism. Only a few drops of urine rather than a continuous flow are voided when the ram urinates. The rectal temperature is normal (39.6°C). The heart is increased at 90 bpm. The BUN concentration is elevated at 29.8 mmol/l (normal range = 2.2–6.6 mmol/l). You suspect partial obstructive urolithiasis and scan the right sublumbar fossa with a 5.0 MHz sector transducer connected to a real-time, B-mode ultrasound machine 5 MHz.

1. Describe the sonogram shown in **Fig. 18.23a**.
2. What action would you take?
3. How could this problem have been prevented?

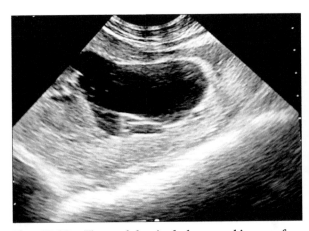

Fig. 18.23a Trans-abdominal ultrasound image of the right sublumbar fossa obtained using a 5 MHz sector scanner.

CASE 24

A depressed ewe is presented during early summer (**Fig. 18.24**). The ewe had lambed approximately 6 weeks previously and was nursing triplets. The shepherd noted the ewe separated from the remainder of the group that morning. The ewe is in poor bodily condition (BCS 1.5) and depressed with toxic mucous membranes. The rectal temperature is raised (40.6°C). The pulse is increased to 120 bpm, the respiratory rate is normal (25 breaths per minute) and there are reduced ruminal sounds. Examination of the udder reveals extensive gangrenous mastitis of the left gland, with associated marked subcutaneous oedema extending to involve the ventral abdominal wall. The sharply demarcated purple areas are cold and firm. There are numerous skin lesions on the medial aspect of both teats.

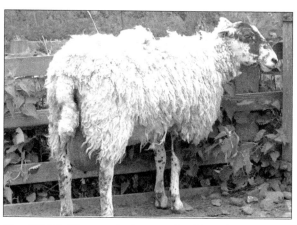

Fig. 18.24 The ewe is depressed with toxic mucous membranes; the rectal temperature is 40.6°C. The pulse is increased to 120 bpm but the respiratory rate is normal.

1. What pathogens could be involved?
2. What is the prognosis?
3. What action should be recommended?

CASE 25

During late April you are presented with an obtunded North Ronaldsay ewe. The rectal temperature is 38.5°C. The ewe has a sluggish menace response in both eyes. There are no cranial nerve deficits. The mucous membranes are jaundiced (**Fig. 18.25**). Rumen contractions are reduced and the abdomen is shrunken consistent with inappetence of several days. There is very little udder development and no vulval discharge. The ewe had been fed approximately 0.25 kg of cattle concentrate daily for 4 weeks

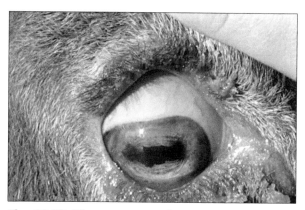

Fig. 18.25 The mucous membranes are jaundiced.

1. What conditions would you consider?
2. Which further tests could be undertaken?
3. What actions/treatments would you recommend?
4. What control measures could be taken?

CASE 26

During October a 4-year-old ewe presents in much poorer body condition (BSC 1.5; scale 1–5) compared with others in the flock (BCS 3.0). The ewe's fleece has an open appearance with poor-quality wool (**Fig. 18.26a**). The ewe is bright and alert and is grazing normally. After gathering the group into the handling pens nearby, the ewe is tachypnoeic (48 breaths per minute) with an obvious abdominal component to her breathing. The rectal temperature is 39.6°C. Auscultation of the chest reveals wheezes distributed dorsally on both sides of the chest. The heart rate is 88 bpm.

1. What conditions would you consider (most likely first)?
2. How would you confirm the diagnosis?
3. What treatment would you administer?
4. What control measures could be attempted in this flock?

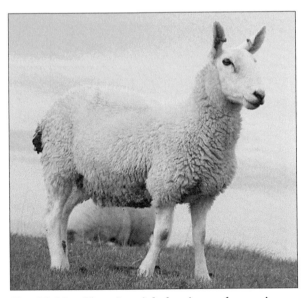

Fig. 18.26a Chronic weight loss in a tachypnoeic 4-year-old ewe. The fleece has an open appearance with poor quality wool.

CASE 27

During July a client complains of poor growth in a large group of 4-month-old lambs on permanent grazing. A large number of the lambs show signs of diarrhoea. The fleeces of some of the lambs are contaminated with faeces and have been dagged. A white drench anthelmintic (1-BZ benzimidazoles) was administered in mid-May to prevent nematodirosis and again 3 weeks ago when the lambs first showed signs of scouring.

1. What are the common causes of poor growth in lambs?
2. How could this problem be investigated?
3. What control measures should be advised?

CASE 28

During February you are presented with a group of housed yearling sheep because they are continually rubbing against pen divisions and abruptly stop eating and nibble at their fleece overlying the dorsal midline, causing fleece damage/loss (**Fig. 18.28**).

1. What conditions would you consider?
2. How would you establish a specific diagnosis?
3. What treatment would you recommend?
4. What control measures would you recommend?

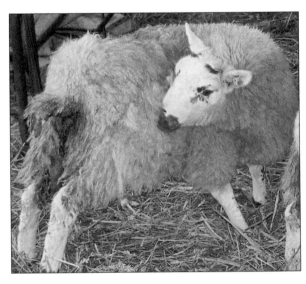

Fig. 18.28 A group of housed yearling sheep present because they continually rub against pen divisions and nibble at their fleece causing fleece damage/loss.

CASE 29

Two 5-month-old pedigree Charollais lambs in the same flock appear unsteady on their limbs. The sheep were normal for the first 8 weeks of life. The lambs have a lowered head carriage, a wide-based stance, ataxia and dysmetria but with preservation of strength. The pelvic ataxia results in the lambs occasionally falling over, especially when turning quickly.

1. Which area of the brain could be involved?
2. What conditions would you consider?
3. What treatment would you administer?
4. What control measures could be adopted?

CASE 30

In an attempt to reduce your client's lamb losses you are anxious that all staff employed to assist over the lambing period are familiar with ensuring colostrum intake.

1. What guidelines would you recommend?
2. What is the most cost-effective method for determining passive antibody transfer?

CASE ANSWERS

ANSWER 1

1. Sheep 1 has normal serum albumin and globulin concentrations >30 g/l and 35-45g/l, respectively.

   Sheep 2 has a serum protein profile typically observed in emaciated ewes without obvious bacterial infection or parasite infestation. Causes include poor molar dentition and lameness.

   Sheep with a protein-losing enteropathy, notably paratuberculosis (very common; sheep 3 and 4), and nephropathy (rare) have profound hypoalbuminaemia (serum concentration <15 g/l) and a normal globulin concentration. Due to immunosuppression, sheep with paratuberculosis often have high faecal egg counts >1000 epg (sheep 4) resulting from increased fecundity of those mature nematodes present; diarrhoea is uncommon. It is exceptional for serum albumin concentrations to fall so low in cases of chronic intestinal parasitism such as haemonchosis.

   Chronic severe bacterial infections (sheep 5) causing weight loss/ill thrift result in significant increases in serum globulin concentration (often >55 g/l) and low serum albumin concentration (18–25 g/l).

   If fed marginal protein levels during late gestation, serum albumin concentrations can fall as immunoglobulins accumulate in colostrum (sheep 6).

   Fasciolosis (sheep 7) results in hypoalbuminaemia; these sheep usually show additional clinical signs such as anaemia and submandibular oedema. In addition, many sheep with subacute and chronic fasciolosis have increased serum globulin concentrations often exceeding 65 g/l. Further specific tests can then be selected based upon the organ system, e.g. serum GLDH and GGT concentrations and faecal fluke egg count for fasciolosis.

ANSWER 2

1. Body condition scores are fine (target 3–3.5) except for two triplet-bearing ewes. Butyrate

concentrations largely reflect energy demands from the developing foetuses, with normal values in the two single-bearing ewes 1 and 2 (target for all sheep <0.8 mmol/l), marginal energy deficiency in twin-bearing ewes and moderate/severe energy deficiency in triplet-bearing ewes. This necessitates nil, 1 MJ and 4–5 MJ/head/day respectively to correct current energy shortfalls. 4 MJ is approximately 300 g of concentrate as fed and costs 4–5 pence/day.

Following correction of these existing energy shortfalls, continuing demands from the developing foetus(es) will necessitate an extra 3, 5, and 7 MJ/day by the end of gestation in a broadly linear relationship for singles, twins and triplets respectively, to maintain energy balance and optimize lamb birth weights.

2. Plasma glucose and non-esterified fatty acid analyses are unnecessary because serum butyrate concentration accurately reflects the balance between lipolysis in response to energy deficiency and dietary supply of propionate and glucogenic amino acids.

3. Urea nitrogen concentrations are normal. Serum albumin concentrations are to the low end of the normal range, but this is a physiological process whereby immunoglobulins are accumulated in colostrum in the udder.

4. Mineral deficiencies are rare when sheep are settled on a correctly formulated ration. Calcium, magnesium and inorganic phosphate analyses would be expensive and provide no useful additional information.

ANSWER 3

1. The most likely conditions to consider would include:
   - Ovine pregnancy toxaemia.
   - Polioencephalomalacia.
   - Listeriosis.
   - Acidosis resulting from excess carbohydrates.
   - Impending abortion.
   - Chronic copper poisoning.
2. The serum 3-OH butyrate concentration is 4.5 mmol/l (>3.0 mmol/l consistent with pregnancy toxaemia). Plasma glucose and

non-esterified fatty acid concentrations are too variable to confirm the presumptive clinical diagnosis.

3. Treatments include a concentrated oral electrolyte and dextrose solution or propylene glycol given per os three times daily. Injection with 4 mg dexamethasone promotes appetite and gluconeogenesis (>16 mg after day 135 of pregnancy will induce abortion which may save the ewe's life). The ewe should be isolated and offered palatable feedstuffs. An elective caesarean operation to remove the foetuses is rarely successful because retained foetal membranes and septic metritis invariably result.

4. Control measures include ultrasound scanning, which would identify ewes carrying multiple foetuses. Correct nutrition during gestation is essential especially for multigravid ewes, which are at most risk from energy deficiency due to foetal demands. Routine monitoring of late gestation nutrition is strongly recommended and the reader is directed to Dr Angus Russel's article (1985), which gives accurate guidelines based upon 3-OH butyrate concentration, foetal number and ewe bodyweight. A veterinary advisory visit undertaken 4–6 weeks before the lambing season is the cornerstone of the flock health programme.

ANSWER 4

1. The most likely conditions to consider would include:
   - *Streptococcus dysgalactiae* polyarthritis.
   - Other bacterial pathogens causing polyarthritis.
2. A recent publication reported 85% of positive bacterial joint cultures yielded *S. dysgalactiae*. Outbreaks of polyarthritis may affect up to 30% of lambs. In addition to the carpus, hock and stifle joints, infection of the atlanto-occipital joint may cause tetraparesis. Early recognition and treatment are essential. Procaine penicillin is cheap, highly effective and no resistance problems have been recorded in streptococci. The lambs should be treated with 44,000 IU/kg procaine penicillin injected intramuscularly

for at least 5 consecutive days with dexametha-sone on day 1. Joint lavage could be undertaken under either alphaxane- or propafol-induced general anaesthesia but this is cost-prohibitive.

3. *S. dysgalactiae* can survive for weeks in bedding material. Ensuring passive antibody transfer often fails to reduce ongoing problems of polyar-thritis. Bacteraemia from the upper respiratory tract and ear notching may explain the appar-ent failure of navel dipping in the control of this problem. The prevalence of polyarthritis caused by *S. dysgalactiae* may justify metaphylactic peni-cillin injection when 24–48 hours old but this is no substitute for good hygiene and husbandry.

ANSWER 5

1. The most likely conditions to consider would include:
   - Infectious keratoconjunctivitis (IKC).
   - Periorbital eczema.
2. The two common causal organisms, *Mycoplasma conjunctivae* and *Chlamydia psittaci*, are each sus-ceptible to a wide range of antibiotics including oxytetracycline. Topical oxytetracycline oph-thalmic ointment or powder should be given twice daily for 3 days; powder adheres to the moist conjunctivae whereas ointment tends to slip off the cornea, especially when the con-tents of the tube are cold. In addition, ewes with bilateral corneal lesions should be injected with long-acting oxytetracycline intramuscularly.
3. Ewes with impaired vision in both eyes must be housed in small groups, thereby ensuring ade-quate feeding to prevent ovine pregnancy tox-aemia. The ewes are markedly photophobic and housing will prevent direct exposure to strong sunlight, especially when there is snow cover on the ground. Confinement also prevents deaths from misadventure. Ewes should be taken off exposed hill ground when storms are forecast but this is not always possible. Occasionally, outbreaks of IKC occur associated with concen-trate/roughage feeding where space allowance is inadequate.

ANSWER 6

1. Abortion/metritis and septicaemia should be considered as the most likely diagnoses. Potential abortifacient agents include:
   - Salmonellosis including *S. montevideo*, *S. typhimurium*.
   - *Campylobacter fetus intestinalis*.
   - *Listeria monocytogenes*.
   - *Chlamydophila abortus* (enzootic abortion of ewes; EAE) but flock closed.
   - *Pasteurella* spp.
2. The abdomen should be carefully balloted to check for foetuses. Transabdominal ultrasound examination of the uterus can be used to check whether the ewe has aborted. Any foetuses and placentae should be sampled for bacteriol-ogy and a blood sample collected for EAE and *Toxoplasma* serology. Vaginal and rectal swabs should be collected if there are no products of abortion.

   Salmonella typhimurium is isolated in pure culture from the vaginal and rectal swabs.
3. The ewe is injected intravenously with oxytet-racycline and a NSAID.
4. The farmer was advised to isolate the ewe for at least 6 weeks. The farmer was advised regarding the zoonotic risk from salmonel-losis and to adopt strict personal hygiene when handling sick sheep. The source of infection was traced to a septic tank overflow that was immediately fenced off and the ewes were moved onto another field. Three more ewes aborted over the next 2 days. All ewes in the group were injected with 20 mg/kg long-acting oxytetracycline at this stage. One more abortion occurred over the next 2 days. No further abortions occurred for 1 week. Two ewes produced autolytic lambs at full term and many of the live lambs were weakly. There is circumstantial evidence that the long-acting oxytetracycline injected intra-muscularly reduced the number of abor-tions in this outbreak although this cannot be proven.

ANSWER 7

1. The most likely conditions to consider would include:
   - *Streptococcus dysgalactiae* infection of the atlanto-occipital joint causing spinal cord compression.
   - Muscular dystrophy (white muscle disease; WMD).
   - Infection tracking to the cervical spinal canal from injection site in the neck muscles.
   - Extradural haemorrhage following trauma C1–C6.
   - Polyarthritis.
2. A rapid response to dexamethasone and penicillin treatment helps to confirm the diagnosis. Compression of the spinal cord causes an increased lumbar CSF protein concentration (>1.0 g/l). Muscular dystrophy causes a 10- to 100-fold increase in serum creatine kinase concentration.
3. There is a rapid and dramatic response to intravenous dexamethasone and intramuscular procaine penicillin injections such that the lamb is ambulatory within 3 hours. A further 10 consecutive days' intramuscular injection of procaine penicillin was administered. Procaine penicillin remains the drug of choice for all streptococcal infections.
4. Hygiene measures in the lambing shed and ensuring passive antibody transfer often fail to reduce ongoing problems of *S. dysgalactiae* polyarthritis. The shepherd had immersed the lamb's navel in strong veterinary iodine on three occasions within the first 6 hours of life. In this situation it was suggested that the *S. dysgalactiae* bacteraemia arose from either the upper respiratory tract or tonsils because there was no gross evidence of omphalitis. The prevalence of polyarthritis caused by *S. dysgalactiae* may become so high, metaphylactic penicillin injection is justified when the lambs are turned out to pasture with their dam at 24–48 hours old.

ANSWER 8

1. Differential diagnoses include:
   - Clostridial disease: pulpy kidney disease, blackleg, black disease, braxy.
   - Acute fasciolosis.
   - Pasteurellosis or other septicaemic disease, possibly secondary to tick-borne fever.
   - Louping-ill.
   - Abdominal catastrophe such as volvulus of the abomasum or small intestine.
   - Poisoning such as nitrate or ammonia.
2. A postmortem examination.

No ticks were present on the carcases. Postmortem examination revealed multiple haemorrhagic tracts within the liver caused by migrating flukes. No volvulus was detected. The kidneys appeared friable but the sheep had been dead for approximately 24 hours in 16–18°C daytime temperatures. A urinary dipstick test was negative for glucose. No other abnormalities were found in the carcases.

A provisional diagnosis of acute fasciolosis was reached.

The farmer was advised to remove the sheep from the pasture and treat them with triclabendazole immediately and again with a flukacide in 2 months' time. More frequent treatment with triclabendazole, then closantel, would be necessary if the new pasture could not be guaranteed free of fluke. If possible, the wet areas of the field should either be drained or fenced off.

ANSWER 9

1. Brisket sores most commonly arise from a poorly fitted harness used to hold marker crayons during the mating period. Lesions may also arise from/are aggravated by prolonged sternal recumbency caused by severe lameness.
2. These lesions prove very difficult to treat and never fully heal. Topical antibiotics will limit secondary bacterial infection. These animals are best kept at pasture to prevent straw adhering to the granulating surface if housed, but they invariably lie in the dirtiest corner of the field. Check constantly for cutaneous myiasis but this is a rare site for strike. Prevention is paramount.

3. Keel marks are used as a management aid to optimize limited accommodation over the lambing period. In most situations it is not necessary to use keel paint for the first 7 days or so of the mating period when up to 80% of the ewes are served. Thereafter, keel paint can be applied to identify the ewes mated after 7 days. Returns after one oestrous cycle can be identified by a colour change at 14 days. If a large number of ewes are identified as returns (>20%) then the fertility of the ram(s) should be questioned.

Alternatives to harnesses include keel paint applied daily during the service period to the fleece immediately cranial to the prepuce when the rams are fed. This method has the advantage that the ram must fully mount the ewe to mark the ewe's tail head, and the extra feeding helps maintain body condition of the rams during the breeding season.

ANSWER 10

1. Chronic debilitating disease affecting dams including:
   * Chronic severe parasitic gastroenteritis, chronic fasciolosis, paratuberculosis and OPA, causing poor placental development and chronic intrauterine growth retardation.
   * Starvation – poor energy supply throughout gestation.
   * Early foetal loss with limited placentomes for remaining foetus(es).
2. Very low lamb birthweights can occur when the dam is affected by one of the severe debilitating diseases listed above over a significant period of gestation. Because the nutritional insult persists over a long period of its development, the lamb is well-formed but very small. Samples collected from two of the three ewes were positive for paratuberculosis.

The possible consequences of energy underfeeding during mid-gestation while the placenta is developing cannot be discounted. A review of farm management during early and mid-lactation would be indicated, especially provision of feed during winter storms. The situation could be monitored by regular condition scoring of ewes every month during pregnancy.

Determination of condition scores of all ewes at weaning time and examination of all lean ewes at that time may give some indication of the prevalence of paratuberculosis in the flock. Postmortem examination of a representative number of emaciated ewes may help to establish an accurate diagnosis of the problem.

ANSWER 11

1. The most likely conditions to consider would include:
   * Nematodirosis.
   * Coccidiosis.
   * Pulpy kidney, and other clostridial diseases if dams unvaccinated or failure of passive antibody transfer.
   * Pneumonic pasteurellosis.
   * Abomasal/intestinal volvulus (single animal only).
2. Sudden hatching of over-wintered infective third stage larvae (L3) of *Nematodirus battus* after a period of cold weather can cause severe diarrhoea and death in young lambs. Such infestation would explain the diarrhoea in other lambs in the group. Pneumonic pasteurellosis can be confirmed at necropsy; pulpy kidney disease would occur only in lambs from unvaccinated dams. Faecal samples are usually negative for worm eggs in acute nematodirosis (not yet patent). Necropsy reveals catarrhal enteritis and acute inflammation of the small intestine with varying numbers of developing and adult worms.
3. Control by means of clean grazing with alternate years of cattle, crops and sheep can rarely be practised on upland farms; prophylactic anthelmintic treatment based upon disease risk forecasts are necessary to avoid costly disease outbreaks. If in doubt use prophylactic anthelmintic treatment early; such treatment can always be repeated if mistimed. Anthelmintic resistance is not a concern with *N. battus* and Group 1 anthelminitics (benzimadazole anthelmintics) can be used that are otherwise largely ineffective due to resistance in other nematode species.

ANSWER 12

1. The most likely conditions to consider would include:
   - Paratuberculosis.
   - Subacute fasciolosis.
   - PGE – haemonchosis.
   - Pleural abscesses or other septic focus.
   - Poor dentition (molars).
   - Intestinal tumour.
2. Sheep with advanced paratuberculosis have profound hypoalbuminaemia (serum values <15 g/l; normal range >30 g/l) and normal globulin concentration, but these protein concentrations may very occasionally be encountered in cases of severe chronic parasitism. In chronic fasciolosis and chronic bacterial infection there is hypoalbuminaemia (<25 g/l) and marked increase in serum globulin concentration (>55 g/l; normal range = <45 g/l). Albumin and globulin values in these ewes were 12.1 g/l and 14.2 g/l, and 39.0 g/l and 40.1 g/l, respectively. These serum protein concentrations are consistent with a diagnosis of paratuberculosis.

   A faecal sample should be checked for fluke eggs, although this may not yet be patent (sedimentation), and strongyle egg counts (modified McMaster technique). Be aware that sheep with Johne's disease may have disproportionately high worm egg counts as a consequence of immune system suppression. It is not unusual to see *Nematodirus battus* eggs, and even lungworm larvae, in McMaster slide preparations.
3. The ewes should be euthanased for welfare reasons. Necropsy findings included an emaciated carcase with gelatinous atrophy of fat depots. The mesenteric lymph nodes were markedly enlarged. There was thickening of the ileum with prominent ridging (**Fig. 18.12b**). The diagnosis is confirmed after ZN staining of gut sections and lymph nodes demonstrates acid-fast bacteria.
4. Vaccination has proven successful in many countries. However, the benefit only outweighs the cost when losses due to paratuberculosis exceed 1.5–2% per annum.

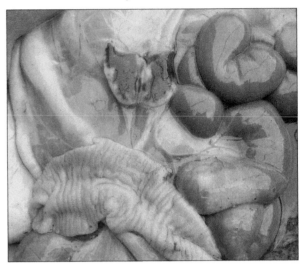

Fig. 18.12b **Necropsy reveals an emaciated carcase with gelatinous atrophy of fat depots in the omentum and enlarged mesenteric lymph nodes.**

ANSWER 13

1. The most likely conditions to consider would include:
   - Hypocalcaemia.
   - Acidosis resulting from carbohydrate overfeed.
   - Mastitis.
   - Metritis.
   - Pneumonia.
   - Listeriosis.
   - Copper poisoning.
   - Hypomagnesaemia.
2. The provisional diagnosis of hypocalcaemia is proven correct after the rapid response to slow intravenous administration of 40 ml of a 40% calcium borogluconate solution. Eructation was heard during the intravenous calcium administration. The ewe stood within 5 minutes of intravenous injection, urinated and suckled her lambs (**Fig. 18.13b**). While it has become standard practice also to administer approximately 40 ml of a 40% calcium borogluconate solution subcutaneously, the usefulness of this 'depot injection' has never been proven. The subcutaneous injection is undoubtedly painful for the sheep and there

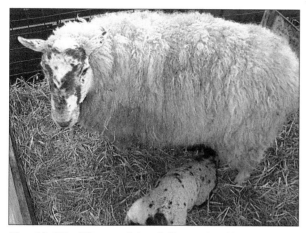

Fig. 18.13b **The provisional diagnosis of hypocalcaemia is proven correct after the rapid response to slow intravenous administration of 40 ml of a 40% calcium borogluconate solution.**

is the risk of localized infection/abscess formation if strict hygiene precautions are not observed. There was no recurrence of hypocalcaemia in this sheep.

3. There are no specific control measures. Hypocalcaemia is more common in 3-crop or older ewes maintained at pasture during late gestation, but also occurs sporadically during early lactation. Hypocalcaemia should always be considered in ewes that show depression/recumbency during late gestation and early lactation. It has been stated that no ewe should die without first being given the benefit of intravenous calcium borogluconate. In sheep recumbent due to hypocalcaemia, serum calcium concentrations are below 1.0 mmol/l.

ANSWER 14

1. A NSAID is injected intravenously. The sheep is injected with a combination of lignocaine plus xylazine at the sacrococcygeal site to allow replacement of the oedematous cervico-vaginal prolapse and insertion of the Buhner retention suture. The first intercoccygeal space is identified by digital palpation during slight vertical movement of the tail, and a 1 inch 19 gauge needle directed at 20° to the tail, which is held horizontally. Correct

position of the needle is determined by the lack of resistance to injection of 2% lignocaine (0.5–0.6 mg/kg injected over 10 seconds; 1.25 ml for 50 kg hogg) and 0.07 mg/kg xylazine (Rompun; Bayer) (0.2 ml for a 50 kg hogg). The hogg is also injected with 44,000 IU/kg of procaine penicillin prior to surgery.

2. Perform a caesarean operation. Any attempt to dilate the cervix using digital pressure over 10–20 minutes would probably cause rupture of the friable vaginal mucosa/cervix.

   Effective flank analgesia is achieved following distal paravertebral block using 2% lignocaine.

3. Two live healthy lambs are delivered by caesarean operation taking 30 minutes from presentation (£80 per hour for your time = £40, plus drugs/suture material, disposables etc = £12 – total £52; market value in 2014 for sheep with single lamb is approximately £150 (the other twin lamb was fostered on to a ewe).

ANSWER 15

1. The most likely conditions to consider would include:
   - Listeriosis.
   - Basilar empyema.
   - Peripheral vestibular lesion with trauma to the right superficial facial nerve.
   - Brain abscess.
   - Acute coenurosis.
   - Sarcocystosis.

2. Gross inspection of lumbar CSF collected under local anaesthesia using a 19 gauge 50 mm hypodermic needle (85 kg ram) reveals no abnormality. Laboratory examination reveals an elevated protein concentration of 1–2 g/l (normal <0.4 g/l), and a slight increase in white cell concentration (pleocytosis) comprised of large mononuclear cells. Serology is not used routinely for diagnosis because many healthy sheep have high listeria titres. In fatal cases, if primary isolation attempts fail, ground brain tissue should be held at 39°F (4°C) for several weeks and recultured weekly.

3. *Listeria monocytogenes* is susceptible to various antibiotics including penicillin (up to 300,000

IU/kg), ceftiofur, erythromycin and trimethoprim/sulphonamide. Emphasis should be placed on administering the maximum dose of penicillin costs will permit at the first visit, rather than the duration of daily penicillin injections thereafter. A single intravenous injection of soluble corticosteroid, such as dexamethasone at a dose rate of 1.1 mg/kg, will reduce the associated severe inflammatory reaction and improve prognosis.

4. Control involves correct fermentation of grass silage through the use of additives and airtight storage. When feeding, discard all spoiled silage, clean troughs daily and discard refusals.

ANSWER 16

1. The most likely conditions to consider would include:
   - Obstructive urolithiasis.
   - Cystitis.
2. The ram should be cast onto its hindquarters and the penis extruded by straightening the sigmoid flexure. A calculus can often be felt within the tip of the vermiform appendage, which is then excised with a scalpel blade. The ram is allowed to stand, when a continuous flow of approximately 500 ml of urine is often produced. The ram must be carefully observed for normal urination and appetite.
3. Blood urea nitrogen (BUN) and creatinine determinations and ultrasonography of the bladder and right kidney could be undertaken. These investigations are not necessary in this case because of the short duration of illness and resolution of the problem after amputation of the vermiform appendix.
4. Early recognition of partial/complete urethral obstruction is essential because irreversible hydronephrosis develops rapidly due to the back pressure within the urinary tract. Reblockage with further calculi is possible. Surgical correction of urolithiasis involves a subischial urethrostomy under caudal block, but is not a simple procedure and is undertaken only as a salvage procedure.

5. Control of urolithiasis involves feeding a correct ration with low magnesium content. The salt concentration of the ration can be increased to increase water intake. Urine acidifiers such as ammonium chloride can also be added to the ration. Good quality roughage should be available *ad libitum*.

ANSWER 17

1. The most likely conditions to consider would include:
   - Photosensitization.
   - Bighead (*Clostridium chauvoei* infection).
   - Dog bite to the face or similar wound/cellulitis.
   - Bluetongue.
2. Photosensitization is most evident in animals with non-pigmented skin. Primary photosensitization results when an ingested photodynamic agent in the animal's body (e.g. hypericin from St. John's wort [*Hypericum perforatum*]), is exposed to ultraviolet light, causing fluorescence and death of cells in the skin. The cell necrosis and dermatitis is characteristically most severe in non-pigmented skin.

   Secondary (hepatogenous) photosensitization results from the liver's inability to excrete phylloerythrin, a breakdown product of chlorophyll. In New Zealand facial eczema is caused by ingestion of the hepatotoxin sporidesmin, produced by the saprophytic fungus *Pithomyces chartarum*.
3. Treatment includes removing the source of photosensitizing agent if identifiable. Animals should be protected from direct sunlight by housing. Parenteral corticosteroids are indicated in the acute erythematous stage of photosensitization, to reduce oedema/inflammation. Topical emollients and antimicrobials may help soften and protect the skin. Systemic antibiotics are indicated in cases of a secondary bacterial dermatitis.
4. In the absence of recognized plant species, primary photosensitization occurs sporadically and there are no specific control measures.

ANSWER 18

1. The most likely conditions to consider would include:
   - Entropion.
   - Infectious keratoconjunctivitis (IKC).
2. Treatment involves eversion of the lower eyelid as soon after birth as possible, with regular inspection to ensure it remains everted. Topical antibiotic application controls secondary bacterial infection and aids movement of the lower eyelid over the cornea, thereby reducing the likelihood of inversion.

   Subcutaneous antibiotic injection (e.g. 0.5–1 ml of procaine penicillin) can be used to evert the lower eyelid (**Fig. 18.18b**). Skin suture(s) can be inserted to evert the lower eyelid but this procedure requires two people, one to restrain the lamb and the other to insert the suture. Eales clip(s) can be inserted in the skin below the lower eyelid to cause eversion when closed; these clips have the advantage of requiring only one operator.
3. Consequences of entropion include rupture of the cornea, with herniation of the lens and loss of the eye in neglected cases.
4. Entropion has a very high hereditary component and rams siring affected progeny should be culled (but this rarely happens).

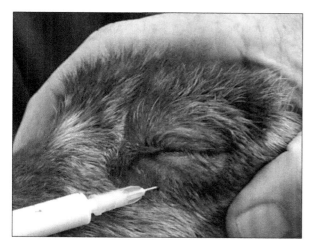

Fig. 18.18b Subcutaneous injection of 0.5 ml of procaine penicillin is used to evert the lower eyelid.

ANSWER 19

1. Differential diagnoses would include:
   - Chronic fasciolosis.
   - Chronic internal parasitism, especially trichostrongylosis.
   - Cobalt deficiency.
   - Poor grazing/poor hay quality.

A provisional diagnosis of fasciolosis was based on the clinical examination and epidemiology; the ewe lambs had been grazing poor pasture during the autumn months.

2. Blood and faecal sampling.

   Routine haematological examination revealed a profound anaemia (PCV 0.07 l/l; total RBC count 1.0 ×10^{12}/l; Hb 20 g/l). The RBCs showed anisocytosis, poikilocytosis and polychromasia. The WBC count was raised at 12.0 × 10^9/l.

   The serum GGT concentration was raised at 97 U/l. There was a profound hypoalbuminaemia (9.9 g/l) and increased globulin concentration (60.9 g/l).

   A faecal sample from the ewe revealed 1200 strongyle epg and a fluke egg count of 350 epg; both values are significant. A pooled faecal nematode egg count from 10 sheep in the group revealed 800 strongyle epg and the fluke egg count was 450 epg.
3. The following day a hogg was found dead in the field and was presented for postmortem examination. The carcase was in very poor bodily condition. On skinning, the carcase appeared jaundiced. The contents of the chest were unremarkable. The liver was enlarged, very friable and bronzed. Cut sections revealed a large number of mature flukes. The gall bladder contained many mature liver flukes (**Fig. 18.19**).

The hoggs were treated with a combined fluke (oxyclozanide) and worm (levamisole) drench. Triclabendazole could have been used as the flukacide but it is considerably more expensive and was thought unnecessary because all the flukes present

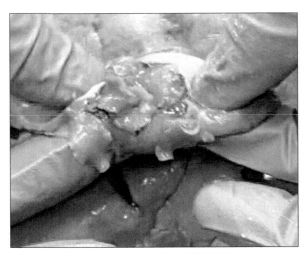

Fig. 18.19 Liver flukes in the gall bladder at necropsy.

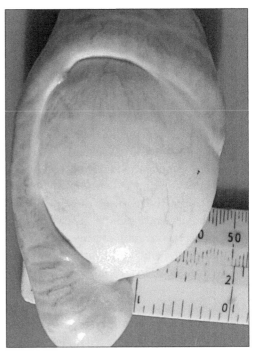

Fig. 18.20b An atrophied testicle shown at necropsy.

would be mature. It was recommended that the ewe lambs should also be treated with a flukacide 3 months later in May. The farmer was advised that it was unlikely the ewe lambs would increase in body condition without supplementary feeding. The farmer fed 250 g of concentrates per head daily as recommended throughout the winter period. At clipping time the sheep were in very good condition but this improvement had only been achieved by a much higher level of supplementary feeding. Fencing off wet areas is rarely affordable on many extensive units.

ANSWER 20

1. The testicle is only 4 cm diameter, appears more hypoechoic than normal and contains many hyperechoic spots. These hyperechoic dots are thought to represent the fibrous supporting architecture now more obvious due to atrophy of the seminiferous tubules. These findings are consistent with testicular atrophy.
2. Fertility assessment by semen collection and examination, whether by electroejaculation or artificial vagina, is unnecessary because of the obvious testicular atrophy. A single semen sample would not indicate serving capacity.
3. Farmers should measure the maximum scrotal circumference of all potential ram purchases using a tape measure. Acceptable values are >36 cm for shearlings and >32 cm for ram lambs.
4. The ram should not be used for breeding for at least 3 months and must be re-examined before turnout with ewes. Without a more detailed history of the ram (e.g. previous illness), it is not possible to advise whether it would be worthwhile keeping the ram one more year until the next breeding season. An atrophied testicle at necropsy is shown in **Fig. 18.20b**.

ANSWER 21

1. The most likely conditions to consider would include:
   - Pasteurellosis or other septicaemic disease.
   - Abdominal catastrophe such as volvulus of either the abomasum or small intestine.
   - Clostridial disease.
   - Peracute mastitis.

- Cowped (found stuck in dorsal recumbency and severely bloated).
- Peracute fluke occurs from September onwards.

2. Postmortem examination reveals necrosis of the whole small intestine containing foetid-smelling material (see **Fig. 18.21**). No volvulus is detected. No other abnormalities are found in the carcase. Despite a correct clostridial vaccination history the gimmer appears to have died from a clostridial-like disease. The farmer was advised to review his vaccination technique such that all sheep are indeed vaccinated correctly. The possibility that death resulted from *Clostridium sordellii* infection (not included in all clostridial vaccines) could not be ruled out.

Further tests revealed a profuse growth of *C. perfringens* suggesting that this ewe may not have received a full vaccination course, although a positive culture is not conclusive for disease. No further losses were recorded in the ewe flock. The cause of the single death could not be readily explained.

ANSWER 22

1. The most likely conditions to consider would include:
   - Infectious polyarthritis caused by *E. rhusiopathiae.*
   - Infectious polyarthritis secondary to tick-born fever.
   - Bacterial endocarditis.
2. *Streptococcus dysgalactiae* affects lambs within the first 2 weeks of life, while *E. rhusiopathiae* tends to affect lambs from several months.
3. Samples of synovial membrane from sacrificed untreated cases are preferable to joint aspirates for bacteriological examination. There is a high seroprevalence to erysipelas in normal healthy sheep.
4. While aggressive antibiotic therapy with penicillin during the very early stages of infection effects a good cure rate in many *E. rhusiopathiae* infections and may render the joints sterile, some chronic infections are not cleared, with the result that progressive and degenerative changes occur within the joint. Indeed, dead bacteria and white blood cells within the joint induce inflammatory changes including proliferation of the synovial membrane and fibrous thickening of the joint capsule. It is these chronic and severe inflammatory changes involving the synovial membrane coupled with loss of articular cartilage that cause the obvious pain and lameness. Such pathology will not respond to further antibiotic therapy and these lambs should be euthanased for welfare reasons.

5. Vaccination of the dam with effective passive antibody transfer protects lambs from erysipelas but may not be available in some countries.

ANSWER 23

1. There is severe hydronephrosis with an enlarged fluid-distended renal pelvis and reduced renal medulla/cortex (**Fig. 18.23b**).
2. Such renal pathology is irreversible and the ram should be euthanased for welfare reasons. Urethral obstruction results in bladder distension and back pressure causing hydroureter and hydronephrosis. The condition is bilateral and there is no requirement to scan the right kidney. Except for uroperitoneum in growing lambs,

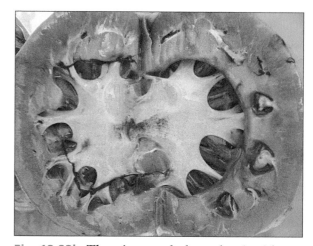

Fig. 18.23b There is severe hydronephrosis with an enlarged fluid-distended renal pelvis and reduced renal medulla/cortex.

leakage from, or rupture of, the bladder is an uncommon event in adult sheep.

3. Hydronephrosis is prevented by prompt identification of the sick ram by the shepherd, with immediate veterinary attention to relieve the urinary tract obstruction.

Correct ration formulation with appropriate mineral supplementation (low magnesium) is the basis for prevention of urolithiasis in intensively-reared sheep. Sodium chloride can be added to rations to promote water intake. Urine acidifiers, such as ammonium chloride, are commonly added to rations. Provision of roughage promotes saliva production and water intake. Fresh clean water must always be available and frequent checks must be made for frozen pipes in subzero temperatures.

ANSWER 24

1. Gangrenous mastitis caused by *Pasteurella* (*Mannheimia*) species and *S. aureus* occurs sporadically during the first 2 months of lactation, and is associated with poor milk supply related to ewe under-nutrition and over-vigorous sucking by the lambs. The condition is commonly reported in ewes nursing triplets and this practice must be actively discouraged unless farmers are prepared to feed the ewes very well (up to 2 kg per head daily) and offer good quality creep feed for the lambs. Staphylococcal skin lesions and CPD virus infection of the ewe's teat(s) often precede mastitis.

2. The prognosis is hopeless.

3. The ewe should be (and was) euthanased for welfare reasons. It would be unacceptable to keep this ewe because, despite antibiotic and supportive therapy, the gangrenous udder tissue will eventually slough and leave a large wound. The granulation tissue will continue to proliferate over the coming months. Ewes cannot be presented at market because the carcase would be condemned at meat inspection.

ANSWER 25

1. The most likely conditions to consider would include:
   - Copper poisoning.
   - Chronic fasciolosis.
   - Hypocalcaemia.
   - Ovine pregnancy toxaemia.
   - Polioencephalomalacia.
   - Plant poisonings including rhododendron.

2. Further tests could include serum liver enzyme assays.

   There are greatly increased GGT (480 IU/l; normal = <10 IU/l) and AST (5560 IU/l; normal = <60 IU/l) concentrations indicating liver damage. The serum copper concentration is elevated above the normal range (69 μmol/l; normal = 9–22 μmol/l).

3. The treatment plan was 1.7 mg/kg ammonium tetrathiomolybdate given by slow intravenous infusion on two occasions 2 days apart (or 3.4 mg/kg injected subcutaneously). The ewe was also given 3 litres of 5% glucose saline intravenously over the next 6 hours. The ewe was found *in extremis* 12 hours after first treatment and was euthanased for welfare reasons. At necropsy the kidney copper concentration is massively elevated at 3900 μmol/kg DM (normal = <314 μmol/kg DM). Liver copper concentrations are usually also elevated but such determinations are not as reliable as kidney copper determination.

4. Breeds such as the Texel, Soay and North Ronaldsay are particularly susceptible to copper poisoning. Sheep must not have access to cattle feed and great care must be taken when considering copper supplementation (to control congenital swayback for example). Copper antagonists, such as molybdenum, may be required when susceptible breeds are fed high levels of concentrates (especially when rearing stud rams), despite content not exceeding 15 mg/kg Cu as fed.

ANSWER 26

1. The most likely conditions to consider would include:
   - Ovine pulmonary adenocarcinoma (OPA).
   - Chronic suppurative pneumonia.
   - Pleuropneumonia/pleural abscess.
   - Mediastinal abscess caused by caseous lymphadenitis (CLA).
   - Maedi.

2. The diagnosis can be readily confirmed following careful ultrasonographic examination of the chest (**Fig. 18.26b**) even using 5MHz linear scanners; sector scanners are not essential. The probe should be placed immediately above the point of the elbow, with the probe head placed in the most cranial intercostal space at this level of the chest wall.

   The production of copious clear frothy fluid from the nostrils when the ewe's hindquarters are raised (positive wheelbarrow test) is also pathognomic for OPA but only in advanced cases; not all positive cases produce this fluid after euthanasia. The wheelbarrow test can greatly exacerbate any dyspnoea, such that affected sheep should be killed immediately afterwards for welfare reasons. Necropsy reveals typical lesions of OPA (**Fig. 18.26c**).

3. The prognosis for OPA is hopeless and affected sheep must be culled immediately for welfare reasons and to limit further disease spread within the flock. Affected sheep must not be sent for slaughter.

4. Control measures include purchase of flock replacements from known OPA-free sources. Many flocks are closed except for purchased rams. These introduced sheep can be examined ultrasonographically after purchase and before introduction into the flock. It is possible to detect early 3–5 cm OPA lesions, reducing the risk of introducing infectious sheep. Purchased introduced sheep should be monitored ultrasonographically every 6–12 months for early lesions and these sheep culled as soon as any lesions are detected.

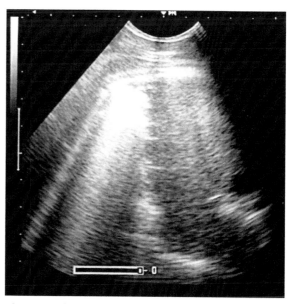

Fig. 18.26b Ultrasonography confirms the provisional diagnosis of OPA, with a sharply demarcated hypoechoic area in the ventral lung lobes.

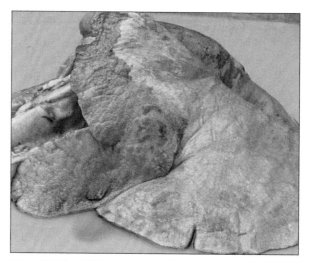

Fig. 18.26c OPA is confirmed at necropsy in the left apical and cardiac lung lobes.

During winter housing when the risk of aerosol transmission is greatly increased, sheep should be grouped in age cohorts not on keel marks (anticipated lambing date) or litter size, to limit spread of OPA to younger sheep. When sheep are grouped by age, infection acquired by older sheep does not present such a problem because these ewes would be voluntarily culled at the end of their productive lives before significant lung pathology had time to develop. Suspected cases should be isolated immediately and culled as soon as the diagnosis has been established.

In endemically-infected flocks, it has been recommended that sheep with early OPA lesions can be detected after a period of driving, with any exercise-intolerant or dyspnoeic sheep culled at this early stage. There is presently no commercially available serological test for OPA. If there is a high prevalence of OPA in one group of sheep that group should be culled. The progeny of all clinical cases of OPA should also be culled.

ANSWER 27

1. Common causes of poor growth in groups of lambs include:
   - Parasitic gastroenteritis.
   - Poor nutrition of ewe, lamb or both, due to either overstocking or poor pasture management.
   - Trace element deficiency (e.g. cobalt or selenium deficiency).
   - Earlier disease episodes leading to poor growth could include coccidiosis and nematodirosis.
   - Trace element deficiency may well exacerbate the effects of parasitic gastroenteritis with respect to poor performance.

2. A provisional diagnosis of parasitic gastroenteritis was based on the clinical findings and flock management.

   Faeces were collected from six diarrhoeic lambs. The geometric mean faecal egg count was 3200 epg (range 1200–4400; interpretation: 400 epg = low, 400–1000 = moderate, >1000 epg = high).

   The high faecal egg count in itself does not indicate benzimidazole resistance; the situation could have simply arisen as a consequence of ill-timed treatment(s). Under the circumstances, testing for the presence of benzimidazole-resistant nematode strains would be prudent. The six lambs were identified for resampling in 10 days.

The six sampled lambs were weighed and drenched with a benzimidazole anthelmintic. The farmer was instructed to collect faeces from these lambs in 10 days and submit them to the surgery. The remaining lambs in the group were drenched with levamisole that contained a cobalt supplement. The cost of supplementing the whole group with oral cobalt sulphate is much cheaper than assaying serum vitamin B12 estimations (2% of cost) which can be of doubtful clinical significance anyway.

The sheep were turned on to a field that had been grazed by cattle only since turnout; there was no safe grazing on this farm. The lambs were treated with cyromazine to prevent cutaneous myiasis.

3. On permanent grassland, parasitic gastroenteritis is very difficult to control by grazing-strategic anthelmintic treatments alone. Every attempt must be made to incorporate management controls such as movement onto safe grazing, for example, silage aftermaths, after weaning.

Typically, lambs on pasture grazed by lambs during the previous season are treated with an anthelmintic once or twice (3 weeks apart) based on the forecast regarding *Nematodirus battus* infestation. Thereafter, those lambs that fail to meet growth targets are treated with an anthelmintic (targeted anhelmintic treatment). There is little advantage to be gained from frequent (every 3–4 weeks) anthelmintic treatments once there has been massive pasture contamination with infective larvae and a move to safe grazing is essential. Repeated anthelmintic treatment greatly increases the selection pressure in favour of resistant nematode strains.

The diarrhoea stopped soon after drenching. The faecal egg reduction test in the six lambs resulted in a 95% reduction in the counts taken 10 days after benzimidazole treatment, implicating mismanagement rather than anthelmintic resistance in this situation. There was a gradual improvement in the lambs' condition over the next 4 weeks.

ANSWER 28

1. The most likely conditions to consider would include:
   - Heavy infestation with the chewing louse *Bovicola ovis*.
   - Psoroptic mange (sheep scab).
   - Both sheep scab and lice infestations.
   - Cutaneous myiasis if summer months.
2. Lice congregate in colonies on the fleece, therefore a minimum of 10–20 fleece partings per sheep to a depth of 10 cm should be examined using a magnifying glass, with a minimum of 10 sheep examined per group. An average count of more than five lice per fleece parting is generally considered a heavy infestation with *B. ovis*. The slow reproductive capacity of *B. ovis* results in a gradual build-up of louse numbers over several months. Skin scrapings (or clear adhesive tape) at the periphery of any lesions are necessary to detect *Psoroptes ovis* mites.
3. Louse infestations can be controlled with topical application of high-cis cypermethrin or deltamethrin. Infested sheep can also be treated by plunge dipping in a synthetic pyrethroid or organophosphate preparation (availability may vary in certain countries).
4. Maintenance of a closed flock and effective biosecurity measures will prevent introduction of louse infestations. Annual dipping practices will eliminate this obligate parasite.

ANSWER 29

1. Involvement of the cerebellum would explain the clinical signs; the lambs appeared normal for the first 8 weeks but have deteriorated over the past 2 months, suggesting a developmental abnormality.
2. The most likely conditions to consider would include:
   - Cerebellar abiotrophy.
   - Cerebellar abscess/focal meningitis.

   Other conditions could include:
   - Delayed swayback.
   - Cervical spinal lesion.
   - Atlanto-occipital joint infection caused by *Streptococcus dysgalactiae*.

   A diagnosis of cerebellar abiotrophy is based upon clinical examination, and lack of intrathecal inflammation (normal CSF parameters).

3. There is no treatment and the lambs were euthanased for welfare reasons.
   At necropsy the cerebellar weight was more than 8% of brain weight indicating no hypoplasia. There was widespread degeneration of Purkinje cells with associated hypocellularity of the granular layer and degeneration of myelin in cerebellar foliae and peduncles. There was widespread loss of Purkinje cells, with individual remaining cells being angular and showing condensed, eosinophilic cytoplasm and loss of nuclear detail but no cytoplasmic vacuolation.
4. Cerebellar abiotrophy is a familial syndrome first described affecting Charollais sheep in the UK in 1994. The inherited nature of this defect stresses the importance of an accurate diagnosis, especially in rams, which contribute significantly to the genetic profile of the flock. Affected lambs should be euthanased for welfare reasons and the sire and dam culled.

ANSWER 30

1. Guidelines to ensure passive antibody transfer include:
   - Feed ewes well during pregnancy with body condition scores and serum 3-OH butyrate concentrations as guidelines.
   - Lambs must ingest sufficient colostrum (200 ml/kg) during the first 24 hours of life and 50 ml/kg within the first 2 hours, if not sooner (**Figs 18.30a**, **18.30b**).
   - Colostrum in the lamb's abomasum immediately caudal to the costal arch can readily be detected by gentle transabdominal palpation. This can be undertaken in the standing lamb or after the lamb has been held up by the forelimbs. (Abdominal

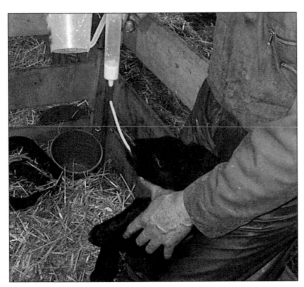

Fig. 18.30a Lambs must ingest sufficient colostrum (200 ml/kg) during the first 24 hours of life, and 50 ml/kg within the first 2 hours.

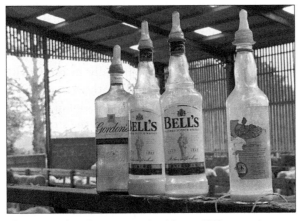

Fig. 18.30b There is no significant difference in absorbed immunoglobulin when colostrum is fed either by bottle and teat or stomach tube.

distension does occur in watery mouth disease but affected lambs are >24 hours old.)

If a ewe has insufficient colostrum, colostrum can be stripped from another ewe with a single lamb or use cow colostrum. Pooled colostrum from four to six vaccinated (clostridial diseases) dairy cows can be used. Wherever possible colostrums from dairy herds free of paratuberculosis should be used, but this is not a real problem in lambs destined for slaughter at 4–6 months old. The risk of anaemia induced by feeding bovine colostrum is very low compared with starvation and bacterial infections. Purchased colostrum supplements are expensive and your clients' money is better spent on ewe feed during late gestation to ensure adequate accumulations within the udder.

2. Total plasma protein concentration determined using a hand-held refractometer is the cheapest method to assess passive antibody transfer in lambs more than 24 hours old. The plasma protein concentration for lambs that have not sucked colostrum is <45g/l compared with >55g/l for lambs that have sucked appropriate volumes of colostrum.

CHAPTER 1: INTRODUCTION

Scott PR, Sargison ND (2007) The potential for improving disease control and welfare standards in the United Kingdom sheep flocks using veterinary flockhealth plans. *Vet J* **173**:522–532.

CHAPTER 4: NEONATAL LAMB DISEASES

Russel A (1985) Nutrition of the pregnant ewe. *In Practice* **7**:23–28.

CHAPTER 11: THE SKIN

Scottish Statutory Instruments (2011) No. 77 Animals. Animal Health, The Sheep Scab (Scotland) Amendment Order 2011.

Printed and bound by CPI Group (UK) Ltd, Croydon, CR0 4YY

24/10/2024

01778285-0013